SEXUALLY TRANSMITTED DISEASES

Guide to Diagnosis and Therapy

Contemporary Patient Management Series

- *Acute Renal Failure,* Edward Kuehnel, M.D., and William Bennett, M.D.

- *Bleeding Disorders,* Jessica H. Lewis, M.D., Joel A. Spero, M.D., and Ute Hasiba, M.D.

- *Stroke,* Lowell G. Lubic, M.D., and Harry P. Palkovitz, M.D.

- *Tuberculosis,* Douglas R. Gracey, M.D., and Whitney W. Addington, M.D.

- *Chronic Obstructive Pulmonary Disease,* Warren C. Miller, M.D.

- *Renal Tubular Dysfunction,* Vardaman M. Buckalew, Jr., M.D., and Michael A. Moore, M.D.

- *Infections in Obstetrics and Gynecology,* Lester T. Hibbard, M.D.

- *Pain: Origin and Treatment,* Benjamin H. Gorsky, M.D.

- *Rheumatoid Arthritis,* edited by Duncan A. Gordon, M.D.

- *Chronic Duodenal Ulcer,* G. Gordon McHardy, M.D.

- *Anxiety: A Guide to Biobehavioral Diagnosis and Therapy for Physicians and Mental Health Clinicians,* Richard J. Goldberg, M.D.

- *Inflammatory Bowel Disease,* Marshall Sparberg, M.D.

- *Headache,* Seymour Diamond, M.D., and Arnold P. Friedman, M.D.

- *Osteoarthritis and Musculoskeletal Pain Syndromes,* edited by Bernard F. Germain, M.D.

- *Peptic Ulcer,* Herman J. Kaplan, M.D.

- *Sexually Transmitted Diseases: Guide to Diagnosis and Therapy,* Third Edition, Robert C. Noble, M.D.

- *Coronary Heart Disease,* Robert M. Davidson, M.D.

SEXUALLY TRANSMITTED DISEASES

Guide to Diagnosis and Therapy

Third Edition

Robert C. Noble, M.D.
Professor, Division of Infectious Diseases
Department of Medicine
University of Kentucky College of Medicine
Lexington, Kentucky

MEDICAL EXAMINATION PUBLISHING COMPANY

Noble, Robert C.
    Sexually transmitted diseases.

    (Contemporary patient management series)
    Includes bibliographies and index.
    1. Venereal diseases. I. Title. II. Series.
[DNLM: 1. Venereal Diseases—diagnosis—handbooks.
2. Venereal Diseases—therapy—handbooks.
WC 39 N751s]
RC200.N62 1984   616.95'1   84-16541
ISBN 0-87488-620-1

To Kenneth L. Vosti, MD
my mentor

Contents

Preface

This book is written for physicians, house staff, and clinic personnel as a handbook for the diagnosis and treatment of sexually transmitted diseases. Such diseases are generally defined as those transmitted principally by sexual intercourse. The traditional list included five diseases: syphilis and gonorrhea as the major venereal diseases and chancroid, lymphogranuloma venereum, and granuloma inguinale as the minor venereal diseases. In recent years this list of sexually transmitted diseases has been expanded to include infectious diseases customarily regarded in other contexts. Some of these are listed in the "Contents" of this book and in Chapter 1.

The propriety of including certain infectious diseases in this book may be questioned. In fact, it is difficult to define what is a sexually transmitted disease in view of the multitude of ways in which pathogenic microorganisms can be transmitted. For example, I suspect most adults get scabies from their children and, for most patients, <u>Candida</u> vaginitis is not a sexually transmitted disease. However, the diseases included in this text do occur in sexually active people, and sexual intercourse appears to be of epidemiologic significance. A line cannot now be drawn between the sexually and nonsexually transmitted infectious diseases.

A number of infectious diseases that are considered by some to be sexually transmitted were not included in the text such as toxic shock syndrome, infectious mononucleosis, urinary tract infection, and group B streptococcal infection. A better perspective on transmission mechanisms of these diseases undoubtedly will be forthcoming, but a sharp definition of a sexually transmitted disease probably will not result from current research.

A substantial portion of the diagnosis of sexually transmitted disease rests with a visual recognition of the disease entity. It is hard to do justice to most of the sexually transmitted diseases with black and white photographs. But the expense of printing high quality color photographs would price this book above the budget of the average medical student or house officer.

No attempt has been made to cover pathophysiology or the most recent laboratory research findings. The end-of-chapter bibliographies lead the curious reader into the current literature. Rapid advances are being made in the understanding of many sexually transmitted diseases. This book will provide the practitioner with access to the relevant information.

Acknowledgments

The photographs in this book came from a number of sources, and I thank the contributors, including Ira P. Mersack, MD, and Ullin W. Leavell, MD, of the Division of Dermatology and Norman L. Goodman, PhD, Deborah E. Powell, MD, and Sylvia L. Avram, C.T. (ASCP) I.A.C., of the Department of Pathology of the University of Kentucky College of Medicine. Photographs marked in the legend with an asterisk (*) are taken from the Portfolio Sexually Transmitted Diseases by Dr. E. Stolz and Mr. J. van der Stek, C.H. Boehringer Sohn, Ingelheim am Rhein, 1977. I wish to express my gratitude to Dr. Stolz for the use of the excellent photos by Mr. van der Stek.

I am indebted to the staff of the Lexington-Fayette County Health Department Venereal Disease Clinic for their help and cooperation. I am also grateful to Mrs. Linda Kimmel, Ms. Judy Rogers and Ms. Sharon Evans for their patience in typing the manuscript. I want to especially thank Dr. G. D. Morrison, Dr. Walter E. Stamm, Dr. Jeff Susman and Dr. A. Balows. Their critical reviews of the second edition of the book brought about a number of changes.

notice

The author and the publisher of this book have made every effort to ensure that all therapeutic modalities that are recommended are in accordance with accepted standards at the time of publication.

The drugs specified within this book may not have specific approval by the Food and Drug Administration in regard to the indications and dosages that are recommended by the author. The manufacturer's package insert is the best source of current prescribing information.

Chapter 1

PATIENT MANAGEMENT

This chapter is a collection of short topics related to general
patient management. The selection of the topics reflects a personal
bias. The suggestions and points are presented in outline form.
Sexually transmitted diseases are seldom regarded as health problems unassociated with moral judgment. This results in one of the
principal difficulties in their management. To presumed monogamous sexual partners, a venereal disease is an unwelcome biological mark of infidelity. The emotional disturbance that surrounds
such a discovery is often a detriment to treatment. Sexually transmitted diseases may never be viewed by the public in the same
sympathetic manner as renal, cardiovascular, or neoplastic diseases. It will be a pleasant day when I answer my door to a solici-
tation for research funds for a sexually transmitted disease.
Because of the prevailing negative views, most patients are highly
anxious that their problems remain in the confidence of a physician.
Tables 1.1 and 1.2 indicate the types of sexually transmitted
diseases and their relative proportions as seen in American and
English clinics.

EPIDEMIOLOGY

1. A patient with one sexually transmitted disease may have
   another one as yet undiagnosed.
2. For every patient there is an infected sexual partner who also
   should be identified and treated.
3. Since the patient's sexual orientation may not be known initially, refer to the patient's sexual partner as such rather than
   specifying a gender.

Table 1.1 Diagnosis of Sexually Transmitted Diseases Among Men and Women Per 100 Visits to Venereal Disease Clinics in the United States[a]

Diagnosis	Men	Women
Gonorrhea	24.0	15.0
Nongonococcal urethritis	24.8	—
Nonspecific vaginitis	—	11.3
Trichomoniasis	—	10.4
Candidiasis	—	6.1
Molluscum contagiosum	1.0	3.4
Venereal warts	4.3	3.0
Herpes genitalis	3.4	1.5
Syphilis	1.7	1.4
Scabies	1.3	0.4
Crab louse infestation	2.9	1.6
Chancroid	0.1	0.1
Lymphogranuloma venereum	0.1	0.0
Granuloma inguinale	0.0	0.0

[a] Ronald K. St. John, MD, Venereal Disease Control Division, CDC, USPHS. From R. K. St. John and O. G. Jones, Nonreported Sexually Transmitted Diseases, American Public Health Association Annual Meeting, Washington, DC, 1977.

Table 1.2 Diagnosis of Sexually Transmitted Diseases Among Men and Women in Hospital Clinics in England Per 100,000 Population[a]

Diagnosis	Men	Women
Gonorrhea	150.49	85.26
Nongonococcal urethritis	383.82	—
Nonspecific vaginitis	—	115.02
Trichomoniasis	8.42	78.62
Candidiasis	40.68	148.53
Molluscum contagiosum	3.32	1.69
Venereal warts	79.20	43.00
Herpes genitalis	27.16	16.34
Syphilis (early)	9.41	1.60
Scabies	7.95	2.05
Crab louse infestation	24.10	10.53
Chancroid	0.17	0.07
Lymphogranuloma venereum	0.10	0.03
Granuloma inguinale	0.07	0.02

[a] From the Annual Report of the Chief Medical Officer of the Department of Health and Social Security for the year of 1981, Br J Vener Dis, 59:206–210, 1983.

4. Patients with histories of sexually transmitted diseases are likely to acquire such diseases a second time.

HISTORY AND PHYSICAL EXAMINATION

1. The sites of sexual contact should be determined in order to know from where to take specimens. Anoscopy is indicated in patients who have rectal symptoms or who practice rectal intercourse.
2. Discretion, attitude, and nonjudgmental phrasing of questions may mean the difference between an adequate and an inadequate history. If you need to know, you must ask the specific question.
3. The patient's right to privacy must be respected during the history and physical examination.
4. Is there local extension of the disease?
5. Are there drug allergies?
6. Is there concurrent liver or renal disease?
7. Is the patient pregnant?
8. Search for a second disease.
9. Recognize that up to 40% of patients visiting venereal disease clinics do not have a sexually transmitted disease despite their concern that they do.
10. Sexual behavior cannot be assumed because of dress or mannerisms.
11. If questions of a personal nature are asked, always supply a reason.
12. Parker et al. have shown that uncircumcised men are twice as likely as circumcised men to develop herpes genitalis or gonorrhea and five times as likely to develop syphilis. Perhaps the defenders of the foreskin will refute this.

The Pelvic Examination

Dr. Joni Magee gives helpful advice to male physicians who have never "experienced" a pelvic examination:

1. Introduce yourself to the patient while she is sitting up and clothed.
2. Explain to her continuously what you are doing.
3. Your finger in the vagina may be used to demonstrate the muscles of the perineal floor. Instead of saying "relax,"

ask the patient to bear down as if she were going to the bathroom.
4. Lubricate the vaginal speculum with warm water.
5. Insert the speculum <u>slowly</u> horizontally just over your fingers, avoiding the top of the vagina and urethra.
6. Give specific instructions such as "Let your belly go soft" rather than "relax."
7. Watch the patient's face during the bimanual examination.

<u>Common Presenting Complaints or Syndromes</u>

Sexually transmitted diseases may be grouped in part according to the patient's presenting complaint. Most patients do not come to the physician with complaints of gonorrhea, scabies, or syphilis. They are more likely to have a urethral discharge, a terrible itch, or a genital ulcer. This chapter points the clinician in the direction of the specific diagnosis by means of presenting lists of etiologic agents that may be associated with a specific complaint, syndrome, or problem-oriented category.

<u>Routine Laboratory Specimens for All Patients (A Suggestion)</u>

1. Serologic test for syphilis (unless negative within the preceding month).
2. <u>Neisseria gonorrhoeae</u> culture of the urethra in men and endocervix in women (other sites: pharynx or rectum if sexual exposure claimed).
3. Papanicolaou smear in women unless they have had a previous negative test within one year. A smear should be performed on any women with an unexplained cervical lesion.
4. <u>Chlamydia trachomatis</u> culture of the urethra in men and endocervix in women (this may not be economically feasible in many sections of the United States and many parts of the world). Nevertheless, <u>C. trachomatis</u> infection is likely the most underdiagnosed of all sexually transmitted diseases.

VAGINAL DISCHARGE

Vaginal discharge is a common and vexing complaint to many women. The characteristics of an abnormal vaginal discharge are shown in Table 1.3.

Table 1.3   Characteristics of an Abnormal Vaginal Discharge

Profuse in amount

Offensive odor

Contains polymorphonuclear leukocytes in large numbers

Contains abnormal vaginal microflora

Accompanied by dysuria, dyspareunia, burning, itching, or vulvar soreness

---

Vaginal discharge has a number of infectious and noninfectious causes. Some of them are outlined in Table 1.4.

<u>Diagnostic Tests</u>

Certain diagnostic tests should be performed on all patients with vaginitis. These include the following:

1. Wet mount. A cotton swab from the anterior or posterior fornix is shaken in 1 ml warm saline, and this suspension is examined at 100× and 400× on a microscopic slide with a glass coverslip. Look for clue cells (<u>Gardnerella</u> vaginitis), a large number of leukocytes (think of trichomoniasis or inflammatory genital focus), trichomonads (trichomoniasis), or yeast or fungal hyphae (candidiasis).
2. Vaginal pH. If indicator paper measures the vaginal pH as greater than 4.5, then suspect trichomonas infection or nonspecific vaginitis. (Menstrual blood and cervical mucous also raise the pH.)
3. Potassium hydroxide preparation—amine test. A drop of 10% KOH is added to the vaginal fluid to destroy the cellular elements and leave the fungal hyphae visible on microscopic examination. If fishy odor is emitted after the KOH addition, think of <u>Gardnerella</u> or anaerobic infection.
4. Gram stain of cervical exudate to look for the gram-negative intracellular diplococci of <u>Neisseria gonorrhoeae.</u>

Table 1.4   Common Causes of Vaginal Discharge

I. Infectious

    A. <u>Trichomonas vaginalis</u>

    B. <u>Candida albicans</u>

    C. <u>Gardnerella vaginalis</u>

    D. <u>Neisseria gonorrhoeae</u>

    E. Herpes simplex virus (discharge alone is rare)

    F. Anaerobic bacteria (curved rods)[a]

II. Noninfectious

    A. Physiologic or normal

        1. Prior to menses

        2. After sexual intercourse or sexual excitement

        3. Following the use of intravaginal birth control creams, foams, or jellies

        4. During pregnancy or use of oral contraceptives

    B. Chemical irritation or allergy from

        1. Contraceptive creams, foams, or jellies

        2. Douches

        3. Deodorants

        4. Rubber in condoms or diaphragms

    C. Atrophic vaginitis in postmenopausal women

    D. Foreign body

        1. Forgotten vaginal tampon

        2. Objects used in sex play or masturbation

        3. Intrauterine device

    E. Neoplasia

---

[a] See Spiegel, CA, et al.   J Infect Dis, 148:817–822, 1983.

5. Cultures for herpes simplex virus, <u>Trichomonas vaginalis</u>, <u>Candida albicans</u>, <u>Gardnerella vaginalis</u> as indicated.
6. Rectal and endocervical culture for <u>Neisseria gonorrhoeae</u>.

Other Considerations in Patients with Vaginitis

1. A fistula may be present (vesicovaginal, rectovaginal, or ureterovaginal).
2. The problem may really be inflammatory rectal disease rather than vaginitis.

URETHRAL DISCHARGE

Dysuria and urethral discharge are a common complaint of men with sexually transmitted diseases. Table 1.5 lists the common causes of urethral discharge in men.

Diagnostic Tests

Certain diagnostic tests should be performed on patients with urethral discharge.

1. Gram stain of the urethral exudate examined microscopically.
2. Culture for <u>Neisseria gonorrhoeae</u> and <u>Chlamydia trachomatis</u>.
3. Examination of the urine should be performed if no discharge is available for microscopic examination. (See Chapter 3.)

The Urethral Culture

1. Have the patient sitting or lying down in case of fainting.
2. Retract the foreskin, and clean the meatus with a gauze pad.
3. You may be able to get the discharge by milking the urethra. Recent urination may have diminished the urethral secretions.
4. The urethral meatus is opened by gentle pressure before inserting the swab about 2 cm.
5. A culture swab should be inserted about 2 cm for diagnosis of <u>Chlamydia</u> (do not rely on the exudate only) as urethral cells are required.

Table 1.5   Common Causes of Urethral Discharge

I. Infectious

    A. Urethritis

        1. <u>Neisseria gonorrhoeae</u>

        2. <u>Chlamydia trachomatis</u>

        3. Herpes simplex virus (discharge alone is uncommon)

        4. <u>Trichomonas vaginalis</u>

        5. <u>Candida albicans</u>

        6. <u>Ureaplasma urealyticum</u>

    B. Infection of the proximal urinary tract

        1. Usually gram-negative enteric floria

        2. There may be an occult prostatic focus

II. Noninfectious

    A. Physiologic or normal such as after sexual excitement or ejaculation

    B. Mechanical or chemical irritation

    C. Foreign body

GENITAL SKIN LESIONS IN PATIENTS WITH SEXUALLY TRANSMITTED DISEASES

Ulcers

Even the best diagnosticians are fooled by genital ulcers. Ulcers from trauma, excoriation, infection, and carcinoma can look confusingly alike. In many cases the cause is never established or is part of a systemic disorder such as Behçet's disease. Some causes of ano-genital ulcers are outlined in Table 1.6

Table 1.6   Sexually Transmitted Diseases That Manifest
as Ulcers

---

1. Herpes genitalis

2. Syphilis

3. Trauma

4. Chancroid

5. Donovanosis

6. Lymphogranuloma venereum

7. Behçet's disease

Certain laboratory studies should be performed on patients
with genital ulcers:

1. Dark-field examination: see Chapter 10. This may be the
   only method of diagnosing syphilis early in its course.
   Acyclovir does not affect the results of the dark-field examination.
2. Serologic test for syphilis: remember that it may be negative
   early in the illness.
3. Tzanck test or, better yet, herpes simplex virus culture.
4. Cervical ulcers can be due to tampon use or mechanical irritation associated with vaginal vibrators.

Laboratory Studies for Patients with a Rash (see Table 1.7)

1. Serologic test for syphilis. A negative test rules out secondary
   syphilis.
2. Skin scrapings for KOH preparation (candidiasis or superficial
   fungal infection) or mineral oil preparation (scabies).
3. Hair examination: nits, pediculosis.

<u>Laboratory Tests for Patients with Papules</u> (see Table 1.8)

1. Serologic test for syphilis
2. Biopsy if required

Tables 1.9 and 1.10 deal with other diseases that cause skin rash or itching.

Table 1.7   Sexually Transmitted Diseases That Manifest as Rashes

---

1. Secondary syphilis

2. Scabies

3. Pediculosis

4. Candidiasis

5. Superficial fungal infections

Table 1.8   Sexually Transmitted Diseases Associated with Papules

---

1. Condyloma acuminatum

2. Molluscum contagiosum

3. Condyloma lata

DYSURIA IN WOMEN (See Table 1.11)

Painful urination is a relatively frequent complaint of women attending sexually transmitted disease clinics, and its differential diagnosis is broad. Nevertheless, there are three general sites

Table 1.9   Other Diseases Causing Skin Rashes Seen in Persons
with Sexually Transmitted Diseases

Allergic

1. Contact dermatitis

2. Drug rash (ampicillin and other drugs)

3. Fixed drug eruption

Other dermatologic conditions (see Chapter 22)

1. Trauma

2. Lichen planus

3. Psoriasis

4. Reiter's syndrome

5. Neurodermatitis

6. Seborrheic dermatitis

7. Balanitis

8. Neoplasm

9. Behçet's disease

10. And many others

---

of infection that can produce dysuria: the vagina, the urethra,
and the bladder.

<u>Vaginitis</u>

Patients complain of external pain on urination in contrast
to the internal pain that occurs with urethritis or cystitis. Usually
there is no frequency, urgency, or hematuria. The common etiologies are <u>Trichomonas vaginalis</u>, <u>Gardnerella vaginalis</u>, <u>Can-
dida albicans</u>, and herpes simplex virus or paraurethral infection.

Table 1.10   Sexually Transmitted Diseases or Other Diseases
of the Genitals Associated with Itching

Skin rash:

> Scabies, neurodermatitis, lichen sclerosis et atrophicus,
> contact dermatitis, pediculosis, leukoplakia, seborrheic der-
> matitis, superficial fungal infections, Paget's disease,
> erythroplasia of Queyrat

Skin papules:

> Fox-Fordyce disease, psoriasis, carcinoma

Vaginal discharge:

> Candidiasis, trichomoniasis, or gonorrhea

Table 1.11   Sexually Transmitted Disease Associated
with Dysuria

---

1. Gonorrhea

2. Nongonococcal urethritis (_Chlamydia_, etc.)

3. Herpes genitalis

4. Urethral syndrome (frequency-dysuria syndrome) in women

5. Any kind of vaginal discharge or vaginitis may cause dysuria
   in women

Urethritis

The pain on urination is internal. The etiologic agents are
most commonly _Chlamydia trachomatis_, _Neisseria gonorrhoeae_,
herpes simplex virus, and _Escherichia coli_ or _Staphylococcus
saprophyticus_. This may also be the "urethral syndrome" or

"frequency-dysuria syndrome," where the bacterial colony counts in urine are less than 10^5/ml.

Cystitis

The symptoms are internal pain, frequency, and suprapubic pain. Hematuria and cloudy urine are frequent. The etiologies are most commonly <u>Escherichia coli</u>, <u>Staphylococcus saprophyticus</u>, <u>Klebsiella</u> species, and <u>Proteus</u> species. The bacterial colony counts in the urine are greater than 10^5. Cystitis seems to be associated with sexual intercourse in some women, but the infecting bacteria are usually the patient's own resident flora, and therefore cystitis is not considered to be a sexually transmitted disease.

Diagnostic Work-Up of Dysuria

1. Rule out the presence of vaginitis and the skin lesions of herpes simplex virus.
   a. Physical examination
   b. Examination of vaginal fluid: as above
   c. Gram stain of cervical mucous
   d. Gonococcal and chlamydial culture
2. Establish the difference between cystitis and frequency-dysuria syndrome.
   a. Pyuria present in both; ≥ 8 white blood cells/ml in an unspun midstream urine specimen
   b. Hematuria present in both
   c. Significant bacteriuria is present in cystitis but not in the urethral syndrome (significant bacteriuria indicates a single organism in counts of greater than 10^5/ml urine).

Tables 1.12, 1.13, and 1.14 give information on pain in the scrotum, pathogens affecting the gastrointestinal tract, and diseases causing enlarged inguinal lymph nodes.

THOUGHTS ON THERAPY OF SEXUALLY TRANSMITTED DISEASES

1. Patient compliance is difficult to predict. Where applicable, single-dose therapies are preferred.
2. Regarding the use of drugs in pregnancy, most physicians would like to avoid all drugs in pregnant women. For most

Table 1.12   Diseases and Conditions That May Cause Pain
in the Scrotum

---

1. Epididymitis

2. Testicular torsion

3. Orchitis

4. Torsion of appendage

5. Testicular tumor

6. Hydrocele, spermatocele, varicocele

7. Hematoma

8. Inguinal hernia

Table 1.13   Sexually Transmitted Pathogens Affecting the
Gastrointestinal Tract (See Chapter 11)

Proctitis:

Neisseria gonorrhoeae

Herpes simplex virus

Chlamydia trachomatis (LGV and non-LGV serotypes)

Treponema pallidum

Proctocolitis:

Campylobacter jejuni

Shigella flexneri

Chlamydia trachomatis (LGV serotypes)

Entamoeba histolytica

Enteritis:

Gardia lamblia

Table 1.14   Sexually Transmitted and Other Diseases Causing
Enlarged Inguinal Lymph Nodes

Syphilis

Genital herpes

Chancroid

Lymphogranuloma venereum

Infectious mononucleosis

Secondary to balanitis, balanoposthitis, vulvitis, urethritis, etc.

Lymphadenopathy in homosexual men (possibly related to acquired
immune deficiency syndrome)

---

    antibiotics, the package insert gives the following advice:
"Safety for use in pregnancy has not been established." Tetracycline and erythromycin estolate are contraindicated during
pregnancy, and metronidazole should be avoided during the
first 16 weeks of pregnancy. Sulfonamides should not be given
during the last 3 months of pregnancy. With the remainder of
the anti-infective agents, the risk of the drug to the mother and
fetus has to be weighed against the adverse consequences of the
disease. Unfortunately, this is an area where data are incomplete.
3. The physician must be prepared to manage anaphylactic shock
or adverse drug reactions. The appropriate equipment and
drugs must be immediately available (see Chapter 24).
4. Patients with syphilis should be reported to the venereal disease control officer of the health department so that an adequate
epidemiologic investigation may be initiated. The adverse
consequences of unreported syphilis exceed those of the other
sexually transmitted diseases.
5. Sexual partners of patients with diagnosed gonorrhea, Chlamydia
infection, or syphilis should be treated with appropriate antibiotics regardless of their laboratory study results.

6. Follow-up examinations for the test of cure should be scheduled
   for 1-2 weeks following the completion of therapy. In certain
   high-risk patient groups, another examination at 6 weeks will
   yield a substantial number of patients with a sexually transmitted disease.

PROPHYLAXIS

1. The condom is the best available method for the prophylaxis of
   venereal diseases. Frequently the people who need it most
   (those with many sexual partners) are the least likely to use
   this method (see Chapter 23).
2. If an antibiotic is given at any stage of a sexually transmitted
   disease, a full therapeutic dose should be administered.
3. Continuous antibiotic or chemical prophylaxis is not practical
   and may have adverse effects.

THE MANAGEMENT OF RAPE VICTIMS AND SEXUAL CHILD ABUSE VICTIMS[1]

The following recommendations are limited to the management
of sexually transmitted infections.

Appropriate management of medical-legal aspects, potential
pregnancy, and physical and psychological trauma also are an integral part of the management of rape and child abuse victims.

There are no firm data with which to estimate the risk of a
sexually assaulted person contracting a sexually transmitted infection. Based on the prevalence of infections in the general population, the most likely diseases for which these patients are at risk
appear to be chlamydial infections, gonorrhea, genital herpes,
cytomegalovirus, and trichomoniasis. If the offender is at high
risk for having syphilis and hepatitis B, there is an increased risk
of the victim acquiring these diseases.

[1] From USDHHS, CDC, USPHS, VD Control Division, Quality Assurance Guidelines for STD Clinics, 1982.

Rape

Initial examination of the rape victim should include the following:

1. Cultures for <u>Neisseria gonorrhoeae</u> from any potentially infected sites.
2. If available, cultures for <u>Chlamydia trachomatis</u> from any potentially infected sites.
3. Examination of vaginal specimens for <u>Trichomonas vaginalis</u> by wet mount and, if available, by culture.
4. A bimanual pelvic examination for women.
5. A serologic test for syphilis.
6. A sample of serum should be frozen and saved for future testing.

The risk of infection after rape, while unknown, is thought to be low. If prophylaxis is to be administered because the physician feels it is indicated or because the patient requests it, the following should be used: tetracycline, 0.5 g by mouth, four times a day, for at least 7 days, or doxycycline, 100 mg by mouth, twice a day, for at least 7 days. Patients who are allergic to tetracycline and pregnant women should be treated with amoxicillin, 3.0 g, or ampicillin, 3.5 g, each given with 1.0 g of probenecid as a single oral dose.

Patients should be seen for medical follow-up in 7 days, and the aforementioned studies, except for the serologic test for syphilis, should be repeated. A serologic test for syphilis, six weeks after the incident, is important in cases of assault by individuals who are at high risk for syphilis.

Every effort should be made to establish whether the assailant is infected with an STD. Victims should receive treatment for exposure to an STD which is documented in the assailant.

Child Abuse

Any sexually transmitted infection in a child should be considered as evidence of sexual abuse until proven otherwise. Any child with a sexually transmitted infection, and any child or teenager who reports sexual abuse, should be reported to the appropriate authorities for investigation of possible sexual abuse. Sexually abused children are best managed by a team of professionals experienced in addressing their physical and psychological needs.

The risk of acquisition of a sexually transmitted infection in child victims of sexual assault or abuse is believed to be lower than in adult victims. Such children should be evaluated for STD pathogens as described under the guidelines for the management of rape victims but with particular sensitivity to clinical procedures which may be traumatic to them.

Treatment is indicated when disease is present. However, prophylactic treatment prior to diagnosis usually is not indicated unless there is evidence that the assailant is infected.

OTHER POSTEXPOSURE MANAGEMENT AND THERAPY OF SEXUALLY TRANSMITTED DISEASES

In handling the spouse of a patient with a sexually transmitted disease, note the following:

1. Tact, consideration, and a nonjudgmental approach are important.
2. If the spouse has had sexual relations with a patient who has an established sexually transmitted disease, then the spouse should be treated. In this case no attempt should be made to conceal the diagnosis or reason for therapy.
3. If the spouse has not had sexual relations with a patient who has an established sexually transmitted disease, then no treatment or contact with the spouse is necessary if the patient is promptly treated. In this case the management of the patient should be as described previously.

PATIENT EDUCATION

1. Many patients are alarmed and disturbed by the knowledge that they have a sexually transmitted disease. Thus they may not be receptive to information about their illness given by the physician during their visit. It is useful to have printed patient handouts that patients may take with them to read at a more convenient time. The handout also may include instructions on administration of medications and explain the necessity for a follow-up examination.
2. Posters or reading material on sexually transmitted diseases in a waiting room indicate to patients that the physician is willing to assist them with problems.

In the United States the American Social Health Association has a number of well-written, patient-oriented pamphlets. Patients may be encouraged to request educational materials on their specific problem such as Herpes, NGU, Women and VD, PID, Gays and STD, etc. The patients should send their request and a self-addressed envelope to

HELP
Post Office Box 100
Palo Alto, CA 94302

They also have a VD National Hotline, toll-free at 1-800-227-8922 or, in California, 1-800-982-5883.

BIBLIOGRAPHY

Blackmore CA, Keegan RA, Cates W. Diagnosis and treatment of sexually transmitted diseases in rape victims. Rev Infect Dis, 4(Suppl.):S877-S882, 1982.

Blackwell A, Barlow D. Clinical diagnosis of anaerobic vaginosis (nonspecific vaginitis). A practical guide. Br J Vener Dis, 58: 387-393, 1982.

Blackwell B. Drug therapy. Patient compliance. N Eng J Med, 289:249-252, 1973.

Chapel TA, Brown WJ, Jeffries C, Stewart JA. How reliable is the morphological diagnosis of penile ulcerations? Sex Transm Dis, 4:150-152, 1977.

Chapel T, Brown WJ, Jeffries C, Stewart JA. The microbiological flora of penile ulcerations. J Infect Dis, 137:50-56, 1978.

Dans PE, Klaus B. Dysuria in women. Johns Hopkins Med J, 138:13-18, 1976.

Fiumara NJ, Cahn T. Traumatic ulceration of the cervix. Case report. Br J Vener Dis, 58:202-203, 1982.

Hart G. The role of preventive methods in the control of venereal disease. U.S. Dept. HEW, Public Health Service, Center for Disease Control, Atlanta, 1976.

Hart G. Epidemiologic treatment for syphilis and gonorrhea. Sex Transm Dis, 7:149-152, 1980.

Judson FN, Maltz, AB. A rational basis for the epidemiologic treatment of gonorrhea in a clinic for sexually transmitted diseases. Sex Transm Dis, 5:89-92, 1978.

Kramer DG, Jason J. Sexually abused children and sexually transmitted diseases. Rev Infect Dis, 4(Suppl.):S883-S890, 1982.

Magee J. The pelvic examination: A view from the other end of the table. Ann Int Med, 83:563-564, 1975.

Mashell R, Pead L, Sanderson RA. Fastidious bacteria and the urethral syndrome: A 2-year clinical and bactcriological study of 51 women. Lancet, 1:1277-1280, 1983.

Nicolle LE, Harding GKM, Preiksaitis J, Ronald AR. The association of urinary tract infection with sexual intercourse. J Infect Dis, 146:579-583, 1982.

Panja SK. Urethral syndrome in women attending a clinic for sexually transmitted diseases. Br J Vener Dis, 59:179-181, 1983.

Parker SW, Stewart AJ, Wren MN, Gollow MM, Straton, JA. Circumcision and sexually transmitted diseases. Med J Aust, 2: 288-290, 1983.

Robertson DHH. The differential diagnosis of genital ulceration. Practitioner 217:734-740, 1976.

Spiegel CA, Eschenbach DA, Ansel R, Holmes KK. Curved anaerobic bacteria in bacterial (nonspecific) vaginosis and their response to antimicrobial therapy. J Infect Dis, 148:817-822, 1983.

Stamm, WE, Running K, McKevitt M, Counts GW, Truck M, Holmes KK. Treatment of the acute urethral syndrome. N Eng J Med, 304:956-958, 1981.

Stamm WE, Wagner KF, Amsel R, et al. Causes of the acute urethral syndrome in women. N Eng J Med, 303:409-415, 1980.

Thomason JL, Schreckenberger PC, Spellacy WN, Riff LJ, LeBeau LJ. Clinical and microbiological characterization of patients with nonspecific vaginosis associated with motile, curved anaerobic rods. J Infect Dis, 149:801–809, 1984.

Vosti KL. Recurrent urinary tract infections: Prevention by prophylactic antibiotics after sexual intercourse. J Amer Med Assoc, 231:934–940, 1975.

Wallin JE, Thompson SE, Zaidi A, Wong K-H. Urethritis in women attending an STD clinic. Br J Vener Dis, 57:50–54, 1981.

Weissberg SM, Dodson MG. Recurrent vaginal and cervical ulcers associated with tampon use. J Amer Med Assoc, 250:1430–1431, 1983.

White ST, Loda FA, Ingram DL, Pearson A. Sexually transmitted diseases in sexually abused children. Pediatrics, 72:16–21, 1983.

Willcox RR. The prophylaxis of nonvenereal conditions: With its application to venereology. J Amer Vener Dis Assoc, 1:113–117, 1975.

Chapter 2

GONORRHEA

ETIOLOGIC AGENT

Gonorrhea is caused by <u>Neisseria gonorrhoeae</u>, a relatively fastidious gram-negative diplococcus naturally pathogenic only in humans. <u>Neisseria meningitidis</u>, the other major pathogen of the <u>Neisseria</u> genus, is routinely distinguished from the gonococcus by sugar utilization reactions. Given various sexual practices, the territoriality of the two species is remarkable. Gonococcal meningitis and meningococcal urethritis are rare. Both species may cause disseminated infections, and both may be isolated from the pharynx of asymptomatic patients. Both the meningococcus and the gonococcus have capsules, the latter being only recently recognized. Both also have surface pili, which may be important in attaching to human epithelium.

Gonococci may be subdivided by means of auxotyping and serotyping. The auxotyping requires a series of chemically defined, complex nutritional media from which selected amino acids or other compounds have been withdrawn. For clinicians, it is relevant that one auxotype requiring arginine, hypoxanthine, and uracil (AHU) has been associated with disseminated gonococcal infections. Gonococci from patients with disseminated infections and gonococci of the AHU auxotype are remarkably sensitive to penicillin when compared to other auxotypes. Certain auxotypes also may be related to the patient's geographic location and race. The AHU auxotype is found more frequently in white patients. A serotyping scheme also has been devised based on major outer membrane proteins of the gonococcus. Neither auxotyping nor serotyping is routinely performed outside of research laboratories.

23

EPIDEMIOLOGY

Since 1965, gonorrhea has been the most frequently reported communicable disease in the United States. Beginning in the early 1960s and until 1975, the number of reported cases of gonorrhea has been on the increase. The causes of this remarkable increase have been attributed to a rise in promiscuity which, in turn, may be influenced by the availability of contraceptive pills for women, the mobility of populations, and the rejection of traditional morality by young people. The leveling off of reported cases since 1975 is thought to be the result of gonorrhea treatment programs started in 1973.

Gonorrhea is also difficult to control because of its rapid incubation period and the presence of large numbers of infected patients with asymptomatic disease. It is estimated that approximately 80% of women and up to one-half of men with gonorrhea have few, if any symptoms. Another complicating factor in the gonorrhea epidemic is the recent development of chromosomally mediated resistance to penicillin, tetracycline, and other antibiotics. Patients infected with these organisms must be treated with spectinomycin, cefoxitin, cefotaxime, or cefurovime.

Penicillinase-producing gonococci were reported for the first time in the United States in August 1976. There is every indication that these organisms will continue to be a problem. Increasing numbers of penicillinase-producing gonococci have been subsequently identified in Europe, Asia, Africa, Oceania, and the Americas. These organisms account for about 30% of all recent gonococcal isolates in the Philippines and 16% of the isolates in the Republic of Singapore. Penicillinase-producing <u>Neisseria gonorrhoeae</u> have become endemic in London, England, and have been reported from all but a handful of the states in the United States. These strains appear to be here to stay and may ultimately result in the adoption of more expensive antibiotics to combat them.

At present gonorrhea appears to be most prevalent in people between the ages of 15 and 30. The incidence of gonorrhea in blacks is higher than that in the white population, and in venereal disease clinics the incidence in men is higher than in women. The risk of acquiring gonorrhea from a single sexual exposure with an infected person is probably less than 25%. Susceptibility to repeated attacks of gonorrhea appears to be the rule, and patients with repeated infections contribute significantly to the current problem.

CLINICAL MANIFESTATIONS

Men

Urethral infections

Men usually develop symptoms within several days of exposure. The first symptom is frequently that of a burning sensation in the anterior urethra. Within a day, a profuse purulent urethral discharge (Fig. 2.1) appears that often stains the patient's underclothes. It is important to remember that asymptomatic gonorrhea may be present in men, and such individuals may be responsible for transmitting the infection to their sexual partners. Asymptomatic infections occur more frequently in men with their first infection than in men with repeated infections. Thus it is imperative to obtain a culture of, and to treat, the male sexual partner of a woman with gonorrhea even if he is asymptomatic. Complications due to direct extension of the infecting organism are unusual, although epididymitis, prostatitis, and seminal vesicle infections have been described. Regional lymphadenopahy has been described

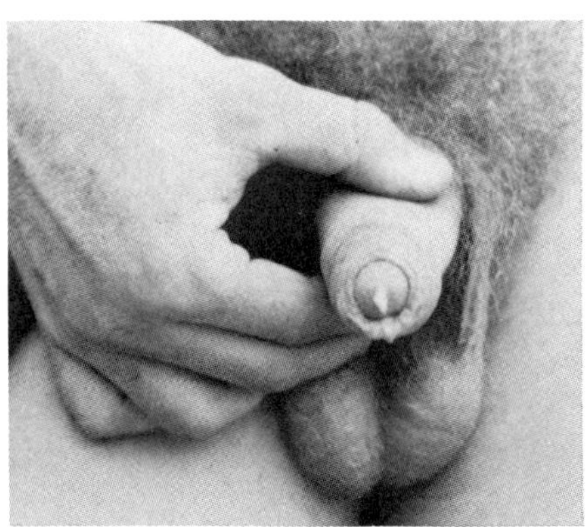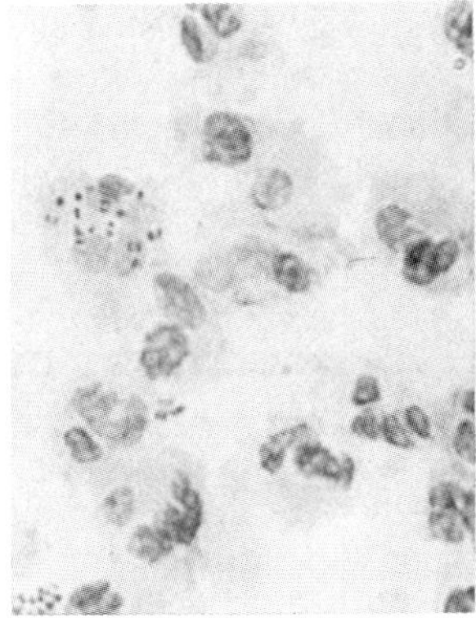

Figure 2.1   Left: Patient with acute gonococcal urethritis. The urethral discharge may be profuse, purulent, and associated with dysuria. Right: Microscopic examination of a Gram-stained discharge (original magnification 240×) reveals numerous polymorphonuclear leukocytes and gram-negative intracelleular diplococci. In men, this is diagnostic of gonorrhea.

in some patients with gonococcal urethritis. It is thought that untreated gonorrhea may be responsible for urethral strictures.

Rectal infections

Gonococcal proctitis may be present in homosexual men and
may be their presenting complaint. Pain on defecation, rectal
itching, tenesmus, or pus or mucous in the stool may all be reasons that a patient with gonococcal proctitis seeks medical aid.
A bloody discharge, however, is unusual. At least two-thirds of
the patients are asymptomatic. Anoscopic examination in symptomatic patients reveals a purulent exudate in the anal crypts.

Pharyngeal infections

Gonococci are present in the pharynx of less than 5% of all
patients who attend venereal disease clinics. Patients most likely
to harbor the organism are those who have orogenital sexual contact. The presence of symptoms is not a reliable indicator of
gonococcal pharyngeal infection, and culture is required for the
diagnosis. Gonococcal pharyngitis may initiate a systemic gonococcal infection. Sugar reactions are necessary to distinguish
Neisseria gonorrhoeae from Neisseria meningitidis in pharyngeal
cultures. Meningococci reacting with glucose only may result in
an inadvertent diagnosis of gonorrhea. This possibility should be
remembered in cultures taken from low-prevalence populations,
and particularly in situations where medical-legal questions may
arise such as in child abuse.

Disseminated gonorrhea

The gonococcal arthritis-dermatitis syndrome is more common in women patients and will be subsequently discussed.

Women

Urethral infections

Gonococcal urethritis rarely occurs as the sole manifestation
of gonorrhea in women. Although the presence of a urethral discharge is not of diagnostic help, women with gonorrhea may complain of dysuria. However, most urethral infections are probably
asymptomatic and occur in association with cervical gonorrhea.

Infections of the Bartholin and Skene's glands are unusual. (See Chapter 22.)

Cervical infections

Gonococcal cervicitis is asymptomatic in approximately 80% of women. Symptoms, when present, may be related to urethritis or the presence of a vaginal discharge. There are no distinctive visual signs on direct examination of the cervix.

Pelvic inflammatory disease

Pelvic inflammatory disease is the most serious complication of gonorrhea in women. The clinical syndrome has multiple causes, and gonococci can be cultured from the cervix of one-half of the patients. Approximately 10-15% of women with gonorrhea develop some form of pelvic inflammatory disease. Symptoms usually begin shortly after or during the menstrual period. Some patients have, in addition, dysuria, vaginal discharge, or abnormal uterine bleeding. Lower abdominal pain, malaise, and fever are present. Peripheral blood polymorphonuclear leukocytosis also may be present in about one-half of the patients. During the pelvic examination, there may be adnexal masses and/or tenderness, and motion of the cervix produces pain. Rebound tenderness is absent. A more complete description is found in Chapter 14.

Gonococcal proctitis

Gonococcal proctitis in women is usually asymptomatic. It is present in approximately 20-60% of women with genital gonorrhea. Approximately 5-10% of women with gonorrhea have infections of the rectum only. Those infections probably result from both rectal intercourse and soiling from vaginal discharge. It is important to culture the anal canal following therapy, because gonococci may persist in the anal canal of 30% of patients who are treatment failures.

Disseminated gonorrhea

The gonococcal arthritis-dermatitis syndrome occurs principally in women and is present in less than 1% of all patients with gonorrhea. The syndrome is due to the presence of gonococci in the bloodstream and their localization distal to the genital tract.

Dissemination frequently occurs following menstruation. The patient may initially note the presence of malaise, headache, fever, myalgias, and anorexia.

The patients frequently seek medical aid because of the appearance of skin lesions in conjunction with tenosynovitis or arthritis (see Figs. 2.2-2.4). This occurrence in a sexually active young person is highly suggestive of disseminated gonorrhea. The skin lesions initially are often painless and do not itch. They are usually present in small numbers (5-20) on the trunk and the extremities, including the palms of the hands and soles of the feet. Gonococcal skin lesions are uncommon on the face. At first the skin lesions are pink, flat, and blanch on pressure. They are usually 1.5 cm or less in size. Within a day, the lesions become raised in the center, where a small pustule develops. Hemorrhage may occur in the pustule, giving it a purple color. The pustule may rupture, forming a shallow ulcer surrounded by an area of erythema. Healing occurs in three or four days, and residual scarring is unusual.

In early cases tenosynovitis, skin lesions, and positive blood cultures are more frequent than arthritis. However, if the disease remains untreated, arthritis will develop with a purulent synovial

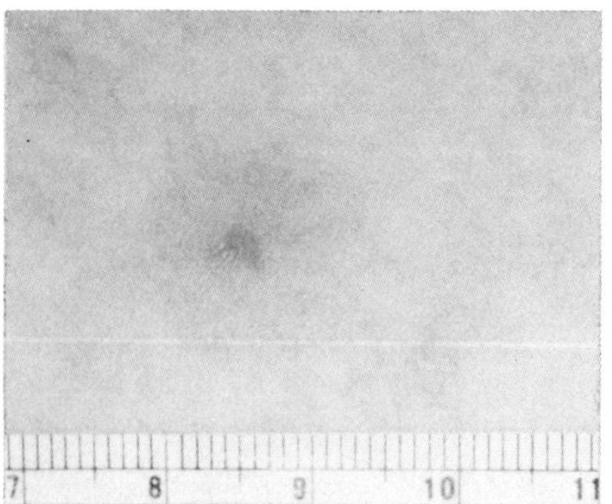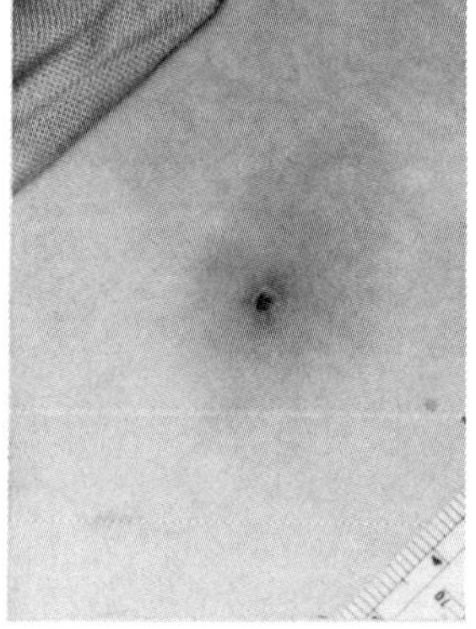

Figure 2.2   Skin lesions of the gonococcal arthritis-dermatitis syndrome. Left: An early lesion with a raised center and an erythematous base, 1.5 cm in diameter. Right: These lesions progress through a pustular state to form shallow ulcers which heal without scarring in a few days.

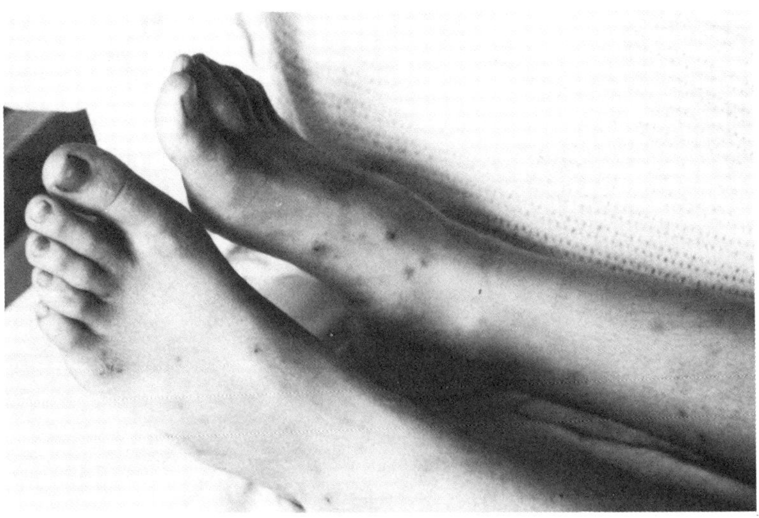

Figure 2.3   Skin lesions of the gonococcal arthritis-dermatitis syndrome. The lesions are few in number and appear most frequently on the extremities and trunk. They are uncommon on the face. Initially they are asymptomatic. This patient was a 23-year-old sexually active college student who noted the onset of skin lesions two days prior to her admission. The lesions were associated with fever, chills, and the appearance of arthritis in her left ankle.

effusion and the possibility of joint damage. The joints most likely to be affected are the wrists, knees, ankles, and small joints of the hands. Upper limbs are more frequently affected than lower limbs. The rash may be confused with that caused by meningococcal sepsis as well as a number of other diseases. Gonococci causing this syndrome are extremely sensitive to penicillin G, and the patients respond rapidly to this and other appropriate antibiotics, usually within 48 hours.

Gonococcal perihepatitis

This is called the Fitz-Hugh-Curtis syndrome and, for the most part, occurs in women. Patients may or may not have concurrent pelvic inflammatory disease, and the principal finding is right upper quadrant tenderness. Fever, nausea, and sometimes

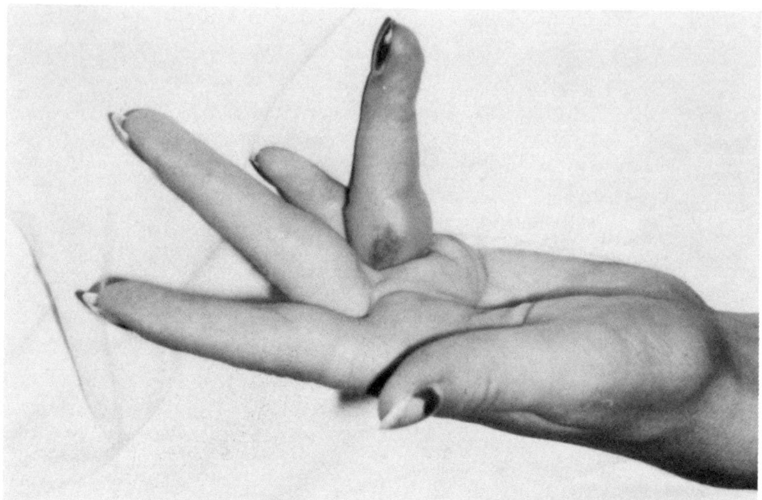

Figure 2.4   Skin lesions of the gonococcal arthritis-dermatitis syndrome. In some patients the lesions may become hemorrhagic pustules. In this young women such a lesion was present on her ring finger in association with a swollen, tender proximal inter-phalangeal joint.

vomiting are present. A perihepatic friction rub may be heard, and transient dysfunction of the gallbladder and elevation of liver enzymes occur. The diagnosis is established by the presence of a positive gonococcal culture in a genital or rectal site. Adhesions may form between the liver surface and the peritoneal coverings of the anterior wall and diaphragm. Chlamydia also may cause this.

Pharyngeal infections

Gonococcal pharyngeal infection occurs in approximately 5% of women with gonorrhea cultured at another site. Pharyngeal gonorrhea is asymptomatic and is more common in pregnant women. The pharynx may be the only culture-positive site in pa-tients who are in their third trimester. This finding may not be universal but should be kept in mind, since pharyngeal gonorrhea is not eradicated by all antibiotic regimens.

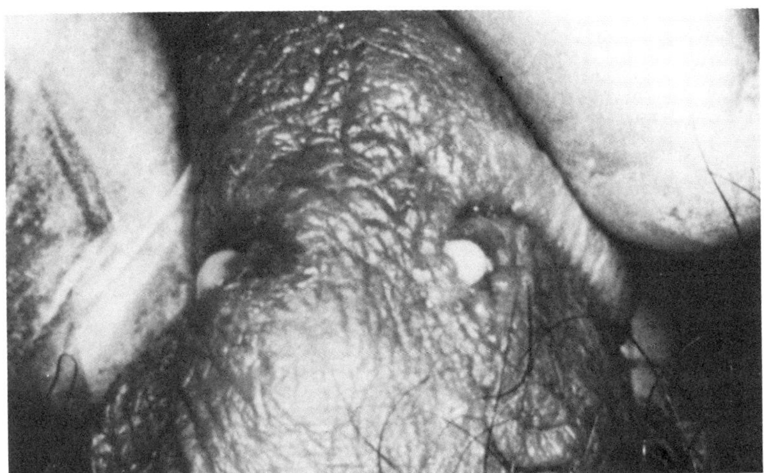

Figure 2.5   Gonococcal infections of Tyson's glands are an uncommon complication of gonorrhea in men.   Tyson's glands are
sebaceous glands of the prepuce which secrete smegma.   In this
photo the examiner's fingers grip the corona of the penis and pus
extrudes from the glands.   (Photograph from the teaching collection of the Venereal Disease Control Division, CDC, USPHS.)

Children

Genital infection

Gonorrhea in girls may cause vulvovaginitis.   The girl may
complain of itching or burning with urination, or the parent may
notice staining on the underpants.   Boys may complain of dysuria.
Outbreaks of gonorrhea among children have been described.   Sexual assault should always be suspected when gonorrhea is found in
a child.   It is wise to always hospitalize a child with gonorrhea,
as it is easier then to get cultures on the appropriate contacts.   It
may be possible for a child to acquire gonorrhea from an adult by
using the same bath towel, but in children greater than 4 years
old, the gonorrhea is most likely from sexual contact.   In children
with gonorrhea from ages 1 to 4, Ingram et al. found evidence of
contact in one-third.   The contact is usually an older male.

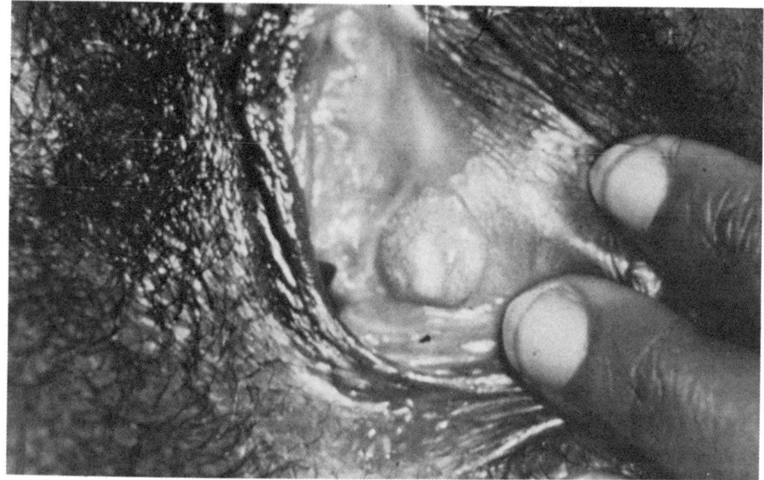

Figure 2.6   Gonococcal infection of the Bartholin glands is an uncommon complication of gonococcal infection in women.   Bartholinitis is not always caused by <u>Neisseria gonorrhoeae</u> (see Chapter 22).   In the photograph the patient has pulled the labium majus to one side, exposing the swollen gland with pus draining from the opening near the vulval entrance.   (Photograph from the teaching collection of the Venereal Disease Control Division, CDC, USPHS.)

Ophthalmia neonatorum

Gonococcal ophthalmia is a relatively uncommon disease among newborns today.   It appears as early as 48 hr after delivery and up to 1 week later.   The affected eye becomes inflamed, with pus appearing between the lids.   The lids are edematous, and the inner surfaces are red.   The conjunctivae are injected.   <u>Chlamydia trachomatis</u> also may be a cause of neonatal ophthalmia.   If untreated, the cornea becomes involved and damage to sight follows.   Silver nitrate applications are not totally effective in the prevention of gonococcal ophthalmia.   The inflammatory response in the eye also may be minimal or absent.

DIAGNOSIS

Use of the Gram Stain in the Diagnosis of Gonorrhea

The Gram stain may be used to evaluate a urethral exudate, a cervical discharge, a conjunctival excudate, or purulent material from the anorectal wall. The Gram stain is used by the physician to decide therapy between gonorrhea and nongonococcal urethritis in a man with a urethral discharge. In cervical, conjunctival, and rectal specimens, a positive Gram stain allows the physician to initiate therapy for gonorrhea before receiving the culture results.

Obtaining the Specimen in Women

Routine specimens in women should include one or two cultures taken from the endocervical canal and inoculated on the same culture plate and a specimen from the anal canal inoculated on the same plate in a separate section (only two cultures per plate). The second endocervical specimen gives an increase in the yield of positive cultures. The anal culture should be performed on patients returning after receiving antibiotics.

The endocervical canal is the site yielding the most positive results in women. The examining speculum is moistened with warm water only. Lubricants are to be avoided, as they may contain antibacterial substances. Insert a cotton-tipped swab into the endocervical canal, and rotate the swab from side to side to allow time enough for the absorption of the endocervical mucus into the cotton. The use of two swabs plated on the same culture plate increases the yield 2-5%. The presence of endocervical mucous or menstrual blood does not seem to affect the culture yield.

Anal canal cultures are performed by inserting a sterile cotton-tipped swab approximately 1 in. into the anal canal. The swab should be moved from side to side in the canal 10-30 sec in order that organisms can be absorbed into the swab. If the swab is contaminated with fecal material, it should be discarded. If the patient is complaining of anal discomfort or has symptoms of proctitis, the area should be visualized with an anoscope before taking the culture. The use of the anoscope greatly improves the yield of the Gram-stained smears and thus hastens the initiation of therapy. The use of the anoscope to collect gonococcal cultures does not give better culture results than does collection by a blind anorectal swab if a selective medium is used.

Urethral or vaginal cultures may be taken in children or in patients who have undergone hysterectomy. The urethra may be stripped toward the orifice in order to express exudate. The specimen may be collected by means of a sterile loop or a cotton swab. Specimens may be obtained from the posterior vaginal vault or from the anterior portion of the vagina in patients in whom the hymen is intact.

Pharyngeal cultures are obtained by swabbing the posterior pharynx and tonsillar crypts with a cotton-tipped swab.

Obtaining the Specimen in Men

The routine specimen in men is the urethral culture and smear. In homosexual men, additional specimens should be taken from the oropharynx and anal canal.

Urethral cultures are obtained by means of a sterile wire loop or a sterile cotton-tipped or calcium alginate swab that is small enough to be easily inserted into the urethra. The swab or loop is inserted only into the anterior 2 cm portion of the urethra. The specimen is collected by gently scraping the mucosa with the wire loop or by rotating the swab. My preference is to have the patient lying down or sitting to prevent a fall in case a vasovagal reaction occurs. For many patients the wire loop is the least painful culture collection method. With spontaneous discharges, simple urethral stripping will obviate the attack on the urethra. If gram-negative diplococci are seen on the Gram stain of the urethral exudate, one may assume that the diagnosis is gonorrhea and save the expense of the culture. Cultures should always be done in asymptomatic male patients and in patients returning for a test of cure or when the Gram stain of the urethral exudate is negative.

Anal canal cultures are taken in men the same way as in women.

Pharyngeal cultures are performed in men the same way as they are performed in women.

Blood Cultures

Blood cultures or synovial fluid cultures should be inoculated into an enriched broth medium such as trypticase soy broth supplemented with 1% IsoVitaleX, 10% horse serum, and 1% glucose.

Inoculating the Specimen

The appropriate medium for the growth of gonococci is modified Thayer-Martin medium or New York City medium, which contain antibiotics capable of suppressing nongonococcal flora present in the vagina, rectum, and pharynx. The culture plates should be brought to room temperature prior to inoculation. The swab should be rolled onto the plate in a Z pattern. The plate should be cross-streaked immediately with a sterile loop or the tip of a fresh swab. Within 15 min following inoculation of the culture plate, the plate should be placed in an atmosphere containing approximately 5% CO_2. This may be a candle jar. The plates should be incubated as soon as possible. However, organisms may survive a few hours without immediate incubation. Incubator temperatures above 36°C may result in loss of viability of the gonococci. The optimum temperature for incubation is between 35 and 36°C.

Other containment systems are available for the selective medium. In one of these, the plates are placed in plastic bags that may be easily sealed. The CO_2 is produced by a special tablet that is activated by the moisture present in the medium. When such systems are used, care must be taken that the tablets are not outdated and that the chambers are closed promptly and tightly sealed prior to incubation.

Clinical and Laboratory Criteria for Diagnosis

Gonococci belong to the genus _Neisseria_, which contains two pathogenic members, _Neisseria gonorrhoeae_ and _Neisseria meningitidis_. All _Neisseria_ species are gram-negative cocci, and they all produce a positive oxidase reaction. Members of the species are differentiated from one another by means of sugar utilization tests. The test sugars include glucose, maltose, fructose, sucrose, and lactose. Gonococci react only with glucose, whereas meningococci react with glucose and maltose. Because the sugar reactions are somewhat time-consuming and therefore expensive to run on a large number of cultures, many clinics and the U.S. Public Health Service recommend that they be done only in certain situations. Sugar reactions should be used to confirm all isolates obtained from other than anal or genital sites. Sugar reactions also should be performed when the diagnosis of gonorrhea is unlikely and when there are special social and medicolegal situations. In most other situations, the presence of oxidase-positive gram-negative diplococci growing on modified Thayer-Martin medium is sufficient for the presumptive diagnosis of gonorrhea. In men, the presence of typical gram-negative intracellular diplococci on the smear of a urethral exudate is sufficient for the diagnosis of gonorrhea. Noncultural identification methods (enzyme-linked immunoassay, monoclonal antibody) may, if sufficiently improved, replace the culture method. However, the predictive value of a positive test is low in women with a low prevalence of gonorrhea.

THERAPY OF GONOCOCCAL INFECTIONS[1]

The following guidelines for the treatment of gonococcal infection in the United States take into account several observations: the increasing incidence of infections due to penicillinase-producing <u>Neisseria gonorrhoeae</u> (PPNG), unpublished reports of the emergence of tetracycline-resistant gonococci in several geographic areas, the high frequency of coexisting clamydial and gonococcal infections, and increased recognition of the serious complications of chlamydial and gonococcal infections. In addition, new antimicrobials, in particular new cephalosporins, that may prove to be effective in treating gonococcal infection are becoming available in the United States. Therefore, these guidelines do not attempt to be a comprehensive list of all possible treatment regimens. Rather, they seek to provide guidance for regimens that meet general criteria of efficacy, safety, ease of administration, and cost.

UNCOMPLICATED INFECTION IN ADULTS

<u>Recommended Regimens</u>

The following order of presentation does not indicate preference.
Tetracycline HCl: 500 mg, by mouth, four times a day for seven days (total dose 14.0 g). Other tetracyclines are not more effective than tetracycline HCl. All tetracyclines are ineffective as a single-dose therapy. Doxycycline hyclate 100 mg by mouth, twice a day for seven days, may be substituted for tetracycline. (See Table 2.1.)
Amoxicillin/ampicillin: Amoxicillin, 3.0 g, or ampicillin, 3.5 g, either with 1.0 g probenecid by mouth. (See Table 2.2.)

[1] This section of the chapter is taken from Centers for Disease Control. Sexually Transmitted Diseases Treatment Guidelines, 1982. Morbid Mortal Weekly Rep, 31:37S-41S, 1982.

Table 2.1   Advantage and Disadvantages of Tetracycline HCl

Advantage	Disadvantages
Effective against coexisting chlamydial infections	1. Requires compliance with multiple doses
	2. May encourage the emergence of tetracycline-resistant strains if the regimen is not strictly followed
	3. Ineffective against anorectal gonococcal infections in men

Table 2.2   Advantage and Disadvantages of Amoxicillin/Ampicillin

Advantage	Disadvantages
Single-dose treatment	1. Ineffective against chlamydial infections
	2. Ineffective against anorectal and pharyngeal gonococcal infections

Aqueous procaine penicillin G: 4.8 million units injected intramuscularly (IM) at two sites, with 1.0 g of probenecid by mouth. (See Table 2.3.)

An important concern in the treatment of gonorrhea is coexisting chlamydial infection, which has been documented in up to 45% of gonorrhea patients for whom adequate chlamydial cultures are done. Patient compliance also can be a problem with

Table 2.3   Advantage and Disadvantages of Aqueous Procaine
Penicillin G

Advantage	Disadvantages
Single-dose therapy	1. Injection
	2. Possible procaine reaction
	3. Possible penicillin anaphylaxis
	4. Ineffective against chlamydial infections

multiple-day tetracycline/doxycycline regimens for gonococcal infections, as can the potential selection of tetracycline-resistant
isolates when incomplete doses are taken. To address these con-
cerns, a single-dose regimen could be administered just before the
tetracycline/doxycycline regimen. On theoretical grounds, this
combined regimen (outlined below) is very attractive, but its efficacy and side effects have not been evaluated. CDC intends to
undertake such an evaluation and encourages others to do the same.
The combined regimen includes the following:

Amoxicillin/ampicillin: Amoxicillin 3.0 g or ampicillin 3.5 g,
either with 1.0 g probenecid by mouth
                         PLUS
Tetracycline HCl: 500 mg, by mouth, four times a day for
seven days (total dose 14.0 g)

Doxycycline hyclate 100 mg, by mouth, twice a day for seven
days may be substituted for tetracycline HCl. (See Table 2.4.)
Special note: Tetracycline or aqueous procaine penicillin G
(APPG) is the preferred therapy for pharyngeal gonococcal infection. Pharyngeal infection is not effectively treated by either the
amoxicillin or ampicillin regimens. A homosexual man with uncomplicated gonococcal infection should be treated with aqueous
procaine penicillin G 4.8 million units, plus 1.0 g probenecid. If
he is allergic to penicillin, use spectinomycin 2.0 g, IM, in one

Table 2.4   Advantages and Disadvantages of the Combined Regimen

Advantages	Disadvantage
1. Provides adequate single-dose treatment for gonorrhea	Efficacy and side effects of this specific combined regimen have not been evaluated
2. Effective against chlamydial infections	

injection. Both these regimens provide adequate treatment for urethral and anorectal gonococcal infection. However, spectinomycin is ineffective in the treatment of pharyngeal gonococcal infection.

Other Considerations

Patients other than homosexual men who are allergic to penicillins or probenecid should be treated with oral tetracycline or doxycycline as above. Penicillin-allergic patients who cannot tolerate tetracyclines may be treated with spectinomycin HCl, 2.0 g, IM, in one injection.

Patients with incubating syphilis (seronegative without clinical signs of syphilis) are likely to be cured by all the above regimens except spectinomycin. All patients treated for gonorrhea should have a serologic test for syphilis.

Patients with gonorrhea who also have syphilis or are established contacts of syphilis patients should be given additional treatment appropriate to the stage of syphilis.

TREATMENT OF SEXUAL PARTNERS

Men and women exposed to gonorrhea should be examined, cultured, and treated at once with one of the regimens above.

FOLLOW-UP

Follow-up cultures should be obtained from the infected site(s) four to seven days after completion of treatment. In addition, cultures should be obtained from the rectum of all women who have been treated for gonorrhea.

TREATMENT FAILURES

The patient in whom gonorrhea persists after treatment with one of the nonspectinomycin regimens above should be treated with 2.0 g spectinomycin IM. (See penicillinase-producing <u>Neisseria gonorrhoeae</u> below.) Recurrent gonococcal infections after treatment with the recommended schedules may be due to reinfection and indicate a need for improved contact tracing and patient education. Since PPNG infection is a cause of treatment failure, post-treatment isolates should be tested for penicillinase production.

DRUGS NOT RECOMMENDED

Although long-acting forms of penicillin (such as benzathine penicillin G) are effective in the treatment of syphilis, they have no place in the treatment of gonorrhea. Oral penicillin preparations such as penicillin V are not recommended for the treatment of gonococcal infection.

PENICILLINASE-PRODUCING
<u>NEISSERIA GONORRHOEAE</u> (PPNG)

Patients with proven PPNG infection or who are likely to have acquired gonorrhea in areas of high PPNG prevalence and their sexual partners should receive spectinomycin 2.0 g, IM, in a single injection. Tetracycline may be added to treat coexistent chlamydial infection. Patients with positive cultures after spectinomycin therapy should be treated with cefoxitin 2.0 g, IM, in a single injection plus probenecid 1.0 g, by mouth, or cefotaxime 1.0 g, IM, in a single injection without probenecid. A daily single dose of nine tablets of trimethoprim/sulfamethoxazole (80 mg/400 mg) for five days should be used to treat pharyngeal gonococcal infection due to PPNG. Spectinomycin and cefoxitin are ineffective in pharyngeal infections.

GONOCOCCAL INFECTIONS IN PREGNANCY

All pregnant women should have endocervical cultures for gonococci as an integral part of the prenatal care at the time of the first visit. A second culture late in the third trimester should be obtained from women at high risk of gonococcal infection.

Drug regimens of choice are amoxicillin or ampicillin, each with probenecid as described above. Women who are allergic to penicillin or probenecid should be treated with spectinomycin 2.0 g, IM. Erythromycin in the dosage recommended under chlamydial infection can be added to treat coexistent chlamydial infection.

Refer to the sections on acute salpingitis and disseminated gonococcal infections for the treatment of these conditions during pregnancy. Tetracycline should not be used in pregnant women because of potential adverse effects for the fetus.

DISSEMINATED GONOCOCCAL INFECTION

<u>Treatment Schedules</u>

Hospitalization is usually indicated, especially for those who cannot reliably comply with treatment, have uncertain diagnosis, or have purulent joint effusions or other complications.

There are several acceptable treatment schedules for the gonococcal arthritis-dermatitis syndrome. These include the following:

Aqueous crystalline penicillin G: 10 million units, intravenously (IV), per day until improvement occurs, followed by amoxicillin 500 mg or ampicillin 500 mg, by mouth, four times a day to complete at least seven days of antibiotic treatment

OR

Amoxicillin/ampicillin: amoxicillin 3.0 g or ampicillin 3.5 g, by mouth, each with probenecid 1.0 g, followed by amoxicillin 500 mg or ampicillin 500 mg, by mouth, four times a day for at least seven days

OR

Tetracycline HCl: 500 mg, by mouth, four times a day for at
least seven days. Tetracycline HCl should not be used for complicated gonococcal infection in pregnant women

OR

Cefoxitin/cefotaxime: cefoxitin 1.0 g or cefotaxime 500 mg,
either given four times a day IV for at least seven days (treatment of choice for disseminated infections caused by PPNG)

OR

Erythromycin: 500 mg, by mouth, four times a day for at
least seven days

Special Considerations

Open drainage of joints other than the hip is not indicated.
Intra-articular injection of antibiotics is unnecessary.

MENINGITIS AND ENDOCARDITIS

Meningitis and endocarditis caused by the gonococcus require
high-dose IV penicillin therapy. Optimal duration of therapy is
unknown, but most authorities treat patients for a month. Therapy
of penicillin-allergic patients must be individualized.

GONOCOCCAL OPHTHALMIA IN ADULTS

Adults with gonococcal ophthalmia should be hospitalized and
treated with aqueous crystalline penicillin G, 10 million units, IV,
daily for five days. For PPNG, use cefoxitin 1.0 g or cefotaxime
500 mg, IV, four times a day. Eyes should be irrigated immediately with saline or buffered ophthalmic solutions and then at least
at hourly intervals as long as necessary to eliminate discharge.
Cases must have careful ophthalmic follow-up to deal with ocular
complications.

INFANTS BORN TO MOTHERS WITH
GONOCOCCAL INFECTION

The infant born to a mother with gonorrhea is at high risk of
infection and requires treatment with a single injection of aqueous
crystalline penicillin G, 50,000 units, IM or IV, for full-term infants

or 20,000 units, IM or IV, for low-birth-weight infants. Topical prophylaxis for neonatal ophthalmia is not adequate treatment for infections at other sites. Clinical illness requires additional treatment. [Neonatal ophthalmia is best prevented with 1% tetracycline ointment or 1% silver nitrate solution. The latter will not prevent chlamydia ophthalmia.]

NEONATAL GONOCOCCAL INFECTIONS

Gonococcal Ophthalmia

Neonates with gonococcal ophthalmia should be hospitalized and isolated for 24 hours after initiation of treatment. Untreated gonococcal ophthalmia is highly contagious and may rapidly lead to blindness. Aqueous crystalline penicillin G, 50,000 units/kg/day, IV, in two doses should be administered for seven days. Eyes should be irrigated immediately with saline or buffered ophthalmic solutions and then at least at hourly intervals as long as necessary to eliminate discharge. Topical antibiotic preparations alone are neither sufficient nor required when appropriate systemic antibiotic therapy is given. Both parents of newborns with gonococcal ophthalmia must be treated.

Penicillinase-Producing Neisseria gonorrhoeae

Neonates should be treated with cefotaxime or gentamicin in appropriate neonatal doses.

Complicated Infection

Neonates with arthritis and septicemia should be hospitalized and treated with aqueous crystalline penicillin G, 75,000-100,000 units/kg/day, IV, in four divided doses for at least seven days. Meningitis should be treated with aqueous crystalline penicillin G, 100,000 units/kg/day, IV, divided into three or four doses and continued for at least ten days.

GONOCOCCAL INFECTIONS OF OLDER CHILDREN
(Also See Child Abuse)

Children who weigh 100 lb (45 kg) or more should receive adult regimens. Children who weigh less than 100 lb should be treated as follows.

Uncomplicated Disease

Uncomplicated vulvovaginitis and urethritis can be treated at one visit with amoxicillin 50 mg/kg plus probenecid 25 mg/kg (maximum 1.0 g), both given orally, or with aqueous procaine penicillin G, 100,000 units/kg, IM, plus probenecid, by mouth, 25 mg/kg (maximum 1.0 g). The latter regimen is recommended for proctitis and pharyngitis.

Penicillinase-Producing Neisseria gonorrhoeae

Children with infection due to PPNG should be treated with spectinomycin or cefotaxime in appropriate doses.

Special Considerations

Topical and/or systemic estrogen therapy are of no benefit in vulvovaginitis. Long-acting penicillins, such as benzathine penicillin G, are not effective. All patients should have follow-up cultures, and the source of infection should be identified, examined, and treated.

Allergy to Penicillins

Children who are allergic to penicillins should be treated with spectinomycin 40 mg/kg, IM. Children older than 8 years may be treated with tetracycline 40 mg/kg/day, by mouth, in four divided doses for five days. For treatment of complicated disease, the alternative regimens recommended for adults may be used in appropriate pediatric dosages.

OTHER CONSIDERATIONS OF GONOCOCCAL THERAPY OUTSIDE THE UNITED STATES

There are some parts of the world where the presence of PPNG gonococci and gonococci with high chromosomal resistance to penicillin G and other antibiotics make the preceding regimens likely to fail or at least have cure rates below 95%. For these locations, the following regimens should be considered.

1. Spectinomycin, 2.0 g by intramuscular injection
2. Cefoxitin, 2.0 g by intramuscular injection with 1.0 g of pro-benecid by mouth

3. Cefotaxime, 1.0 g by intramuscular injection with 1.0 g of probenecid by mouth
4. Ceftriaxone, 250 mg by intramuscular injection
5. Norfloxacin, 1200 mg divided into two equal oral doses four hours apart
6. Kanamycin, 2.0 g by intramuscular injection
7. Thiamphenicol, 2.5 g by mouth
8. Trimethoprim (80 mg)/sulfamethoxazole (400 mg), ten tablets by mouth daily for three days

The last three regimens may have considerable geographic variation in their efficacy but they are all active against PPNG.

BIBLIOGRAPHY

Alfonso E, Friedland B, Hupp S, et al. Neisseria gonorrhoeae conjunctivitis. An outbreak during an epidemic of acute hemorrhagic conjunctivitis. J Amer Med Assoc, 250:794–795, 1983.

Belsey EM. Diagnosis of gonorrhea in women. A national survey. Br J Vener Dis, 59:59–62, 1983.

Berg SW, Kilpatrick ME, Harrison WO, et al. Cefoxitin as a single-dose treatment for urethritis caused by penicillinase-producing Neisseria gonorrhoeae. N Eng J Med, 301:509–511, 1979.

Bonin P, Tanimo TT, Hansfield HH. Isolation of Neisseria gonorrhoeae on selective and nonselective media in a sexually transmitted disease clinic. J Clin Microbiol, 19:218–220, 1984.

Center for Disease Control. Penicillinase-producing Neisseria gonorrhoeae. Morb Mort Week Rep, 25:251, 1976.

Center for Disease Control. Criteria and techniques for the diagnosis of gonorrhea. USPHS Publication Number 96–552, 1979.

Center for Disease Control. Sexually transmitted diseases treatment guidelines, 1982. Morb Mort Week Rep, 31:37S–41S, 1982.

Eisenstein BI, Masi AT. Disseminated gonococcal infection (DEI) and gonococcal arthritis (GCA): I. Bacteriology, epidemiology, host factors, pathogen factors, and pathology. Seminars in Arthritis and Rheumatism, 10:155–172, 1981.

Faur YC, Weisburd MH, Wilson ME, et al. A new medium for the isolation of pathogenic Neisseria (NYC Medium). Health Laboratory Science, 10:44-74, 1973.

Handsfield HH, Hodson A, Holmes KK. Neonatal gonococcal infection. I. Orogastric contamination with Neisseria gonorrhoeae. J Amer Med Assoc, 225:697-701, 1973.

Handsfield HH, Lipman TO, Harnisch JP, et al. Asymptomatic gonorrhea in men. Diagnosis, natural course, prevalence and significance. N Eng J Med, 290:117-123, 1974.

Handsfield HH, Wiesner PJ, Holmes KK. Treatment of the gonococcal arthritis-dermatitis syndrome. Ann Int Med, 84:661-667, 1976.

Holmes KK, Counts GW, Beaty HN. Disseminated gonococcal infection. Ann Int Med, 74:979-993, 1971.

Ingram DL, White ST, Durfee MF, Pearson AW. Sexual contact in children with gonorrhea. Amer J Dis Child, 136:994-996, 1982.

Jaffee HW, Schroeter AL, Reynolds GH, et al. Pharmokinetic determinants of penicillin cure of gonococcal urethritis. Antimicrob Agent Chemother, 15:187-191, 1978.

Jaffee HW, Biddle JW, Johnson SR, Wiesner PJ. Infections due to penicillinase-producing Neisseria gonorrhoeae in the United States: 1976-1980. J Infect Dis, 144:191-197, 1981.

Jephcott AE, Dickgiesser N, McClean AN. Penicillinase-producing gonococci in Britain. Lancet, 2:247-248, 1981.

Judson FN, Maltz AB. A rational basis for the epidemiologic treatment of gonorrhea in a clinic for sexually transmitted diseases. Sex Transm Dis, 5:89-92, 1978.

Judson FN, Werness BA. Combining cervical and anal-canal specimens for gonorrhea on a single culture plate. J Clin Microbiol, 12:216-219, 1980.

Kaufman RE, Johnson RE, Jaffee HW, et al. National gonorrhea therapy monitoring study. Treatment results. N Eng J Med, 294: 1-4, 1976.

Keiser H, Rubin FL, Wolinsky E, et al. Clinical forms of gonococcal arthritis. N Eng J Med, 279:234-240, 1968.

Klein EJ, Fisher LS, Chow AW, Guge LB. Anorectal gonococcal infection. Ann Int Med, 86:340-346, 1977.

Kleris GS, Arnold AJ. Differential diagnosis of urethritis: Predictive value and therapeutic implications of the urethral smear. Sex Transm Dis 8:110-116, 1981.

Lebedeff DA, Hochman EB. Rectal gonorrhea in men: Diagnosis and treatment. Ann Int Med, 92:463-466, 1980.

Lossick JG, Smeltzer MP, Curran JW. The value of the cervical gram stain in the diagnosis and treatment of gonorrhea in women in a venereal disease clinic. Sex Transm Dis, 9:124-127, 1982.

McCormack WM, Reynolds GH. Effect on menstrual cycle and method of contraceptive on recovery of Neisseria gonorrhoeae. J Amer Med Assoc, 247:1292-1294, 1982.

Martin JE Jr., Armstrong JH, Smith PB. New system for cultivation of Neisseria gonorrhoeae. Appl Microbiol, 4:802-805, 1974.

Masi AT, Eisenstein BI. Disseminated gonococcal infection (DGI) and gonococcal arthritis (GCA): II. Clinical manifestations, diagnosis, complications, treatment, and prevention. Seminars in Arthritis and Rheumatism, 10:173-197, 1981.

Nelson JD, Mohs M, Dajani AS, et al. Gonorrhea in preschool and school-aged children. J Amer Med Assoc, 236:1359-1364, 1976.

O'Brien JP, Goldenberg DL, Rice PA. Disseminated gonococcal infection: A prospective analysis of 49 patients and a review of pathophysiology and immune mechanisms. Medicine, 62:395-406, 1983.

Oxtoby MJ, Arnold AJ, Zaidi AA, Kleris GS, Kraus SJ. Potential shortcuts in the laboratory diagnosis of gonorrhea: A single stain for smears and nonremoval of cervical secretions before obtaining test specimens. Sex Transm Dis, 9:59-62, 1982.

Podgore JK, Holmes KK. Ocular gonococcal infection with minimal or no inflammatory response. J Amer Med Assoc, 246:242-243, 1981.

Sandström E, Danielsson D. Serology of Neisseria gonorrhoeae. Classification by co-agglutination. Acta Path Microbiol Scand Sect B, 88:27-38, 1980.

Siegel MS, Thornsberry C, Biddle JW, et al. Penicillinase-producing Neisseria gonorrhoeae: Results of surveillance in the United States. J Infect Dis, 137:170-175, 1978.

Stamm WE, Cole B, Fennell C, et al. Antigen detection for the diagnosis of gonorrhea. J Clin Microbiol, 19:399-403, 1984.

Stamm WE, Guinan ME, Johnson C, et al. Effect of treatment regimens for Neisseria gonorrhoeae on simultaneous infection with Chlamydia trachomatis. N Eng J Med, 310:544-549, 1984.

Thin RN, Barlow D, Eykyn S, Phillips I. Imported penicillinase-producing Neisseria gonorrhoeae becomes endemic in London. Br J Vener Dis, 59:364-368, 1983.

Thompson SE, Jacobs NF, Zacarias F, et al. Gonococcal tenosynovitis-dermatitis and septic arthritis. Intravenous penicillin vs. oral erythromycin. J Amer Med Assoc, 244:1101-1102, 1980.

Washington AE. Update on treatment recommendations for gonococcal infections. Rev Infect Dis, 4(Suppl.):S758-S771, 1982.

Wiesner PJ, Tronca E, Bonin P, et al. Clinical spectrum of pharyngeal gonococcal infection. N Eng J Med, 288:181-185, 1973.

William DC, Felman YM, Riccardi NB. The utility of anoscopy in the rapid diagnosis of symptomatic anorectal gonorrhea in men. Sex Transm Dis, 8:16-17, 1981.

Zaidi AA, Aral SO, Reynolds GH, Blount JH, Jones OG, Fichtner RR. Gonorrhea in the United States: 1967-1979. Sex Transm Dis, 10:72-76, 1983.

Chapter 3

NONGONOCOCCAL URETHRITIS, MUCOPURULENT CERVICITIS, AND OTHER CHLAMYDIAL INFECTIONS

ETIOLOGIC AGENT

Nongonococcal urethritis (NGU) is likely to be caused by more than one micro-organism. Strains of Chlamydia trachomatis cause approximately 40% of cases of NGU. Chlamydia share many properties with both bacteria and viruses. The chlamydiae exist in two forms: the infectious, extracellular elementary body and the intracellular metabolically active, replicating form of the organism, the initial body. Like viruses, the Chlamydia must develop within the cellular material of the host. Like bacteria, the Chlamydia maintains its cellular identity throughout its developmental cycle and utilizes its own ribosomes and enzymes for the synthesis of proteins. The latter properties probably are the reason these organisms are susceptible to antibiotic agents.

Chlamydia trachomatis differs markedly from Chlamydia psittaci, the other Chlamydia species, which may cause respiratory and other human disease. Chlamydia trachomatis has been divided into 15 serotypes based on a microimmunofluorescence test. One group of serotypes, A, B, Ba, and C, is generally associated with trachoma. Another group of serotypes, D, E, F, G, H, I, J, and K, is generally associated with inclusion conjunctivitis of both newborns and adults, nongonococcal urethritis, cervicitis, salpingitis, proctitis, epididymitis, and pneumonia of the newborn. A final group of serotypes, L-1, L-2, and L-3, is associated with lymphogranuloma venereum. Infection with chlamydia produces both cellular and humoral antibody responses, which are ineffective in preventing recurrent infection.

Ureaplasma urealyticum (T-strain mycoplasma) infections also have been associated with urethritis in men. Their significance as a causative agent in NGU is currently not clear. However, men with chlamydia-negative, ureaplasma-positive, NGU will respond to antibiotic therapy directed toward the ureaplasma. Data suggest that Ureaplasma urealyticum is acquired by sexual contact and may be part of the vaginal flora of sexually active women. A small percentage of NGU may be caused by herpes simplex virus, Trichomonas vaginalis, Neisseria meningitidis, Neisseria flava, and Branhamella catarrhalis. Anaerobes do not seem to be an important etiology of nongonococcal urethritis.

EPIDEMIOLOGY

Nongonococcal urethritis may be one of the most common of the sexually transmitted diseases. Information on the incidence and epidemiology is incomplete, as reporting is not required and diagnostic criteria are not universally accepted. However, from limited data it appears that the incidence of NGU is increasing in the United States. In 1974 statistics from the U.S. Navy indicated that NGU was more frequently reported than gonorrhea. Public venereal disease clinics during the same year had varying experiences with NGU as a cause of urethritis in their patients. NGU accounted for 62% of all cases of urethritis in Seattle, Washington, and 20% of all cases of urethritis in Albuquerque, New Mexico. Such differences may reflect different radical composition of the clinics rather than specific geographic differences. In a number of studies in venereal disease clinics, white men with urethritis are more likely to have NGU, while black men are more likely to have gonorrhea. It also is probable that private physicians treat more patients with NGU than patients with gonorrhea. In college students in the United States, it is thought that a high percentage of cases of urethritis are nongonococcal and that most of the nongonococcal urethritis is caused by Chlmaydia trachomatis. For some unknown reason, NGU and Chlamydia-positive NGU are less common in homosexual than heterosexual men.

CLINICAL MANIFESTATIONS

NGU is, in general, a milder disease in men than gonorrhea. The onset is less abrupt, and the duration of symptoms is frequently longer in patients with NGU than in patients with gonorrhea. Stamm et al. found that whereas 10% of men with gonococcal urethral infection lacked signs or symptoms of urethritis, nearly 25% of men with chlamydial urethral infection had no signs or symptoms. Men generally complain of dysuria, frequency of urination, and a mucoid discharge. Discharge also may be present in the absence of symptoms. The discharge of NGU is commonly less copious and more mucoid or watery than is the discharge of patients with gonorrhea. A profuse, spontaneous discharge is more common in gonorrhea. Patients with NGU may have a recognizable discharge only upon arising in the morning. Although such symptoms and findings may be suggestive in distinguishing NGU from gonorrhea, they are not entirely reliable. Therefore, an examination and culture of the urethral exudate must be performed in order to establish the diagnosis.

DIAGNOSIS

Gram-stained smears and cultures of the urethral exudate should be performed to eliminate the possibility of gonorrhea as described in the chapter on gonorrhea. Despite the general lack of accessibility to chlamydia culture facilities, the chlamydial culture is important in the correct diagnosis of chlamydial infection. Stamm et al. found that 33% of his patients lacked abnormal numbers of leukocytes on the urethral Gram stain, and one-half of the patients were identified and treated solely on the basis of a screening culture. Noncultural identification methods (enzyme-linked immunoassay, monoclonal antibody) may, if sufficiently improved, replace the culture method. However, the predictive value of a positive test is low in women with a low prevalence of chlamydia.

After a culture swab is withdrawn from the urethra, the calcium alginate urethral swab is rolled once on a microscope slide to cover a 1 × 2 cm area. The specimen is Gram stained, and the greatest concentration of polymorphonuclear leukocytes is located with a low power microscope lens. The area is then examined under high power, and the mean number of polymorphonuclear leukocytes in five high-power (970×) fields is determined. According to Swartz et al. and Bowie, this correlates with the diagnosis of urethritis. If the Gram stain of the exudate contains polymorphonuclear leukocytes, and bacteria or gram-negative intracellular diplococci are absent, then the diagnosis of nongonococcal urethritis is likely. If less than four polymorphonuclear leukocytes per high-power field are seen in a symptomatic patient, a first voided urine may be examined early in the morning.

If urethritis is present, then the patient usually will have 15 or more polymorphonuclear leukocytes per high-power field in a first voided (first 15 ml) urine sediment. Kraus points out that collecting and spinning down urine is time-consuming in a busy clinic, and he suggests the following. Patients who have no objective urethral discharge and less than four polymorphonuclear leukocytes per high-power field should be reevaluated after 1 week's abstinence from intercourse. If the culture is negative for gonococci, and there is still no urethral discharge and fewer than four polymorphonuclear leukocytes per high-power field, then the patient is not treated (Fig. 3.1). Urine cultures may be performed to rule out urinary tract infection or prostatitis.

If the culture does not grow <u>Neisseria gonorrhoeae</u>, then the diagnosis of NGU is established. If laboratory facilities are available, both <u>Chlamydia</u> and ureaplasma organisms may be isolated. Cultures should be taken from men by inserting a calcium alginate swab 2 cm into the urethra. Urethral or cervical swabs for mycoplasma isolation may be plated directly on special media. For chlamydial isolation, the swabs should be placed in special transport media and then inoculated into a tissue culture composed of irradiated or otherwise treated McCoy cells. A microimmunofluorescence test to measure <u>Chlamydia trachomatis</u> antibody in serum and local secretions is available only as a research procedure.

Patients with urinary tract infections, prostatitis, or Reiter's syndrome must be excluded. Urethral exudate is not present in cystitis or pyelonephritis, and patients with uncomplicated urethritis generally do not have an enlarged or tender prostate.

Urinary tract infections may be distinguished by the presence of gram-negative rods on microscopic examination of a centrifuged urine specimen or the presence in a urine culture of greater than 10^5 bacterial colonies per milliliter from a clean catch specimen. The presence of prostatitis may be suggested by discovery of an enlarged and tender prostate by rectal examination or a predominance of leukocytes in the terminal urine specimen, as compared to the first portion of the voided specimen. There may be overlap of the entities, prostatitis, and urethritis in the male. Reiter's syndrome consists of urethritis, conjunctivitis, nonsuppurative polyarticular arthritis, and mucocutaneous lesions.

TREATMENT

Tetracycline is the drug of choice in the treatment of NGU. The dosage is 500 mg orally four times per day for seven days.

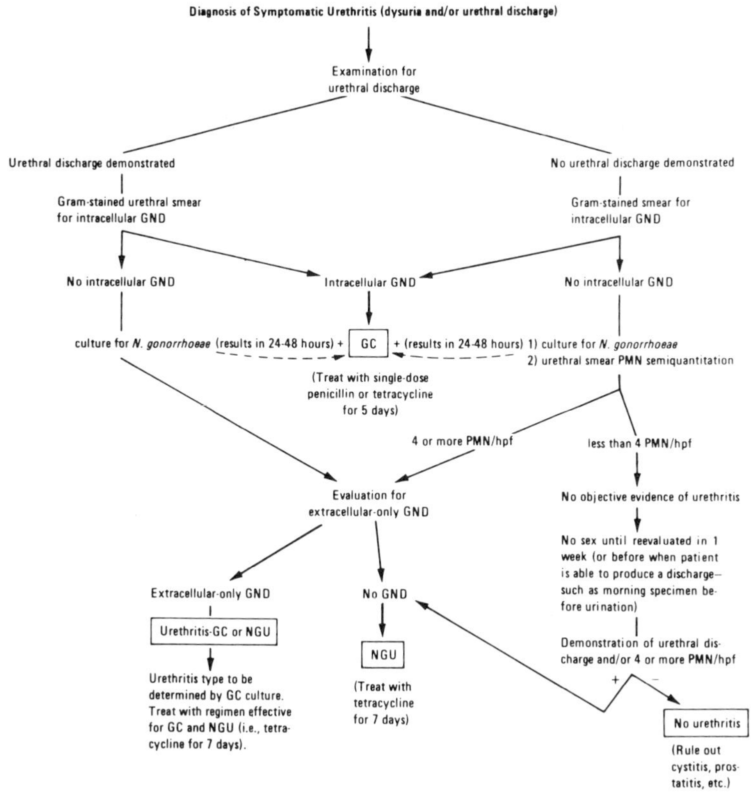

Diagnosis of Symptomatic Urethritis (dysuria and/or urethral discharge)

Examination for urethral discharge

Urethral discharge demonstrated

Gram-stained urethral smear for intracellular GND

No intracellular GND

Intracellular GND

culture for *N. gonorrhoeae* (results in 24-48 hours) + | GC | + (results in 24-48 hours)

(Treat with single-dose penicillin or tetracycline for 5 days)

No urethral discharge demonstrated

Gram-stained smear for intracellular GND

No intracellular GND

1) culture for *N. gonorrhoeae*
2) urethral smear PMN semiquantitation

4 or more PMN/hpf

less than 4 PMN/hpf

Evaluation for extracellular-only GND

No objective evidence of urethritis

No sex until reevaluated in 1 week (or before when patient is able to produce a discharge—such as morning specimen before urination)

Demonstration of urethral discharge and/or 4 or more PMN/hpf

Extracellular-only GND

| Urethritis-GC or NGU |

Urethritis type to be determined by GC culture. Treat with regimen effective for GC and NGU (i.e., tetracycline for 7 days).

No GND

| NGU |

(Treat with tetracycline for 7 days)

+   −

| No urethritis |

(Rule out cystitis, prostatitis, etc.)

Figure 3.1   Flowchart showing the steps to be followed in the diagnosis and treatment of urethritis. Abbreviations: GND = gram-negative diplococci, GC = gonococcal urethritis, PMN/hpf = polymorphonuclear leukocytes per high-power field (970×), and NGU = nongonococcal urethritis. (From SJ Kraus, Sex Transm Dis, 9: 52–55, 1982.)

Treatment is recommended for the sexual partner as well as the patient. This therapy should result in a cure rate of approximately 80%. If relapse occurs, the patient and the sexual partner should be treated with oral tetracycline for 14–21 days. (Some physicians give half the dose during the second and third weeks to reduce side effects.) Both ureaplasma and chlamydia urethritis respond to tetracycline. Alternative tetracyclines, minocycline, and doxycycline are effective in a dosage of 100 mg orally twice daily for seven days. Dizziness is an unpleasant side effect of both drugs. Patients who are allergic or who do not respond to tetracycline should be treated with erythromycin in the same dosage as is used for tetracycline. Chlamydia urethritis may respond to sulfisoxazole, 500 mg orally four times per day for ten days. Ureaplasma urethritis has been shown to respond to a single dose of spectinomycin, 2 g intramuscularly. However, the latter drug has not been cleared for use by the U.S. Food and Drug Administration for this purpose. A patient is cured when he becomes culture negative and is free from pyuria.

In patients who do not respond to therapy, the diagnosis of Trichomonas infection should be considered. Trichomonas organisms are difficult to detect in the urethra of men. Examination of the female sexual partner may be helpful in making a presumptive diagnosis. Trichomonas infections (see Chapter 5) should be treated in both sexual partners by the administration of metronidazole, 250 mg three times a day for ten days or by giving 2 g in a single dose. Herpes virus infections are an infrequent cause of urethritis. Tetracycline-resistant Ureaplasma urealyticum has been reported as a cause of nongonococcal urethritis, and in such individuals erythromycin therapy is suggested.

MUCOPURULENT CERVICITIS

Chlamydia trachomatis can be recovered in a large proportion of women attending venereal disease clinics. Chlamydia isolation from the cervix is more frequent in black women and in women who use oral contraceptives and intrauterine devices. Many women with cervical infection are without symptoms and have no visible consequences of the disease. In others, Chlamydia infection results in a mucopurulent cervical inflammation with edema and ectopy of the cervix. Women with hypertrophic ectopy and endocervical mucopus have a higher frequency of Chlamydia isolation than those without those signs. Judson reviewed the epidemiology of NGU and genital chlamydial infections and found that the isolation rates of Chlamydia trachomatis from the cervix in women were highest in contacts of men with chlamydial urethritis (46-68%). About 27-63% of women with endocervical gonorrhea were infected with Chlamydia, and about 22-37% of women contacts of men with NGU were infected with Chlamydia. Judson believes that the most cost-effective strategy for controlling chlamydial infection in women is to treat all women who have endocervical gonorrhea with tetracycline and to trace and treat female contacts of men with NGU.

Women with cervical chlamydial infection have a higher incidence of Class II or III papanicolaou smears. Women with neoplasia have an excess prevalence of antibody to <u>Chlamydia trachomatis</u>. The meaning of these findings is unclear.

Infection with <u>Chlamydia trachomatis</u> also is associated with postpartum fever and postpartum endometritis. Endocervical infection with <u>Chlamydia trachomatis</u> also has been associated with prematurity and excess perinatal mortality. In addition, 25-65% of infants of mothers infected with <u>Chlamydia trachomatis</u> are likely to acquire this disease in the form of inclusion conjunctivitis or infections of the nasopharynx or pneumonia.

When taking a culture from women with mucopurulent cervicitis, do the chlamydial culture after the gonococcal culture has been performed or insert one or two swabs into the cervical os, rotate them, and discard them before the specimen has been taken. This will decrease the contamination and increase the yield of Chlamydia. Since urethral cultures also are frequently positive in these women, it is worthwhile to culture both sites.

The therapy of mucopurulent cervicitis in nonpregnant women is tetracycline in the same dosage and administration as for men with NGU. Optimal therapy for pregnant women has not been established. Thompson and Dretter recommend for these women 500 mg of generic oral erythromycin four times daily on an empty stomach for seven days. There are no good alternative regimens available to women who are allergic to erythromycin or who are unable to tolerate it. Sulfisoxazole four times daily for two weeks may be tried, but this drug should be avoided during the last weeks before delivery and for the first 2 months after delivery if breast feeding is planned. Sulfonamide administration may cause kernicterus in premature infants. Patients who are treatment failures should be treated with erythromycin base for 2 weeks. This antibiotic, unfortunately, is prone to cause nausea, vomiting, and stomach discomfort in patients who may already have these symptoms as a result of pregnancy. There are four oral forms of erythromycin: base, sterate salt, estolate (propionyl lauryl ester), and ethylsuccinate ester. The estolate form appears to be the most toxic of the four and should be avoided in pregnant women.

OTHER SEXUALLY TRANSMITTED DISEASES
CAUSED BY <u>CHLAMYDIA</u>

In addition to its role in nongonococcal urethritis and lympho-granuloma venereum, <u>Chlamydia</u> are responsible for other sexually transmitted diseases including salpingitis, Fitz-Hugh-Curtis syndrome, Bartholin duct infection, enteritis, proctitis, and epididymitis. <u>Chlamydia</u> also are an important cause of the acute urethral syndrome in women (Chapter 1). The role of <u>Chlamydia</u> in acute and chronic prostatitis is unsettled. These diseases are covered in separate sections of this book, and the reader should refer to the index and table of contents.

<u>Chlamydia</u> also are responsible for conjunctival infection, respiratory tract colonization, and pneumonia in newborns and infants. Neonatal chlamydial infection may represent a poorly recognized public health problem for pregnant women.

BIBLIOGRAPHY

Arya OP, Alergant CD, Annels EH, et al. Management of non-specific urethritis in men. Evaluation of six treatment regimens and effect of other factors including alcohol and sexual intercourse. Br J Vener Dis, 54:414-421, 1978.

Arya OP, Mallison H, Goddard AD. Epidemiological and clinical correlates of chlamydial infection of the cervix. Br J Vener Dis, 57:118-124, 1981.

Arya OP, Mallison H, Pareek SS, Goddard AD. Post-gonococcal cervicitis and post-gonococcal urethritis. A study of their epidemiological correlation and the role of <u>Chlamydia trachomatis</u> in their aetiology. Br J Vener Dis, 57:395-399, 1981.

Becker Y. The chlamydia: Molecular biology of procaryotic obligate parasites of eucaryocytes. Microbiol Rev, 42:274-306, 1978.

Bowie WR, et al. Differential response of chlamydial and urea-plasma-associated urethritis to sulphfurzaole (sulfisoxazole) and aminocyclitols. Lancet, 2:1276-1278, 1976.

Bowie WR, Wang SP, Alexander ER, et al. Etiology of nongono-coccal urethritis, evidence for Chlamydia trachomatis and Urea-plasma urealyticum. J Clin Invest, 59:735-742, 1977.

Bowie WR, Yu JS, Fawcett A, et al. Tetracycline in nongono-coccal urethritis. Comparison of 2 g and 1 g daily for seven days. Br J Vener Dis, 56:332-336, 1980.

Bowie WR, et al. Therapy for nongonococcal urethritis. Double-blind randomized comparison of two doses and two durations of minocycline. Ann Int Med, 95:306-311, 1981.

Bruce AW, Chadwick P, Willett WS, O'Shaughnessy MO. The role of chlamydiae in genitourinary disease. J Urol, 126:625-630, 1981.

Brunham RC, Kuo C-C, Stevens CE, Holmes KK. Therapy of cervical chlamydial infection. Ann Int Med, 97:216-219, 1982.

Burney P, Marson WS, Evans M, Forsey T. Chlamydia tracho-matis and lower urinary tract symptoms among women in one gen-eral practice. Br Med J, 186:1550-1552, 1983.

Carr MC, Hanna L, Jawetz E. Chlamydia cervicitis, and abnor-mal Papanicolaou smears. Obstet Gynecol, 53:27-30, 1979.

Cevenini R, Costa S, Rumpianesi F, et al. Cytological and histo-pathological abnormalities of the cervix in genital Chlamydia trachomatis. Br J Vener Dis, 57:334-337, 1981.

Davies JA, Rees E, Hobson D, Karayiannis P. Isolation of Chlamydia trachomatis from Bartholin's ducts. Brit J Vener Dis, 54:409-413, 1978.

Desai K, Robson HG. Comparison of the Gram-stained urethral smear and first-voided urine sediment in the diagnosis of nongono-coccal urethritis. Sex Transm Dis, 9:21-25, 1982.

Doren GV, Grantz NM. Isolation of Branhamella (Neisseria) catarrhalis from men with urethritis. Sex Transm Dis, 10:202-204, 1982.

Embil JA, Thiébaux J, Manuel R, Pereira LH, MacDonald SW. Sequential cervical specimens and the isolation of Chlamydia trachomatis: Factors affecting detection. Sex Transm Dis, 10: 62-66, 1983.

Felman YM, Nikitas JA. Nongonococcal urethritis. A clinical review. J Amer Med Assoc, 245:381-386, 1981.

Fontaine EA, Taylor-Robinson D, Hanna NF, Coufalik ED. Anaerobes in men with urethritis. Br J Vener Dis, 58:321-326, 1982.

Grayson JT, Wang S. New knowledge of chlamydia and the diseases they cause. J Infect Dis, 132:87-105, 1975.

Hare MJ, Thin RN. Chlamydial infection of the lower genital tract of women. Br Med Bull, 39:138-144, 1983.

Hobson D, Holmes KK (eds). Nongonococcal Urethritis and Related Infections. American Society for Microbiology, Washington, DC, 1977.

Holmes KK, Handsfield HH, Wang SP, et al. Etiology of nongonococcal urethritis. N Eng J Med, 292:1199-1237, 1975.

Jacobs NF, Kraus SJ. Gonococcal and nongonococcal urethritis in men. Clinical and laboratory differentiation. Ann Int Med, 82: 7-12, 1975.

Jaffe H. Nongonococcal urethritis: Treatment of men and their sexual partners. Rev Infect Dis, 4(Suppl.):S772-S777, 1982.

Johannisson G, Löwhagen G-B, Lycke E. Genital Chlamydia trachomatis infection in women. Obstet Gynecol, 56:671-675, 1980.

Judson FN. Epidemiology and control of nongonococcal urethritis and genital chlamydial infections: A review. Sex Transm Dis, 8: 117-126, 1981.

Kaufman RE, Wiesner PJ. Current concepts. Nonspecific urethritis. N Eng J Med, 291:1175-1177, 1974.

Kinghorn GR, Waugh MA. Oral contraceptive use and prevalence of infection with Chlamydia trachomatis in women. Br J Vener Dis, 57:187-190, 1981.

Kraus SJ. Semiquantitation of urethral polymorphonuclear leukocytes as objective evidence of nongonococcal urethritis. Sex Transm Dis, 9:52-55, 1982.

Kuberski T. Trichomonas vaginalis associated with nongonococcal urethritis and prostatitis. Sex Transm Dis, 7:135-136, 1980.

Lee Y, Tarr PI, Schumacher JR. Re-evaluation of the role of T-mycoplasmas in nongonococcal urethritis. J Amer Vener Dis Assoc, 3:25-28, 1976.

Lee Y, Rosner B, Alpert S, et al. Clinical and microbiological investigation of men with urethritis. J Infect Dis, 138:798-803, 1978.

Mårdh P-A, Weström L, Colleen S, Wølner-Hanssen P. Sampling, specimen handling, and isolation techniques in the diagnosis of chlamydial and other genital infections. Sex Transm Dis, 8:280-285, 1981.

Martin DH, Koutsky L, Eschenbach DA, et al. Prematurity and perinatal mortality in pregnancies complicated by antepartum maternal Chlamydia trachomatis infections. J Amer Med Assoc, 247:1585-1588, 1982.

McCormack WM, Almeida PC, Bailey PE, et al. Sexual activity and vaginal colonization with genital mycoplasmas. J Amer Med Assoc, 221:1375-1377, 1972.

McCormack WM, Braun P, Lee YH, et al. The genital mycoplasms. N Eng J Med, 228:78-89, 1973.

McNeil PJ, Fiumara NJ, Caliando JJ, et al. Evaluation of doxycycline hyeclate in the treatment of nongonococcal urethritis. Sex Transm Dis, 8:127-131, 1981.

Melton LJ. Comparative incidence of gonorrhoeae and nongonococcal urethritis in the United States Navy. Amer J Epidemiol, 104:535-542, 1975.

Nilsson S, Johannisson G, Lycke E. Isolation of Chlamydia trachomatis from the urethra and from the prostatic fluid in men with signs and symptoms of acute urethritis. Acta Dermatovener (Stockholm), 61:456-459, 1981.

Oriel JD, Ridgway GL. Comparison of tetracycline and minocycline in the treatment of nongonococcal urethritis. Br J Vener Dis, 59:245-248, 1983.

Paavonen J. Chlamydial infections. Microbiological clinical and diagnostic aspects. Med Biol, 57:135-157, 1979.

Paavonen J, Kousa M, Saikku P, et al. Examination of men with nongonococcal urethritis and their sexual partners for Chlamydia trachomatis and Ureaplasma urealyticum. Sex Transm Dis, 5:93-96, 1978.

Root TE, Edwards LD, Spengler PJ. Nongonococcal urethritis: A survey of clinical and laboratory features. Sex Transm Dis, 7: 59-65, 1980.

Saltz GR, Linnemann CC, Brookman RR, Rauh JL. Chlamydia trachomatis cervical infections in female adolescents. J Pediatr, 6:981-985, 1981.

Schacter J. Chlamydial infections. N Eng J Med, 298:428-435, 490-495, 540-549, 1978.

Schacter J, Hill EC, King EB, et al. Chlamydia trachomatis and cervical neoplasia. J Amer Med Assoc, 248:2134-2138, 1982.

Scheibel JH, Kristensen JK, Hentzer B, et al. Treatment of Chlamydial urethritis in men and Chlamydia trachomatis-positive female partners: Comparison of erythromycin and tetracycline in treatment courses of one week. Sex Transm Dis, 9:128-131, 1982.

Stamm WE, Koutsky LA, Benedetti JK, Jourden JL, Brunham RC, Holmes KK. Chlamydia trachomatis urethral infections in men. Prevalence, risk factors and clinical manifestations. Ann Int Med, 100:47-51, 1984.

Stimson, JB, Hale J, Bowie WR, et al. Tetracycline-resistant Ureaplasma urealyticum: A cause of persistent nongonococcal urethritis. Ann Int Med, 94:192-194, 1981.

Svensson L, Westrom L, Moardh P-A. Chlamydia trachomatis in women attending a gynecological outpatient clinic with lower genital tract infection. Br J Vener Dis, 57:259-262, 1981.

Swartz SL, Kraus SJ, Herrmann KL, et al. Diagnosis and etiology of nongonococcal urethritis. J Infect Dis, 183:445-454, 1978.

Tait IA, Rees E, Hobson D, Byng RE, Tweedie MCK. Chlamydial infection of the cervix in contacts of men with nongonococcal urethritis. Br J Vener Dis, 56:37-45, 1980.

Tarr PI, Lee YH, Alpert S, et al. Comparison of methods for the isolation of genital mycoplasmas from men. J Infect Dis, 133: 419-423, 1976.

Taylor-Robinson D, McCormack WM. The genital mycoplasmas. N Eng J Med, 302:1003-1010, 1063-1067, 1980.

Thambar IV, Simmons PD, Thin RN, et al. Double-blind comparison of two regimens in the treatment of nongonococcal urethritis. Seven-day vs. 21-day course of triple tetracycline (Deteclo). Br J Vener Dis, 55:284-288, 1979.

Thompson SE, Dretler RH. Epidemiology and treatment of Chlamydial infections in pregnant women and infants. Rev Infect Dis, 4(Suppl.):S747-S757, 1982.

Thompson SE, Washington AE. Epidemiology of sexually transmitted Chlamydia trachomatis infections. Epidemiol Rev. 5:96-108, 1983.

Volk J, Kraus SJ. Nongonococcal urethritis, a veneral disease as prevalent as epidemic gonorrhoea. Arch Int Med, 134:511-514, 1974.

Willcox RR. Epidemiological importance of concealed nongonococcal urethritis. Br J Vener Dis, 55:149-153, 1979.

Wong JL, Hines PA, Brasher MD, et al. The etiology of nongonococcal urethritis in men attending a venereal disease clinic. Sex Transm Dis, 4:4-8, 1977.

Chapter 4

GARDNERELLA VAGINALIS VAGINITIS

ETIOLOGIC AGENT

Gardnerella (Haemophilus) vaginalis is a small (0.4-0.6 to 1-2 μm), nonmotile, nonencapsulated pleomorphic gram-variable rod associated with leukorrhea and vaginitis. Its presence in the vaginal flora of some women is one of the few undisputed facts about the micro-organism. The micro-organism had been previously designated Haemophilus vaginalis and Corynebacterium vaginale. In 1980 the micro-organism was reclassified into a new genus. Its new name, Gardnerella vaginalis, recognizes the work of Gardner, who showed its relationship to nonspecific vaginitis.

EPIDEMIOLOGY

G. vaginalis can be cultured from approximately one-third of normal women. Isolation rates are higher, but not significantly so, in sexually experienced women in comparison to sexually inexperienced women. Up to 90% of the male sexual partners of infected women also harbor G. vaginalis in the urethra. G. vaginalis often is cultured from patients with other sexually transmitted diseases.

There is a significant association between the presence of G. vaginalis, increased numbers of anaerobic bacteria, and the presence of nonspecific vaginitis. The role of anaerobic bacteria in conjunction with G. vaginalis to produce disease recently has been recognized. The odor from a positive amine test is caused by anaerobic bacteria rather than G. vaginalis. Women who are clinically cured of their nonspecific vaginitis may still harbor G. vaginalis in low numbers.

CLINICAL MANIFESTATIONS

G. vaginalis is thought to be the major cause of nonspecific
vaginitis. The vaginal disease caused by G. vaginalis generally
results in only mild inflammatory changes in the vaginal mucosa,
and the term "vaginal leukorrhea" might be the more proper desig-
nation. Patients usually have a gray-colored, malodorous vaginal
discharge which is increased in quantity. One-third of patients
will complain of itching or burning, and one-fifth will have redness
and edema of the vulva. The vaginal discharge has the consistency
of a thin flour paste, and it adheres to the vaginal wall in a thin
film. In about 10% of patients, erythema or petechiae are present
in the vaginal wall. The presence of nonspecific vaginitis is correlated with a history of sexual activity, a history of prior trichomonas infection, and current use of nonbarrier contraceptive
methods, particularly intrauterine devices.

G. vaginalis has been isolated in blood cultures from neonates,
postpartum patients, and patients following gynecologic surgery.
The organism also is an uncommon cause of septic abortion and
postpartum endometritis. It has been isolated in vaginal abscesses,
Bartholin cyst infections, postoperative abdominal wounds, and
peritoneal fluid. G. vaginalis is an unusual cause of urinary tract
infection in both men and women. Urethral carriage in men may
be present without symptoms of urethritis. Dawson et al. found
carriage of G. vaginalis to be higher among heterosexual men
(14.5%) than among homosexual men (4.5%). They found no evidence of rectal or subpreputial carriage. On the other hand, Kinghorn et al. identified G. vaginalis in 7.2% of 194 unselected men
attending a Department of Genitourinary Medicine. G. vaginalis
was found more frequently in preputial swabs than in urethral
swabs. G. vaginalis in concert with Bacteroides species may
cause balanoposthitis in men.

DIAGNOSIS

The diagnosis of nonspecific vaginitis reflects the uncertainty
of its cause. At the moment there is no entirely satisfactory diagnostic criteria. One set of criteria was proposed by Amsel et al.
They believe that the diagnosis of nonspecific vaginitis may be
established by the presence of three or four criteria: (1) vaginal
pH above 4.5, (2) characteristic vaginal discharge as described
above, (3) positive potassium hydroxide odor test, and (4) clue

cells on saline wet mount. The difficulty with this set of criteria is that it may overdiagnose the condition, as asymptomatic disease was found in 50% of patients meeting their criteria.

The pH of the vaginal secretions on the tip of the speculum may be measured with indicator paper or a pH meter. However, the presence of semen, cervical discharge, or mucous or menstrual blood also will raise the pH of vaginal secretions. The vaginal discharge of nonspecific vaginitis is generally thin with a milk-like consistency, and women frequently complain of a bad vaginal odor.

The vaginal contents are collected with a cotton swab, avoiding the cervix. The swab is carefully rolled on a glass slide prior to Gram staining. A wet mount is made by placing a second swab in a tube containing 1 ml physiologic saline. The swab is agitated and then squeezed out by rotating it on the side of the tube above the liquid. The diluted vaginal secretions are then microscopically examined for the presence of "clue cells." (See Figs. 4.1-4.3.)

After microscopic examination of the vaginal fluid, a drop of 10% potassium hydroxide should be added to the wet mount specimen.

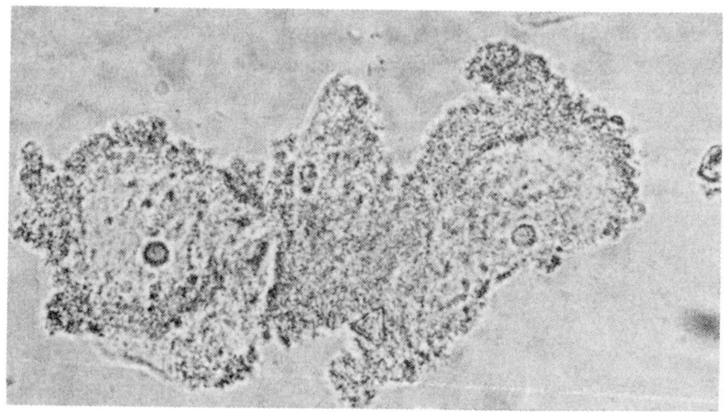

Figure 4.1   Clue cell. This is a diagnostic feature of infection with _Gardnerella vaginalis_. The clue cell is a vaginal epithelial cell with a granular appearance as the result of adherence of these pleomorphic bacteria. From H. L. Gardner and C. D. Dukes, _Haemophilus vaginalis_ vaginitis: A newly defined specific infection previously classified "nonspecific" vaginitis. Amer J Gynecol, 69:962-976, 1955.

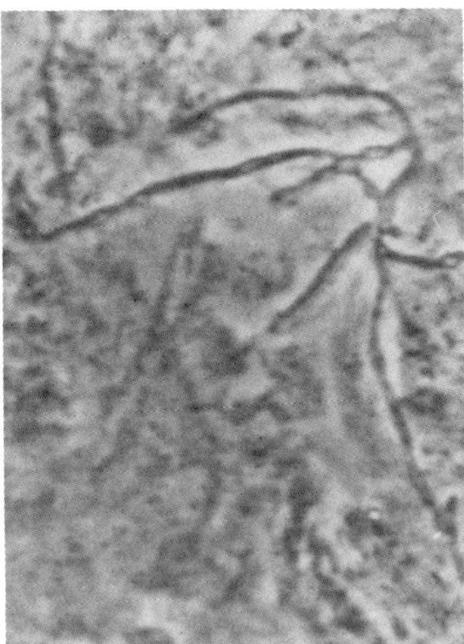

Figure 4.2 Candida vaginitis. Pseudohyphae of C. albicans in a wet mount from a patient with Candida vaginitis.

In patients with G. vaginalis infection, this maneuver results in the appearance of a "fishy" smell (amine test).

Successful culture of the organism requires a special effort on the part of the diagnostic laboratory. The identification of G. vaginalis is highly dependent on the type of growth medium utilized. The bacterial colonies may be overlooked, because they are only pinpoint size after 48 hr incubation on sheep blood agar. Both Columbia colistin-nalidixic acid agar, pepton-starch-dextrose agar, and human blood agar containing antibiotics described by Totten have been suggested as favorable growth media. If the specimen taken on a swab cannot be plated immediately, a transport medium is recommended. As previously mentioned, G. vaginalis may be present in asymptomatic patients, and therefore its presence may not have diagnostic significance. Thus the diagnosis of G. vaginalis remains, to some extent, one of exclusion, i.e., it involves the presence of a positive criteria in a patient without another explanation for the vaginitis.

Future diagnostic methods may be more biochemical in nature, i.e., they may detect metabolic end products of the infecting bacteria. Certain organic acids and abnormal amines have been detected by means of physical and biochemical methods in women with nonspecific vaginitis.

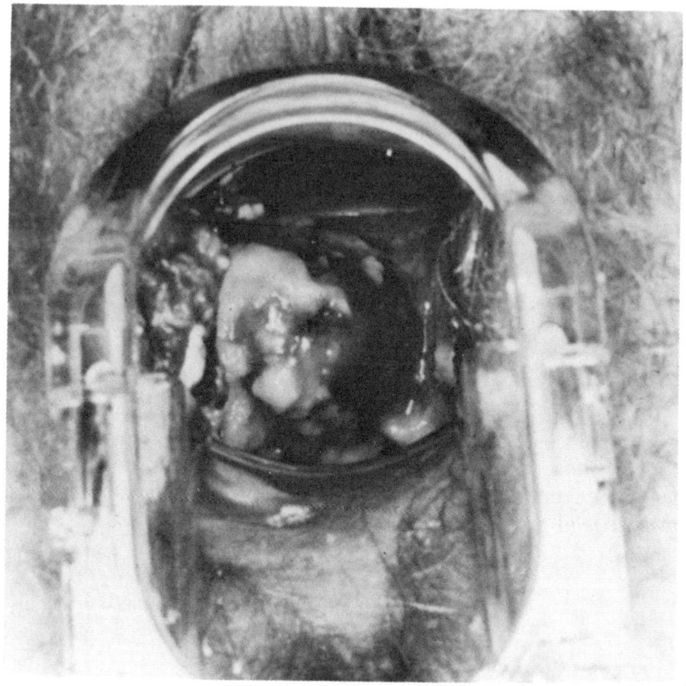

Figure 4.3   A patient with <u>Candida</u> vaginitis has a vaginal discharge with a thick, curdlike consistency. The discharge often is present in white patches on the vaginal wall. The photograph of a vaginal examination shows the white patchy discharge partially covering the cervix. Photograph courtesy of Venereal Disease Control Division, CDC, USPHS.

THERAPY

The treatment of choice is metronidazole, 400-500 mg orally twice daily for seven days. This therapy, although not approved by the U.S. Food and Drug Administration, is the most successful of all antibiotic therapies studied to date. Metronidazole also may be given as a single 2 g dose. A related drug, tinidazole, also is effective in a single 2 g dose given after a meal. Sexual partners also should receive therapy. For a more complete discussion of metronidazole see Chapter 6. Ampicillin, 500 mg orally four times daily for seven days, is less effective but may be an alternative therapy. Sulfa creams and oral erythromycin are ineffective. Clindamycin has in vitro activity but has not been studied to date in a clinical trial. In patients with systemic infections, intravenous ampicillin or chloramphenicol may be effective. In one trial, nonspecific vaginitis was treated with 2 g metronidazole with a 95% cure rate. Tinidazole also may be given in a 2 g single dose after a meal. Sexual partners also should be treated.

In vitro, metronidazole is only moderately active against G. vaginalis in contrast to its 2-hydroxy-methyl metabolite. It is possible that the in vitro effectiveness of metronidazole is a result of its breakdown product rather than the parent antibiotic.

BIBLIOGRAPHY

Amstel R, Totten PA, Spiegel CA, et al. Nonspecific vaginitis. Diagnostic and microbiologic and epidemiologic associations. Amer J Med 74:14-22, 1983.

Bailey RK, Voss JL, Smith RF. Factors affecting the isolation and identification of Haemophilus vaginalis (Corynebacterium vaginale). J Clin Microbiol 9:65-71, 1979.

Balsdon MJ, Taylor GE, Pead L, et al. Corynebacterium vaginale and vaginitis: A controlled clinical trial of treatment. Lancet, 1:501-504, 1980.

Barton A, Kerr M. Vaginitis associated with vaginal malodour. Med J Aust, 2:245-246, 1981.

Blackwell A, Barlow D. Clinical diagnosis of anaerobic vaginosis (nonspecific vaginitis). A practical guide. Br J Vener Dis, 58: 387-393, 1982.

Carmona O, Silva H, Acosta H. Vaginitis due to Gardnerella vaginalis: Treatment with tinidazole. Curr Ther Res, 33:898-904, 1983.

Carney FE. Hemophilus vaginalis septicemia. Obstet Gynecol, 41:78-79, 1973.

Chen KCS, Amsel R, Eschenback DA, Holmes KK. Biochemical diagnosis of vaginitis: Determination of diamines in vaginal fluid. J Infect Dis, 145:337-345, 1982.

Dukelberg WE. <u>Corynebacterium vaginale</u> Review. Sex Transm Dis, 4:69-75, 1977.

Durfee MA, Forsyth PS, Hale JA, et al. Ineffectiveness of erythromycin for treatment of <u>Haemophilus vaginalis</u>-associated vaginitis: Possible relationship to acidity of vaginal secretions. Antimicrob Agent Chemother, 16:635-637, 1979.

Easmon CSF, Ison CA, Kaye CM, Timewell RM, Dawson SG. Pharmacokinetics of metronidazole and its principal metabolites and their activity against <u>Gardnerella vaginalis</u>. Br J Vener Dis, 58:246-249, 1982.

Gardner HL. <u>Haemophilus vaginalis</u> vaginitis after twenty-five years. Am J Obstet Gynecol, 137:385-391, 1980.

Gardner HL, Dukes CD. <u>Haemophilus vaginalis</u> vaginitis. A newly defined specific infection previously classified "nonspecific" vaginitis. Amer J Obstet Gynecol, 69:962-976, 1955.

Goldberg RL, Washington JA. Comparison of isolation of <u>Haemophilus vaginalis</u> (<u>Corynebacterium vaginale</u>) from peptone-starch-dextrose agar and Columbia colistin-nalidixic acid agar. J Clin Microbiol, 4:245-247, 1976.

Greenwood JR, Pickett MJ. Salient features of <u>Haemophilus vaginalis</u>. J Clin Microbiol, 9:200-204, 1979.

Greenwood JR, Pickett MJ. Transfer of <u>Haemophilus vaginalis</u> (Gardner and Dukes) to a new genus Gardnerella. Int J System Bacteriol, 30:170-178, 1980.

Josey WE, Lambe DW. Epidemiologic characteristics of women infected with <u>Corynebacterium vaginale</u> (Haemophilus vaginalis). J Amer Vener Dis Assoc, 3:9-13, 1976.

Kinghorn GR, Jones BM, Chowdury FH, Geary I. Balanoposthitis associated with <u>Gardnerella vaginalis</u> infection in men. Br J Vener Dis, 58:127-129, 1982.

Lee L, Schmale JD. Ampicillin therapy of Corynebacterium vaginale (Haemophilus vaginalis) vaginitis. Amer J Obstet Gynecol, 115:786-788, 1973.

Lewis JF, O'Brien SM, Ural JM, et al. Corynebacterium vaginale vaginitis. Review of the literature and presentation of data based on vaginal cultures from 1,008 patients. Amer J Obstet Gynecol, 112:87-90, 1972.

Levison ME, Trestman I, Quach R, et al. Quantitative bacteriology of the vaginal flora in vaginitis. Amer J Obstet Gynecol, 133: 139-144, 1979.

Lossick JG. Gardnerella vaginalis-associated leukorrhea: The disease and its treatment. Rev Infect Dis, 4(Suppl.):S793-S800, 1982.

McCarthy LR, Mickelsen PA, Smith EG. Antibiotic susceptibility of Haemophilus vaginalis (Corynebacterium vaginale) to 21 antibiotics. Antimicrob Agent Chemother, 16:186-189, 1979.

McCormack WM, Hayes CH, Rosner B, et al. Vaginal colonization with Corynebacterium vaginale (Haemophilus vaginalis). J Infect Dis, 136:740-745, 1977.

Monif GRG, Baer H. Haemophilus (Corynebacterium) vaginalis septicemia. Amer J Obstet Gynecol, 12:1041-1045, 1974.

Pheifer TA, Forsyth PS, Durfee MA, et al. Nonspecific vaginitis Role of Haemophilus vaginalis and treatment with metronidazole. N Eng J Med, 298:1429-1434, 1978.

Piot P, van Dyck E, Goodfellow M, et al. A taxonomic study of Gardnerella vaginalis (Haemophilus vaginalis). Gardner and Dukes 1955. J Gen Microbiol, 119:373-396, 1980.

Piot P, van Dyck E, Totten PA, Holmes KK. Identification of Gardnerella (Haemophilus vaginalis). J Clin Microbiol, 15:19-24, 1982.

Platt MS. Neonatal Hemophilus vaginalis (Corynebacterium vaginale) infection. Clin Ped, 10:513-516, 1971.

Ragamey C, Schoenknecht FD. Puerperal fever with Haemophilus vaginalis septicemia. J Amer Med Assoc, 225:1621-1623, 1973.

Ralph ED, Amatnieks YE. Relative susceptibilities of <u>Gardnerella vaginalis</u> (<u>Haemophilus vaginalis</u>), <u>Neisseria gonorrhoeae</u>, and <u>Bacteroides fragilis</u> to metronidazole and its two major metabolites. Sex Transm Dis, 7:157-160, 1980.

Ratnam S, Fitzgerald BC. Semiquantitative culture of <u>Gardnerella vaginalis</u> in laboratory determination of nonspecific vaginitis. J Clin Microbiol, 18:344-347, 1983.

Rein MF. Current therapy of vulvovaginitis. Sex Transm Dis, 8:316-320, 1981.

Rodgers HA, Hesse FE, Pulley HC, et al. <u>Haemophilus vaginalis</u> (<u>Corynebacterium vaginale</u>) vaginitis in women attending public clinics. Response to treatment with ampicillin. Sex Transm Dis, 5:18-21, 1978.

Sanderson BE, White E, Balsdon MJ. Amine content of vaginal fluid from patients with trichomonas and gardnerella associated nonspecific vaginitis. Br J Vener Dis, 59:302-305, 1983.

Shaw CE, Forsyth ME, Bowie WR, Black WA. Rapid presumptive identification of <u>Gardnerella vaginalis</u> (<u>Haemophilus vaginalis</u>) from human blood agar media. J Clin Microbiol 14:108-110, 1981.

Smith RF, Rodgers HA, Hines PA, et al. Comparisons between direct microscopic and cultural methods for recognition of <u>Corynebacterium vaginale</u> in women with vaginitis. J Clin Microbiol, 5:268-272, 1977.

Spiegel CA, Amsel R, Eschenbach D, et al. Anaerobic bacteria in nonspecific vaginitis. N Eng J Med, 303:601-607, 1980.

Spiegel CA, Amsel R, Holmes KK. Diagnosis of bacterial vaginosis by direct Gram stain of vaginal fluid. J Clin Microbiol, 18:170-177, 1983.

Tabaqchali S, Wilks M, Thin RN. <u>Gardnerella vaginalis</u> and anaerobic bacteria in genital disease. Br J Vener Dis, 59:111-115, 1983.

Taylor E, Blackwell AL, Barlow D, Phillips I. <u>Gardnerella vaginalis</u>, anaerobes, and vaginal discharge. Lancet, 1:1376-1379, 1982.

Totten PA, Amsel R, Hale J, Piot P, Holmes KK. Selective differential human blood bilayer media for isolation of Gardnerella (Haemophilus) vaginalis. J Clin Microbiol, 15:141-147, 1982.

Venkataramani TK, Rathburn HK. Corynebacterium vaginale (Haemophilus vaginalis) bacteremia: Clinical study of 29 cases. Johns Hopkins Med J, 139:93-97, 1976.

Yong DCT, Thompson JS. Rapid microbiological method for identification of Gardnerella (Haemophilus) vaginalis. J Clin Microbiol, 16:30-33, 1982.

Chapter 5

TRICHOMONAS INFECTIONS

ETIOLOGIC AGENT

Man is host to three trichomonas species: T. hominis,
T. tenax, and T. vaginalis. T. vaginalis is found in the vagina
and is thought to be the only species in humans causing disease.
T. hominis is found in the intestine, and T. tenax, in the mouth.
T. vaginalis has an ellipsoidal or ovoid-shaped body with average
dimensions of 7×10 μm. The body is not rigid and can form
pseudopods for attachment or feeding purposes. There are four
anterior flagella approximately 7-18 μm in length which originate
from the anterior basal granule complex. Also arising from this
complex is an undulating membrane which is shorter than the body
and extends down one side. The motion of the membrane and the
flagella assist in the identification of the parasite. (See Figs. 5.1
and 5.2.)

Different strains of Trichomonas appear to have different
pathogenic abilities based on correlations between symptomatic
disease in women and an experimental mouse model. Trichomonads may produce an exotoxin resulting in an inflammatory
response in the human host. A recent study has correlated beta-
hemolytic activity of T. vaginalis with virulence in women, in an
animal model, and in tissue culture. Viable gonococci have been
demonstrated within T. vaginalis, and it is not known whether this
may result in antibiotic treatment failures in patients given single
injections of penicillin.

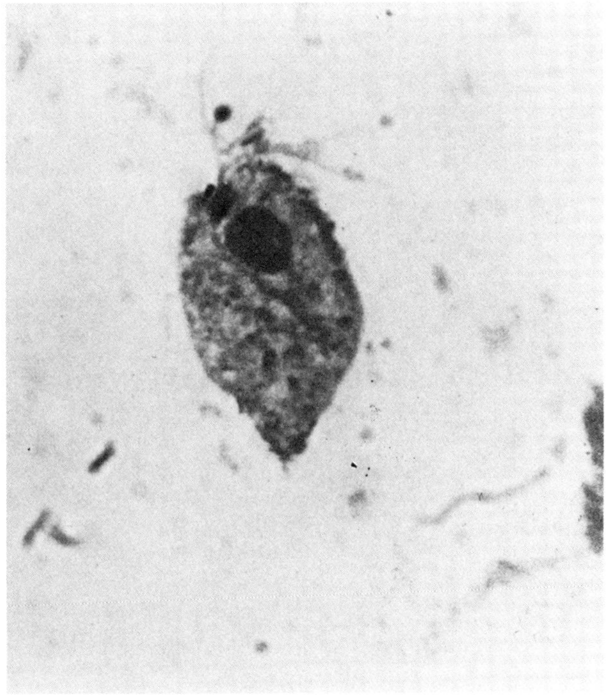

Figure 5.1   A Giemsa-stained vaginal specimen showing a _Trichomonas vaginalis_ organism. Photograph courtesy of E. Stolz and J. van der Stek.*

EPIDEMIOLOGY

T. vaginalis is transmitted by sexual intercourse. Infections also may occur after communal bathing or contact with contaminated bath or toilet articles. In studies performed in women's prisons, fomite transmission did not appear to be important. Infants may acquire _Trichomonas_ from an infected mother. Surveys show that trichomonas infections are present in approximately 20% of women. A number of observations indicate that trichomoniasis is a sexually transmitted disease.

The incidence is highest between ages 16 and 35. Infestation in common in prostitutes and uncommon in virgins. Infestation in sexual partners is common. The female partners of infected males almost always harbor _T. vaginalis_. The incidence in women

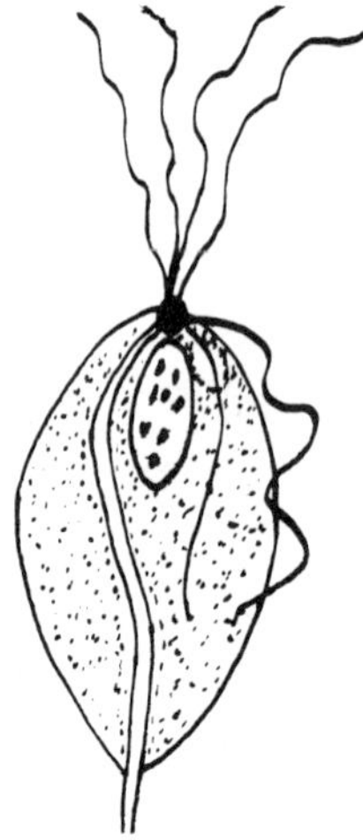

Figure 5.2 Drawing of T. vaginalis. Note the undulating membrane on the right and the flagella at the top.

is at least 12 times that in men. There are, however, technical difficulties in detecting the parasite in the male urethra, possibly because they are present in lower numbers.

CLINICAL MANIFESTATIONS

Many women with Trichomonas infections may be asymptomatic. In studies of women attending clinics, one-fourth of the patients harboring Trichomonas had no symptoms. In another fourth, itching was their major symptom. The itching may be so severe that patients excoriate the vulva and perineal area. In one-half of women patients with trichomoniasis, a vaginal discharge accompanies the itching. The discharge is foamy, foul-smelling, and yellow in color. It may be so profuse that the patient wears a sanitary pad. The patient's symptoms frequently worsen during menstruation. Menstruation results in an elevation of the pH of vaginal secretions, and this favors the proliferation of T. vaginalis. Patients with trichomoniasis often complain of dysuria. On physical examination, the external genitalia of women with the disease may be erythematous, edematous, and excoriated. A vaginal discharge may be present. The vagina and cervix may be inflamed, and erosions may be present on the cervix. Punctate hemorrhages often are present on the vaginal wall.

Most trichomonas infections in men are asymptomatic. T. vaginalis is rarely a cause of nongonococcal urethritis. Male sexual partners of women with trichomonas have trichomonas demonstrated in the urethra in up to 80% of cases. T. vaginalis also has been identified as one cause of prostatitis. Trichomonas infection of the conjunctiva in infants in uncommon.

DIAGNOSIS

Trichomonads are present in the vagina, urethra, and para-urethral glands. Infections that do not concurrently involve the vagina are uncommon. The simplest method of diagnosis is to make a wet mount of the vaginal discharge. The discharge should be taken from the posterior fornix, where it frequently forms a pool. The specimen should be collected with a papanicolaou smear paddle or some other nonabsorbent device. A drop of the discharge should be mixed with a drop of saline on a glass slide. The specimen should be covered with a cover slip and examined immediately, in that the motility of trichomonads is quickly lost. If the specimen is collected with a cotton swab, the swab should be placed in a tube containing 0.5-1.0 ml warm saline, rotated, and squeezed on the side of the tube prior to removal. A drop of the suspension then may be rapidly examined as previously described.

Trichomonads (10 × 17 μm) are a little larger than polymorphonuclear leukocytes and are pear-shaped. The anterior undulating membrane and flagella give them independent locomotion. This is best observed through a "high-dry" objective or 400× magnification. Locomotion is increased in warm temperatures (hence the warm saline). At death, the trichomonads round up and are difficult to distinguish from leukocytes. The presence of a single trichomonad in a vaginal discharge is enough to establish the diagnosis. If there are more than 10 white blood cells per high-powered field on the wet preparation, the patient is at increased risk for trichomoniasis.

Giemsa stains may be used if the slides are not to be read immediately. Although Trichomonas infections may be detected by the pap smear, the sensitivity of this method is in dispute. Acridine-orange stain also is used to detect T. vaginalis, but this method is no better than examining wet mounts immediately after collection. Wet mounts of the urine sediment or urethral and prostatic discharge must be examined in men, but the yield is lower than in women. The wet mount in women is thought to detect at least three-fourths of infections. Culture techniques, where available, are thought to detect 90% of infections. A variety of culture media may be used. Vaginal trichomoniasis may result in dysplasia detected by cervical cytology specimens. Biopsy of the cervix should be delayed until after treatment. A serologic test for diagnosis is not available. To date serologic tests to determine Trichomonas antibody are hot helpful in diagnosis.

THERAPY

Metronidazole is the only effective therapy available in the United States for the treatment of trichomoniasis. Metronidazole, introduced in 1959, is a nitroimidazole derivative that has activity against T. vaginalis, Entamoeba histolytica, and anaerobic bacteria including Bacteroides fragilis. The precise mechanism of drug action is unknown, but the drug probably inhibits protein synthesis and cell multiplication. Cells are arrested in interphase 1 hr after exposure to 1-4 μg/ml metronidazole. Cell death occurs in 8-18 hr. Drug resistance of T. vaginalis to metronidazole has been reported in isolated cases. At the present time, drug resistance is not thought to be a common cause of treatment failure.

Metronidazole is administered orally and is absorbed in the small intestine. Biologically active drugs are present in the serum, urine, saliva, vaginal secretions, and semen. The drug may be present in the milk of nursing mothers, and it also crosses the placental barrier. Peak blood levels of 3-6 μg/ml appear in the blood 1-3 hr after a 250 mg oral dose. All but 1% of parasites are destroyed within 24 hr at a drug concentration of 2.5 μg/ml. Less than 20% of the drug is excreted unchanged in the urine in 24 hr. There is very little protein binding. Some patients receiving the drug develop dark or reddish brown urine due to the presence of breakdown products or metabolites.

Both patient and sexual partner should be treated concurrently for Trichomonas infection. The standard therapy for women is metronidazole, 250 mg three times daily for seven days. For refractory cases in women, a repeat course is advisable. Treatment failures are most commonly due to reexposure to an infected partner, poor intestinal absorption, or possible destruction of the drug by means of micro-organisms in the vagina. Treatment failures are best detected following the menstrual period.

Single-dose metronidazole therapy for both sexual partners is
a convenient method of antitrichomonal therapy. This is accomplished by the administration of eight 250 mg tablets orally while
observing the patient. Cure rates approaching that of conventional
therapy are possible. When both partners are simultaneously
treated, a cure rate of approximately 95% is expected.

Metronidazole is not without side effects. Gastrointestinal
effects are the most common and consist of anorexia, epigastric
distress, abdominal cramps, nausea, vomiting, and diarrhea.
The tongue may become coated, and patients may complain of a
dry mouth or the presence of a bitter metallic taste. Central nervous system effects are rare but are ample reason for stopping the
drug. Skin allergic reactions and monilial vaginitis also have
been reported. The latter may be due to the activity against anaerobic gram-negative rods with resulting <u>Candida</u> overgrowth. Neutro-
penia has been observed following use, and patients who are
retreated should have a leukocyte count prior to therapy.

Metronidazole has been used in research studies for the
treatment of alcoholism because of its disulfiram- (Antabuse)-like
activity. For this reason, patients taking the drug should be
cautioned against drinking alcohol.

Patients who are taking warfarin for anticoagulation may
develop bleeding when treated with metronidazole. The proposed
mechanism is that the microsomal enzymes responsible for the
metabolism of warfarin are inhibited by metronidazole. This results in higher blood levels of warfarin and an enhanced anticoagulation effect. This reaction has been shown to be stereo-selective
in nature (related to the optical rotation of the stereo-isomers of
warfarin). The interaction of racemic warfarin can be lessened or
even avoided by use of the R(+) warfarin alone for long-term therapy. Unfortunately, this compound is not commercially available.

There has been some concern about experiments showing
that metronidazole administration may produce cancer in mice.
This occurs following administration for 2 years of five times the
usual daily dose used in humans. The U.S. Food and Drug Administration presently does not believe that the risk to humans warrants removal of the drug from the market. Metronidazole is the
only drug in the United States which has been demonstrated to be
effective in eradicating trichomonads from vaginal and extravaginal
sites.

A number of other antitrichomonal drugs are available or
are under investigation in European countries. These include

nimorazole, ornidazole, carnidazole, tinidazole, and nifuratel.
At the moment, none appears to be superior to metronidazole.
The nitroimidazoles all have similar structures, and many have
been shown to induce mutations in bacteria resistant to their killing
activity. They are considered to be weak mutagens. Results of
studies indicate that compounds (nitroimidazole derivatives) with
antitrichomonal activity also are able to induce mutations in <u>Sal-
monella typhimurium</u>. Nitroimidazole compounds inactive against
trichomonads are not mutagenic.

Despite the fact that no teratogenic complications have been
described, metronidazole should not be given during the first 16
weeks of pregnancy. During this time, symptoms may be controlled by the gentle administration of acid douches. A number of
proprietary preparations are available, but the patient should first
try a twice daily dilute vinegar douche. This is prepared by the
addition of 2 tablespoons of vinegar to a quart of warm water.
After the sixteenth week of pregnancy, metronidazole may be used
in a single (2 g) dosage given to both the patient and her sexual
partner.

BIBLIOGRAPHY

Beard CM, Noller KL, O'Fallon WM, et al. Lack of evidence for
cancer due to use of metronidazole. N Eng J Med, 301:519-522,
1979.

Dykers JR. Single-dose metronidazole for trichomonal vaginitis.
N Eng J Med, 293:23-24, 1975.

Edwards DI. Mechanisms of selective toxicity of metronidazole
and other nitroimidazole drugs. Br J Vener Dis, 56:285-290,
1980.

Eriksson G, Wanger L. Frequency of <u>N. gonorrhoeae</u>, <u>T. vaginal-
is</u> and <u>C. albicans</u> in female venerological patients. A one-year
study. Br J Vener Dis, 51:192-197, 1975.

Fluery FJ, van Bergen WS, Prentice R, et al. Single dose of two
grams of metronidazole for <u>Trichomonas vaginalis</u> infection.
Amer J Obstet Gynecol, 128:320-322, 1977.

Forsgren A and Forssman L. Metronidazole-resistant Trichomonas vaginalis. Br J Vener Dis, 55:351-353, 1979.

Goldman P. Metronidazole: Proven benefits and potential risks. Johns Hopkins Med J, 147:1-9, 1980.

Greenwood JR, Kirk-Hillaire K. Evaluation of acridine orange stain for detection of Trichomonas vaginalis in vaginal specimens. J Clin Microbiol, 14:699, 1981.

Hager WD, Brown ST, Kraus SJ, et al. Metronidazole for vaginal trichomoniasis. J Amer Med Assoc, 244:1219-1220, 1980.

Heyworth R, Simpson D, McNeillage GJC, et al. Isolation of Trichomonas vaginalis resistant to metronidazole (letter). Lancet, 2:476-478, 1980.

Hillstrom L, Pettersson L, Palsson E. Comparison of ornidazole and tinidazole in single-dose treatment of trichomoniasis in women. Br J Vener Dis, 53:193-194, 1977.

Hipp SS, Kirkwood MW, Gaafer HA. Screening for Trichomonas vaginalis infection by use of acridine orange fluorescent microscopy. Sex Transm Dis, 6:235-238, 1979.

Jirevec O, Petru M. Trichomonas vaginalis and trichomoniasis. Adv Parasitol, 6:117-188, 1968.

Kazmier FJ. A significant interaction between metronidazole and warfarin. Mayo Clinic Proc, 51:782-784, 1976.

Korner B, Jensen HK. Sensitivity of Trichomonas vaginalis to metronidazole, tinidazole and nifuratel in vitro. Br J Vener Dis, 52:404-408, 1976.

Krieger JN, Poisson MA, Rein MF. Beta-hemolytic activity of Trichomonas vaginalis correlates with virulence. Infect Immun, 41:1291-1295, 1983.

Kuberski T. Evaluation of the indirect hemagglutination technique for study of Trichomonas vaginalis infection, particularly in men. Sex Transm Dis, 5:97-102, 1978.

Kulda J, Vojtechovska, Tachezy J, Demes P, Kunzova E. Metronidazole resistance of Trichomonas vaginalis as a cause of treatment failure in trichomoniasis. Br J Vener Dis, 58:394-399, 1982.

Lindmark DG, Muller M. Antitrichomonad action, mutagenicity and reduction of metronidazole and other nitroimidazoles. Antimicrob Chemother, 10:476-482, 1976.

Lossick JG. Treatment of Trichomonas vaginalis infections. Rev Infect Dis, 4(Suppl.):S801-S818, 1982.

Mason PR, Super H, Fripp PJ. Comparison of four techniques for the routine diagnosis of Trichomonas vaginalis infection. J Clin Pathol, 29:154-157, 1976.

Mathews HM, Healy GR. Evaluation of two serological tests for Trichomonas vaginalis infection. J Clin Microbiol, 17:840-843, 1983.

McCann JS. Comparison of direct microscopy and culture in the diagnosis of trichomonas. Br J Vener Dis, 50:450-452, 1974.

McCann JS, Horner T, Shepard I, et al. Two-day treatment of trichomoniasis with nimorazole. Br J Vener Dis, 50:375-376, 1974.

McLellan R, Spence MR, Brockman M, Raffel L, Smith JL. The clinical diagnosis of trichomoniasis. Obstet Gynecol, 60:30-34, 1982.

Mengassner JG, Thurner J. Strain of Trichomonas vaginalis resistant to metronidazole and other 5-nitroimidazoles. Antimicrob Agent Chemother, 15:254-257, 1979.

Morton RS. Metronidazole in the single-dose treatment of trichomoniasis in men and women. Br J Vener Dis, 48:525-527, 1972.

Nielsen MH. In vitro effect of metronidazole on the ultrastructure of Trichomonas vaginalis. Donne Acta Pathol Microbiol Scand Sect B, 84:93-100, 1976.

Norn MS, Lundvall F, Paerregaard P. May Trichimonas vaginalis provoke conjunctivitis? Acta Ophthalmol (Kbh), 43:574-578, 1976.

Notowicz A, Stolz E, de Koning GAJ. First experiences with single-dose treatment of vaginal trichomoniasis with carnidazole (R 25831). Br J Vener Dis, 53:129-131, 1977.

O'Reilly RA. The stereoselective interaction of warfarin and metronidazole in man. N Eng J Med, 295:354-357, 1976.

Ovcinnikov HM, Delektorskij EN, Turanova EN. Further studies of Trichomonas vaginalis with transmission and scanning electron microscopy. Br J Vener Dis, 51:357-375, 1975.

Pereyra AJ, Lansing JD. Urogenital trichomoniasis. Treatment with metronidazole in 2002 incarcerated women. Obstet Gynecol, 24:499-508, 1964.

Ralph ED, Clark JT, Libke RD, et al. Pharmacokinetics of metronidazole as determined by bioassay. Antimicrob Agent Chemother, 6:691-696, 1974.

Ralph ED, Darwish R, Austin TW, Smith EA, Pattison FLM. Susceptibility of Trichomonas vaginalis strains to metronidazole: Response to treatment. Sex Transm Dis, 10:119-122, 1983.

Rein MF. Current therapy of vulvovaginitis. Sex Transm Dis, 8:316-320, 1981.

Ripa T, Westrom L, Mardh P-A, et al. Concentration of tinidazole in body fluids and tissues in gynecological patients. Chemother, 23:227-235, 1977.

Roy RB, Laird SM, Heasman L. Treatment of trichomoniasis in the female. A comparison of metronidazole and nimorazole. Br J Vener Dis, 51:281-284, 1975.

Skole M, Gnarpe H, Hillstrom L. Ornidazole: A new antiprotozoal compound for treatment of Trichomonas vaginalis infection. Br J Vener Dis, 53:44-48, 1977.

Smith RF, DiDomenico A. Measuring the in vitro susceptibility of Trichomonas vaginalis to metronidazole: A disk broth method. Sex Transm Dis, 7:120-124, 1980.

Spence MR, Hollander DH, Smith J, et al. The clinical and laboratory diagnosis of Trichomonas vaginalis infection. Sex Transm Dis, 7:168-171, 1980.

Street DA, Taylor-Robinson D, Ackers JP, Hanna NF, McMillan A. Evaluation of an enzyme-linked immunosorbent assay for the detection of antibody to Trichomonas vaginalis in sera and vaginal secretions. Br J Vener Dis, 58:330-333, 1982.

Thin RNT, Atia W, Parker JDJ, et al. Value of Papanicolaou-stained smears in the diagnosis of trichomoniasis, candidiasis and cervical Herpes simplex virus infections. Br J Vener Dis, 51: 116-118, 1975.

Thin RH, Symonds AE, Booker R, et al. Double-blind comparison of a single dose and a five day course of metronidazole in the treatment of trichomoniasis. Br J Vener Dis, 55:354-356, 1979.

Thorburn AL. Alfred Francois Donne, 1801-1878, discoverer of Trichomonas vaginalis and of leukemia. Br J Vener Dis, 50: 377-380, 1974.

Wilson A, Ackers JP. Urine culture for the detection of Trichomonas vaginalis in men. Br J Vener Dis, 56:46-48, 1980.

Chapter 6

CANDIDA VAGINITIS

ETIOLOGIC AGENT

Candida vaginitis results from infections by Candida species,
organisms belonging to the family Cryptococcacea, Fungi Imper-
fecti (Deuteromycetes). Of the Candida species, Candida albicans
most frequently causes human disease. Candida glabrata,
another fungus of the family Cryptococcacea, has been isolated
from women with vaginal discharges. C. glabrata exists only as
a yeast, but Candida species have the ability to form both yeast
and pseudohyphae. Pseudohyphae may be produced on nutritionally
poor media and are more often seen in clinical specimens.

EPIDEMIOLOGY

Yeasts are frequently isolated from the mouth, throat, large
intestine, and vagina in normal patients. Yeasts are isolated
from the vagina in 20-50% of women attending venereal disease or
other outpatient clinics. More than three-fourths of the yeast isolated are C. albicans. Candida infection is said to be the most
common condition diagnosed in women attending British venereal
disease clinics. C. glabrata often is the second most frequent
yeast isolated (0-20%). C. krusei, C. parapsilosis, and other
Candida species account for the remainder.
In one study of 300 women attending a venereal disease clinic,
Candida species were found in the vagina in 28%, in the rectum in
39%, and in the mouth in 48%. In this and other studies, there was
a significant association between positive vaginal and positive rectal cultures which must be kept in mind in patients with treatment
failures.

<u>Candida</u> vaginitis is more common in women who have recently taken antibiotics or who are pregnant. There is a rapid decrease in <u>Candida</u> isolation in vaginal secretions following delivery. <u>Candida</u> vaginitis also may be a problem in diabetics or patients receiving corticosteroids or immunosuppressive drugs. Less clear predisposing factors include obesity, hypoparathyroidism, hypothyroidism, and hypoadrenalism. Tight-fitting clothing, jeans, and nylon or other synthetic underwear probably predispose to candidiasis. Women on estrogenic anovulants have <u>Candida</u> more frequently in vaginal cultures than do women not on birth control pills or women taking progestagenic anovulants. However, not all studies have found this association.

Vaginal candidiasis is not, strictly speaking, a sexually transmitted disease. However, yeasts have been cultured from the skin of the penis in 14% of circumcised and 17% of uncircumcised men. Symptoms were more common in the uncircumcised men. Eighty percent of the women contacts of the yeast-positive men had yeast infections, while 32% of the women contacts of the yeast-negative men were affected. Balanoposthitis has been described in 10% of men who are sexual contacts of women with vaginal yeast infections. <u>Candida</u> has been cultured from one-half of the male consorts of women with positive vaginal cultures. Similar associations have been observed in the homosexual male when rectal and penile cultures were examined.

CLINICAL MANIFESTATIONS

Up to two-thirds of women are asymptomatic despite the presence of a <u>C. albicans</u> in cultures of their vaginal secretions. Women with symptomatic candida vulvovaginitis complain of vulvar itching, vaginal irritation, pruritus ani, and vaginal discharge. Some patients complain of dyspareunia or dysuria. A white, irritating discharge may be present. The vulva may be edematous and reddened with white patches and fissures. In performing the vaginal examination, the passage of the speculum may be painful. The vaginal discharge usually is white with a thick curdlike consistency. The discharge is often present in white patches on the reddened vaginal wall. Such white plaques in the vagina may be more common in pregnant women. In some women the perineal and perianal skin may be involved with reddened, scaling, and pruritic lesions.

Genital Candida infections in men also may be asymptomatic. As noted in the prior section, C. albicans may be present on the skin of the penis. Symptomatic disease is more common in uncircumcised men. In these men, Candida is found beneath the prepuce. In men with candidiasis, the prepuce may be difficult to retract because of edema or fissuring. A white discharge may be present. The inner surface of the prepuce and the glans may be reddened and inflamed with white patches similar to those seen in the vagina. In circumcised men the glans penis may be glazed, erythematous, and dry in appearance. Scaling, pruritic lesions may be present on the skin of the penis and scrotum. Intertriginous candidiasis may be seen on opposing surfaces of the scrotum and thighs. The early lesions may be vesicular or pustular with round borders and peripheral extension. Perianal lesions may be present in the homosexual male. Candida urethritis is uncommon.

LABORATORY DIAGNOSIS

Candida species or other yeasts may be seen by microscopic examinations of material taken directly from patients. The specimens should be mixed with a drop of saline or 10% sodium hydroxide in water, placed on a glass slide, and covered with a cover slip. A 400× power or greater magnification should be used. Candida yeast forms are unicellular, oval, or spherical cells about 3-5 μm in diameter. Pseudohyphae may be present in clinical specimens in both symptomatic and asymptomatic patients. Candida are gram-positive when stained with Gram stain.

The most sensitive method of identifying patients with Candida infection is by culture. Cultures may be taken with swabs and sent directly to the diagnostic laboratory. In males without obvious skin lesions, a culture is performed with a saline-moistened swab rolled around the posterior border of the glans penis. Candida are easily grown on Sabouraud's or Nickerson's medium. On culture, they form budding cells (blastospores), round, oval, or oblong, 2.5 by 3 to 14 μm, single or in clusters or chains. Pseudohyphae usually are produced on nutritionally poor media, along with secondary blastospores that are characteristic of the species. C. albicans and C. stellatoidea produce germ tubes and spherical chlamydospores. Candida are aerobic and grow optimally between 25 and 35°C. Candida species are differentiated by means of oxidative or fermentative reactions on culture media containing different carbohydrates. Unless specifically sought, <u>C. albicans</u> may not be identified in routine bacterial cultures which are frequently discarded at 48 hr. At that time the colonies of <u>C. albicans</u> may be very tiny and escape detection.

At present, serologic tests to detect <u>Candida</u> species infection are not useful. Secretory immunoglobulin A that reacts with <u>Candida</u> antigen is produced locally in the vaginal secretions. Some of this IgA antibody also may be found in the circulation of women with chronic <u>Candida</u> vaginitis. <u>Candida</u> antigen skin tests also have no diagnostic value in <u>Candida</u> infections but are currently used in a battery of skin tests to assess cutaneous anergy. Some of the <u>Candida</u> species that have been isolated from the vagina include <u>C. albicans</u>, <u>C. krusei</u>, <u>C. parapsilosis</u>, <u>C. tropicalis</u>, <u>C. stellatoidea</u>, and <u>C. guilliermondi</u>. As previously mentioned, <u>Candida glabrata</u> may also be found in vaginal secretions.

TREATMENT

Genital <u>Candida</u> infections may be treated with a number of different topical antifungal agents. As an initial step in patients with yeast vaginitis, the vulva and introitus should be gently cleansed with mild soap and water, rinsed, and dried. Topical creams are applied to external skin and mucous membrane lesions, and the vaginal lesions are treated by means of the insertion of creams with an applicator or the insertion of vaginal suppositories. Men may be treated topically with creams or ointments.

In cases resistant to treatment, consideration should be given to treating the sexual partner or eliminating the rectal focus of the yeast infection by means of oral preparations, such as Nystatin oral suspension (400,000-600,000 units) four times daily or Nystatin tablets (500,000 units) three times daily until cultures of the rectum are negative. Milne and Warnock did not find any difference in cure or relapses in patients treated with and without oral Nystatin in addition to intravaginal clotrimazole. Patients who do not respond to therapy also should be investigated as to the possibility of an underlying metabolic disorder, including diabetes mellitus (see the section on epidemiology above). A cure is generally considered to be a vaginal culture negative for yeasts 2 weeks following the completion of any of the following therapies.

The following drugs have demonstrated effect in the treatment of genital yeast infections; there are few, if any, contraindications, except for the possible development of hypersensitivity or irritation following application:

Miconazole Nitrate

Miconazole is a synthetic imidazole derivative which alters cell membrane permeability with resulting adverse effects on the yeast cells. Small amounts of the drug are absorbed and may be identified in the patient's serum following intravaginal application. Miconazole may be used in the second and third trimesters of pregnancy. It is available in a 2% cream and 100 mg suppositories. Five grams of the cream or one suppository is inserted into the vagina daily at bedtime for seven days. Miconazole cream is more effective and convenient than Nystatin cream, which requires twice daily applications. Cure rates of 80-90% may be expected. Some patients complain of a burning sensation after application of miconazole. This side effect may require discontinuation of therapy. Miconazole coated tampons are another form of therapy. They are used twice daily for 1 week. The cure and recurrence rate is not significantly different from the clotrimazole therapy. The vaginal tampons are not associated with leakage of the medicine from the vagina. Econazole, another imidazole derivative, appears as effective as miconazole or clotrimazole.

Clotrimazole

Clotrimazole is a synthetic antifungal imidazole derivative that is structurally related to miconazole. It acts by binding phospholipids on the cell membrane of fungi and altering their permeability. Small amounts of clotrimazole are absorbed after topical therapy. It is effective against yeast and dermatophyte fungi. Irritation and local reactions have been described in less than 2% of both women and their sexual partners. Clotrimazole vaginal tablets may be given in the second and third trimesters of pregnancy. The cream (1%) is applied once daily at bedtime for seven to fourteen days. Vaginal tablets containing 100 mg of clotrimazole are inserted once daily for seven days. Equal results have been obtained with the insertion of two tablets daily for three days. The three-day therapy is not as effective in pregnant women as is the seven-day therapy. A single 500 mg clotrimazole pessary also is effective but unavailable in the United States.

Nystatin

Nystatin is an amphoteric polyene macrolid antifungal antibiotic produced by <u>Streptomyces noursei.</u> Nystatin acts by binding to sterols in the fungal cell membrane. It is not absorbed from intact skin and is available in several different preparations: cream or ointment, 100,000 units/g; vaginal suppositories, 100,000 units/tablet; oral suspension, 100,000 units/ml; oral tablets, 500,000 units/tablet; and topical powder, 100,000 units/g. The topical preparations are applied twice daily, and the vaginal suppositories are inserted once daily for 2 weeks. The therapy should be continued during menstration, and there is no contraindication to therapy during pregnancy.

Candicidin

This is a heptaene antifungal antibiotic derived from a soil actinomycete, <u>Streptomyces griseus</u>. It is ineffective against bacteria, and its exact mode of action is unknown. It may be used in pregnant patients. The daily therapeutic dose is 6 mg, and this is delivered in a single vaginal tablet or 5 g of vaginal ointment twice daily. Treatment is for fourteen days.

Other

Amphotericin ointment and methylrosaniline chloride (gentian violet) are alternate therapies but are less acceptable because they produce stains on clothing. Two other drugs, natamycin and econazole, are not currently licensed in the United States. Both show promise for therapy of vaginal candidiasis.

A preliminary report has been published on the efficacy of boric acid, 600 mg, in gelatin capsules inserted into the vagina nightly for 2 weeks. This therapy is inexpensive and not associated with significant side effects.

Ketoconazole 400 mg orally per day for three days also has been used to treat vaginal candidosis. The drug should not be used in pregnant women and, because of its potential for hepatotoxicity, it should not be a first choice for therapy.

BIBLIOGRAPHY

Ainsworth JWL, Rutherford AM. Clinical efficacy of Pimafucin (natamycin) vaginal tablets in a ten day course for vaginal candidiasis. N Zealand Med J, 1:420-421, 1980.

Anyon CP, Desmond FB, Eastcott DF. A study of Candida in one thousand and seven women. N Zealand Med J, 73:9-13, 1971.

Balsdon MJ. Comparison of miconazole-coated tampons with clotrinazole vaginal tablets in the treatment of vaginal candidiasis. Br J Vener Dis, 57:275-278, 1981.

Bergstein NAM. Treatment of vulvovaginal candidal infection with miconazole-coated tampons. Br J Vener Dis, 56:408-411, 1980.

Catterall RD. Candida albicans and the contraceptive pill. Lancet, 2:830-831, 1966.

Davidson F. Yeasts and circumcision in the male. Br J Vener Dis, 53:121-122, 1977.

Davidson F, Mould RF. Recurrent genital candidosis in women and the effect of intermittent prophylactic treatment. Br J Vener Dis, 54:176-183, 1978.

Davis JE, Frudenfeld JH, Goddard JL. Comparative evaluation of monistat and mycostatin in the treatment of vulvovaginal candidiasis. Obstet Gynecol, 44:403-406, 1974.

Elegbe IA, Botu M. A preliminary study on dressing patterns and the incidence of candidiasis. Amer J Pub Hlth, 72:176-177, 1982.

Farkas J. Zum klinischen Bild und zur Klassifikation der Balanitis candiomycetica und der Candidiasis follicularis scroti et perigenitalis. Derm Mschr, 161:201-208, 1975.

Fredricsson B, Frisk Å, Hagstrom B, et al. Vaginal mycosis: Aspects on diagnosis and their treatment with econazole nitrate. Curr Ther Res, 27:309-322, 1980.

Fregoso-Dueñas F. Ketoconazole in vulvovaginal candidosis. Rev Infect Dis, 2:620-622, 1980.

Gabriel G, Thin RNT. Clotrimazole and econazole in the treatment of vaginal candidosis. A single blind comparison. Br J Vener Dis, 59:56-58, 1983.

Hilton AL, Warnock DW. Vaginal candidiasis and the role of the digestive tract as a source of infection. Br J Obstet Gynecol, 82: 922-926, 1975.

Justin RG. Do oral contraceptives need to be interrupted in order to treat vaginal candidiasis? J Amer Med Women's Assoc, 28:198-200, 1973.

Masterton G, Sengupta SM, Schofield CBS. Natamycin in genital candidosis in men. Br J Vener Dis, 51:210-212, 1975.

Mathur S, Virella G, Koistinen J, et al. Humoral immunity in vaginal candidiasis. Infect Immunol, 15:287-294, 1977.

Miles MR, Olsen L, Rogers A. Recurrent vaginal candidiasis: Importance of an intestinal reservoir. J Amer Med Assoc, 238: 1836-1837, 1977.

Milne JD, Warnock DW. Effect of simultaneous oral and vaginal treatment on the rate of cure and relapse in vaginal candidosis. Br J Vener Dis, 55:362-365, 1979.

Milson I, Forssman L. Treatment of vaginal candidosis with a single 500 mg clotrimazole pessary. Br J Vener Dis, 58:124-126, 1982.

Morris DF, Sugrue DL. Miconazole nitrate compared with chlordantoin in the treatment of vaginal candidiasis. Br J Vener Dis, 51:123-124, 1975.

Oriel JD, Partridge BM, Denny ML, et al. Genital yeast infections. Br Med J, 4:761-764, 1972.

Parker JDJ. Urethral candidosis in a male treated with amphotericin B instillation. Br J Vener Dis, 46:43-45, 1970.

Pedersen GT. Yeast flora in mother and child, a mycological-clinical study of women followed up during pregnancy, the puerperium and 5-12 months after delivery, and of their children on the 7th day of life and at the age of 5-12 months. Dan Med Bull, 16: 207-220, 1969.

Robertson WH. A concentrated therapeutic regimen for vulvo-vaginal candidiasis. J Amer Med Assoc, 244:2549-2550, 1980.

Rodin P, Kolator B. Carriage of yeasts on the penis. Br Med J, 1:1123-1124, 1976.

Rutherford AM. Gynodaktarin (miconazole nitrate) for vulvo-vaginal candidiasis. N Zealand Med J, 84:9-10, 1976.

Silva-Hunter M, Cooper BH. Medically important yeasts. Chapter 56 in E. H. Lennette, E. H. Spaulding, J. P. Truant (eds.), Manual of Clinical Microbiology (2nd ed.), American Society for Microbiology, Washington, D.C., 1974.

Sousa HM de, van Uden N. The mode of infection and reinfection in yeast vulvovaginitis. Amer J Obstet Gynecol, 80:1096-1100, 1960.

Van Slyke KK, Rein MF. Boric acid treatment of vulvovaginal candidiasis (Abstract No. 230). 20th Interscience Conference on Antimicrobial Agents and Chemotherapy, New Orleans, Louisiana, September 22-24, 1980.

Waldman RH, Cruz J, Rowe DS. Immunoglobulin levels and antibody to Candida albicans in human cervicovaginal secretions. Clin Exp Immunol, 10:427-434, 1972.

Wallenburg HCS, Wladimiroff JW. Recurrence of vulvovaginal candidosis during pregnancy, comparison of miconazole vs. nystatin treatment. Obstet Gynecol, 48:491-494, 1976.

Warnock DW, Speller DCE, Milne JD, et al. Epidemiological investigation of patients with vulvovaginal candidosis. Application of a resistogram method for strain differentiation of Candida albicans. Br J Vener Dis, 55:357-361, 1979.

Waugh MA. Clinical presentation of candidal balanitis—its differential diagnosis and treatment. Chemother, 28(Suppl. 1):56-60, 1982.

Waugh MA, Evans EGV, Nayyar KC, et al. Clotrimazole (Canesten) in the treatment of candidal balanitis in men. Br J Vener Dis, 54:184-186, 1978.

Willimott FE. Genital yeasts in female patients attending a V.D.
clinic. Br J Vener Dis, 51:119-122, 1975.

Winner HI, Hurley R. <u>Candida albicans</u>. Little, Brown, Boston,
1964.

Chapter 7

GENITAL HERPESVIRUS INFECTIONS

ETIOLOGIC AGENT

Herpesviruses are DNA viruses that infect humans. They
include herpes simplex virus, varicella-zoster virus, cytomegalovirus, and the Epstein-Barr virus (the cause of infectious mononucleosis). Herpes simplex virus is composed of two immunological variants, type 1 and type 2. The types can be distinguished by
certain biologic differences as well as by certain antibody tests,
despite the presence of cross-reactive antigen. In general, type 1
virus is isolated above the waist and type 2 virus is isolated below
the waist (Figs. 7.1-7.6). Type 1 infections occur most frequently
during childhood, and type 2 infections, at the onset of sexual activity. Approximately 90% of genital herpes infections are caused
by type 2 virus.

EPIDEMIOLOGY

Herpes simplex virus is found in all parts of the world, and
the type 1 virus infections vary inversely with the socioeconomic
status of the population. Most children in lower socioeconomic
groups have antibody to type 1 virus. Antibody to type 2 virus is
uncommon in the celibate and most common in sexually active
lower socioeconomic groups. The appearance of the type 2 antibody increases with age.

Type 2 herpes simplex virus (HSV-2) infection is probably
the most common causative agent of ulcerative lesions in the female genital tract in patients attending venereal disease clinics in
the United States.

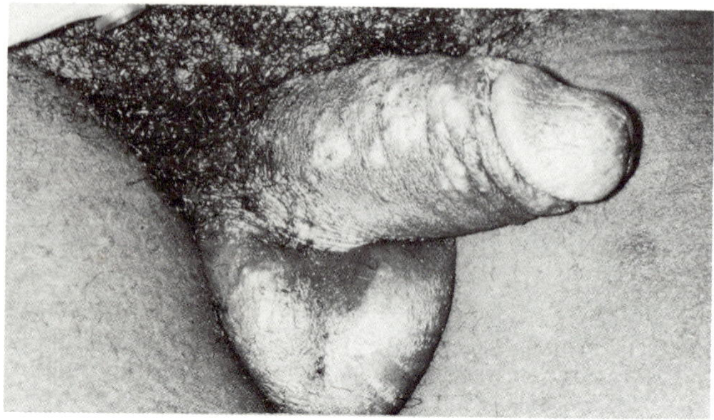

Figure 7.1 Herpes genitalis. A 22-year-old black man noted the onset of painful, burning vesicular lesions four days prior to the photograph. He had enlarged, tender inguinal lymph nodes. There was no prior history of genital herpesvirus infections.

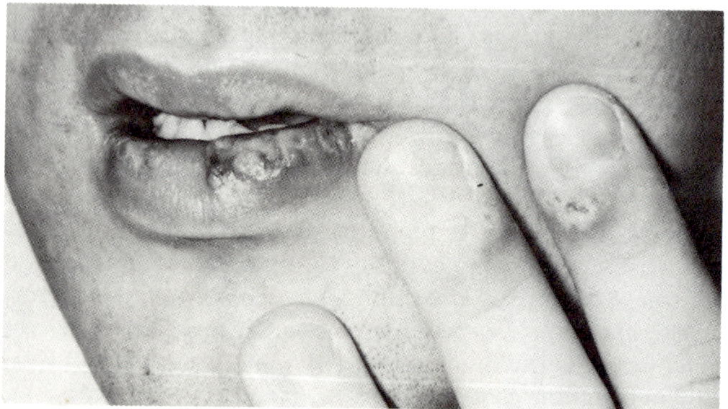

Figure 7.2 Herpes stomatitis and herpes whitlow. A pediatric resident developed painful lesions on his lips, tongue, buccal mucosa, and pharynx three days following resuscitation of an infant later discovered to be infected with herpes simplex virus, type 2. Herpes whitlows developed on his fingers at the sites of cracks and fissures in his skin. At the time of the photograph, he had been ill six days with oral lesions, a painful pharyngitis, and daily fevers to 103° F.

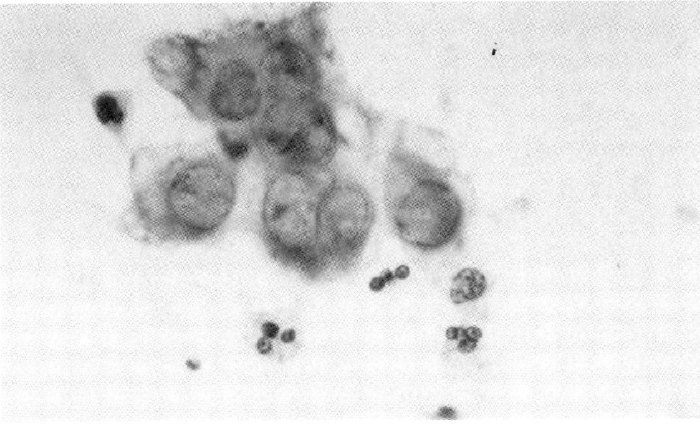

Figure 7.3   Herpes cervicitis.   Cervical cytology from a patient with herpes cervicitis.   Note the multinucleated giant cells with inclusion bodies, and also note their size in relation to the polymorphonuclear leukocytes.

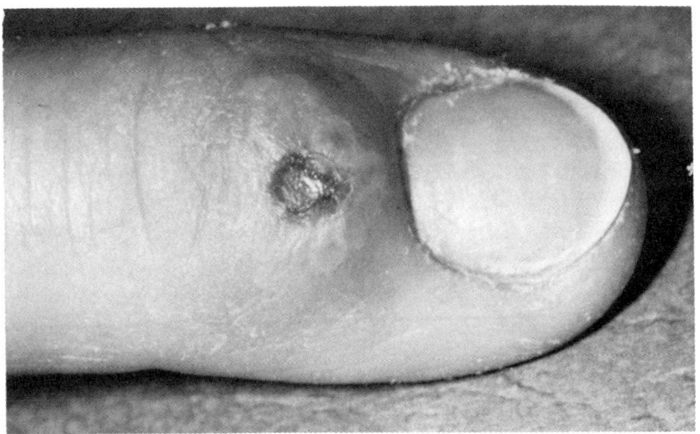

Figure 7.4   Herpes whitlow.   This may be a sexually transmitted disease.   The photograph shows a three-day-old lesion on the index finger of an intensive care nurse.   It consists of a group of circular pustules with an erythematous base.   A Gram stain of material pustule revealed only polymorphonuclear leukocytes and no bacteria. Giemsa stain showed multinucleated giant cells with inclusions. Complete healing is slow and may take ten days or more.

Based on serologic evidence of previous HSV-2 infection, approximately 10% of women attending private gynecology clinics and 20% of women attending public gynecology clinics show evidence of previous infection. Active infection is present in about 5% of all men and women attending venereal disease clinics. The virus is rarely isolated from genital cultures from patients who are celibate or who are monogamous. However, HSV-2 was found in 15% of 273 samples taken from men attending a urology clinic. The samples included urethral swabs, prostatic fluid, vas deferens, and prostatic biopsy specimens. The prostatic biopsy specimens had a two to four times higher recovery rate than the urethral swabs. This study indicated that HSV-2 may be asymptomatically present in the deeper tissue of the male genitourinary tract.

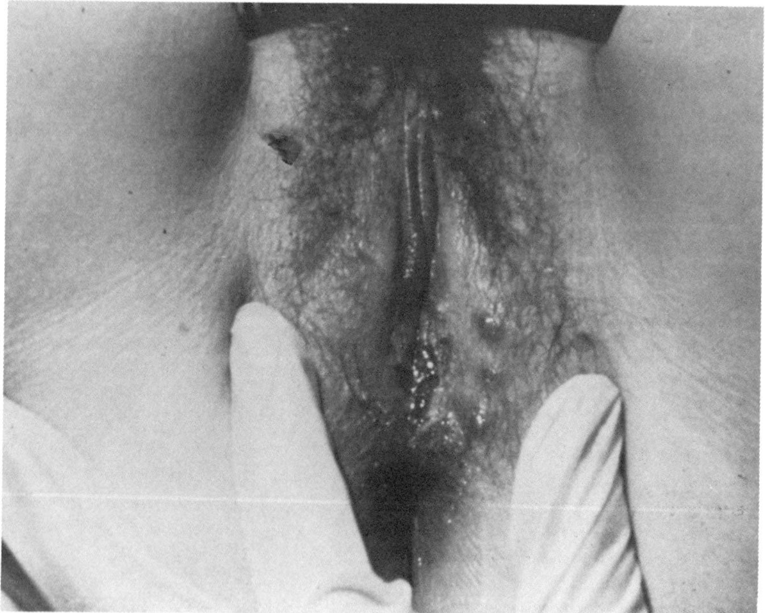

Figure 7.5 Herpes genital infection in a young woman. This woman has a number of vesicular lesions and a painful shallow ulcer secondary to unroofed coalesced vesicles. Photograph courtesy of the Venereal Disease Control Division, CDC, USPHS.

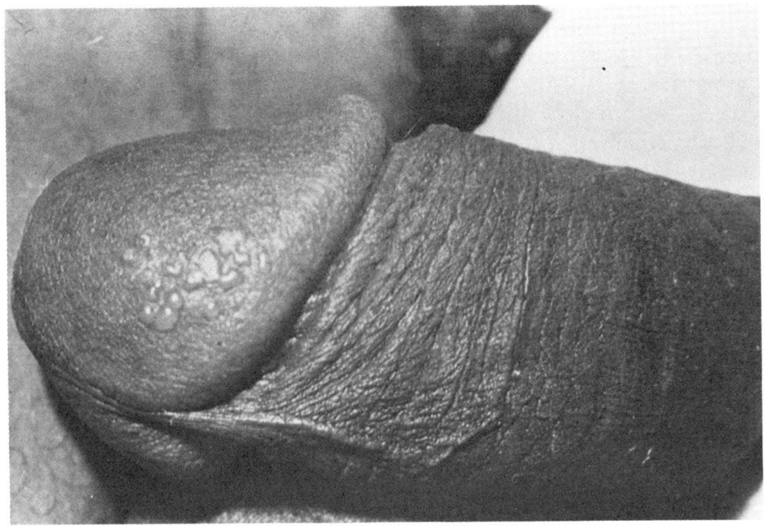

Figure 7.6   Herpes genital infection in a man.   The small vesicles are located on the corona of the penis.   Photograph courtesy
of E. Stolz and J. van der Stek.*

Asymptomatic men may be able to spread the virus to sexual
partners. Women may have asymptomatic infections of the vulva
and cervix, and this was demonstrated in 8% of women attending
one venereal disease clinic. The risk of transmission from such
patients to uninfected sexual partners is unknown. The majority
of primary herpes genital infections are found in sexually active
people. Patients with HSV-2 infections also may have coexistent
venereal disease. In some upper and middle class populations,
genital herpesvirus infection may be more frequent than gonococcal infections. If both primary and recurrent infections are considered, genital herpesvirus infection may be the most common
venereal disease in these groups.

CLINICAL MANIFESTATIONS

Genital herpes infections may be primary, latent, or recurrent in nature. Some infections are subclinical, that is, HSV-2

antibody may be present in patients with no history of genital herpes. The lesions may appear on the penis, scrotum, vulva, perineum, perianal region, vagina, or cervix. In patients with primary herpesvirus infections, symptoms usually begin within three to seven days following contact. Initially, patients complain of pain, itching, or burning sensations or paresthesias at the site of inoculation. Multiple small vesicles surrounded by an erythematous base rapidly rupture to form shallow, moist ulcerations. The vesicles are intraepithelial or intraepidermal, and infectious viral particles are present within the vesicles in large quantity. Multinucleated giant cells and cells with intranuclear inclusions are present on the base of the vesicle. The lesions are usually less than 0.5 cm in diameter. Vesicles may coalesce to form larger bulla or more irregular ulcerations.

In women, the vesicles may not be seen, and the patient may present with only painful ulcerations. External dysuria in women may result from ulcers near the urethral meatus. Ninety percent of women with primary HSV-2 infections have cervical infections as well. The cervical infection may result in a vaginal discharge. Necrotic ulceration of the cervix is present in patients with severe cervicitis.

Urethritis is present in 10-15% of men with primary HSV infections. This can be the only manifestation of herpes infection. The dysuria, which can be severe, may precede the appearance of the genital lesions by a few days and result in a mucoid urethral discharge.

With the appearance of the vesicles, pain and tenderness become more prominent. The pain may be severe and associated with vulvar edema. Women with such involvement often walk with a straddling gait. The virus spreads via lymphatics into regional lymph nodes. The inguinal lymph nodes become enlarged and tender. The primary lesions are generally present for 2-4 weeks. Although most symptoms have resolved within 2 weeks, new crops of vesicles sometimes occur 2-3 weeks after the appearance of the first vesicles. Crusting occurs, and the erosions epithelialize. When lesions are present at moist sites, the crusting step does not take place, and epithelialization takes place directly. Virus may be cultured from crusted lesions in a small quantity, but virus generally is not present after epithelialization. Bacterial infection of the ulcers is rare. Although some discoloration of the skin may be present, scarring at the site of the lesions is rare.

Patients with primary HSV-2 infections often have systemic symptoms including low-grade fever, headache, and generalized

malaise. A severe HSV pharyngitis can accompany genital lesions
in patients who engage in oral-genital sexual contact. Inoculation
of the virus into the fingers (paronychia) or eye is possible and can
occur at extragenital sites such as the buttocks, groin, thigh, or
face. Urinary retention, constipation, impotence, sacral anes-
thesia, and bowel dysfunction may occur, perhaps as a result of
transverse myelitis or sacral radiculopathy. Ano-rectal herpes
and herpes proctitis in homosexual men may be associated with
severe ano-rectal pain, itching, perianal ulcerations tenesmus,
constipation, fever, inguinal adenopathy, sacral paresthesias, and
difficulty in urinating. Vesicles may spread to the natal cleft. In
a small percentage of patients with genital HSV-2 infection, meningitis occurs. This may be quite mild.

In some patients the virus remains latent and the patient never
experiences a recurrence. Other less fortunate individuals have
recurrences over a duration of years. Recurrences usually take
place within 1-3 months following the initial episode and generally
take place five to eight times per year. HSV-2 infections recur
more frequently than infections with HSV-1. Certain situations
are said to be associated with recurrences. Among these are
stress, sexual activity, sunburn, and fever. Recurrences generally take place at the same site and, in some instances, multiple
lesions may be present. Preceding the recurrences, the patient
may note neuralgia or a burning or itching sensation. The vesicles
reach a maximum in size in about three days and in recurrent disease are completely healed within 1-2 weeks. The clinical manifestations are milder and of shorter duration than with the primary
infection. Systemic symptoms and regional lymphadenopathy are
uncommon with recurrences.

Patients are thought to be noninfectious from individual
lesions following the epithelialization of the ulcers. However, as
previously noted, herpesvirus may be present in the vagina and
cervix of asymptomatic women. Between recurrences, the virus
is thought to be latent, possibly in sacral nerve root ganglia.
Most women with recurrent herpesvirus infections who have vulvar
lesions usually will not have positive cervical cultures, and the
cervix will appear normal. In one study of 250 episodes of HSV-2
positive recurrent genital herpes, in only 8% was virus grown from
the cervix. The presence of type 1 antibody does not prevent
infection with type 2 virus , but these infections may be milder.
Second primary infections with type 2 virus are possible.

If herpesvirus infections in women occur early in pregnancy,
there is an increased change of spontaneous abortion. If the

infection takes place late in pregnancy, this increases the risk of infection to the infant. Most infections in infants are acquired by passage through the mother's infected genital tract. If, during labor, active infection is present, the infant should be delivered by caesarean section. This should be performed if the membranes are intact or if the membranes have been ruptured for less than 6 hr. Unfortunately, even these precautions may not prevent the infant from being infected although, fortunately, transplacental infections do not seem to be common. Herpesvirus infection in the infant produces a very severe visceral disease, and the consequences of infection are grave. There is no generally agreed upon strategy to manage pregnant women with recurrent herpes. Physicians in hospitals with access to viral laboratories may elect to do weekly HSV cultures of the cervix prior to delivery. At the onset of labor, cervical scrapings can be examined for evidence of herpesvirus infection with cytological and immunological techniques. If there is no evidence of viral infection, then the baby can be delivered vaginally.

Epidemiologic evidence has linked genital herpesvirus infections in women with carcinoma of the cervix. Carcinoma of the cervix is more frequent in women of lower socioeconomic classes. The occurrence of this cancer is low in celibate women and is increased in women who have intercourse at an early age and in women who have had multiple sex partners. Increased cervical anaplasia is seen in women with herpes infections detected by cytologic methods. Also, HSV-2 antibody is more common in patients with carcinoma of the cervix in comparison to control groups. Cervical cultures of women with cervical cancer have yielded predominantly HSV-2. Genital herpes is acquired in the second and third decades in women, and cervical carcinoma appears in the fourth and fifth decades. A recent study has established an association between HSV-2 and squamous-cell carcinoma in situ of the vulva in nine of ten patients whose lesions were studied for the presence of HSV-2 nonstructural protein antigens.

These observations are consistent with the hypothesis that HSV-2 may initiate a process that results in cancer following a latent period of several years. Women who have had genital herpesvirus infection should have annual Papanicolaou tests of the cervix. At present, it cannot be stated with certainty that herpesvirus causes cervical cancer. However, the association appears to be valid. Because of these observations, genital herpes infections may be the most frightening of all of the sexually transmitted diseases in women.

DIAGNOSIS

The diagnosis of herpesvirus infections of the genitalia is usually made on the clinical picture. The Tzanck test is a direct examination performed on cells scraped from the base of the vesicle with a curette. The cells are smeared onto a glass slide and then stained with Wright's or Giemsa stain. This preparation is positive if multinucleated giant cells are present with intranuclear inclusions. The Tzanck test is of limited value, as it does not distinguish between varicella zoster and herpes simplex virus infections. Cells obtained in a similar manner and fixed with acetone may be stained with fluorescent-labeled antibody to herpesvirus, or the cells may be tested by indirect immune peroxidase staining. The latter two tests are more sensitive and more specific than the Tzanck test. The availability of monoclonal antibodies for diagnosis more than likely will improve the reliability of these immunologic tests. The immunologic tests are the most rapid route to a definitive answer, should one be required. Electron microscopic examination of vesicular fluid is of limited value because of the inability to distinguish herpes simplex virus from varicella zoster.

Viral culture of the vesicular fluid is the most reliable diagnostic method. Vesicular fluid may be collected on a cotton or dacron swab or by means of a small bore needle and syringe. Calcium alginate swabs may be inferior to dacron swabs in that calcium alginate binds directly to the herpesvirus type 2 viron, rendering it noninfectious. The best results are obtained when the material is inoculated directly into tissue cultures. The virus should not be frozen prior to inoculation. Stuart's medium is a convenient transport medium, should there be a delay. Consultation with the virus diagnostic laboratory prior to collection of the specimen will increase the chance of a positive result. The late ulcerative lesions have a poorer diagnostic yield than material taken from the early vesicles. A number of tissue culture cell lines, including WI-38 fibroblasts, are useful in growing the virus. Cytopathic effects usually are detected within 1 week after inoculation. Herpesvirus isolates are best distinguished (HSV-1 or HSV-2) by their reaction with commercially available specific antisera.

Serologic diagnosis, from blood samples taken from the patient, is not advisable because of cross-reactions between HSV-1 and HSV-2. In addition, antibody rises may not occur in patients with recurrent infection with HSV-2.

TREATMENT

The skin lesions of herpesvirus infections are self-limited and will heal unless secondary bacterial infections supervene, and this rarely takes place. Some women with primary genital infections seem to have a propensity for vaginal superinfection with Candida during their second week of illness. The self-limiting nature of the disease is of little comfort to a patient suffering the discomfort of genital lesions, and treatment of primary disease is always indicated.

The most promising treatment of genital herpes to date is acyclovir, a pruine analog that is a substrate for viral thymidine kinase. This drug is available in a topical, oral, and intravenous formulation. In the United States, the topical acyclovir (5% ointment in polyethylene glycol) and the intravenous acyclovir are licensed by the Food and Drug Administration. Topical acyclovir is applied to the external lesions four to six times daily for seven to fourteen days or until all of the ulcers have formed crusts. This drug is effective in reducing the duration and intensity of the symptoms in patients with their first attack of genital herpes. It has no effect on dysuria, vaginal discharge, or the systemic complications.

Intravenous acyclovir given at 5 mg/kg body weight every 8 hr for five days markedly shortens the time of viral shedding and the systemic symptoms. This therapy results in a 60% reduction in time to healing (median nine days versus twenty-one days in controls of one study). Oral acyclovir, currently under investigation, may not be as effective at reducing the systemic symptoms as the intravenous preparations, but the oral preparation may be of value in recurrent herpes.

Acyclovir therapy in patients with first attacks of genital herpes does shorten the initial illness but does not prevent or reduce the frequency of recurrences. The topical preparation is not recommended for patients with recurrent genital herpes. Corey, however, suggests a slight benefit in early application of the ointment in recurrent disease in men with large lesions (50–150 mm^2). Acyclovir in all forms has not been approved by the Food and Drug Administration for use in pregnant women. Clearly, the final chapter on genital herpes therapy has yet to be written.

Patients with recurrent disease may be treated with symptomatic therapy. This includes genital hygiene, topical anesthetics such as 2% lidocaine jelly, loose-fitting undergarments, and cool tapwater compresses or sitz bath followed by blow drying with a hair drier. Analgesia with aspirin or codeine may be required.

Therapies which are of unproven benefit include idoxuridine, cytosine arabinoside, alcohol, ether, chloroform, povidone iodine, and interferon inducers. Other unproven therapies include smallpox, BCG, oral polio, and herpesvirus vaccines.

Photoinactivation therapy was a popular method of treatment. A heterotricyclic dye, such as neutral red or proflavine, was painted on the unroofed vesicles. Viral DNA was bound by the dye. Subsequent exposure to any ordinary fluorescent light was thought to disrupt the viral nucleic acid inactivating the virus. However, tissue culture and hamster transplantation experiments indicated that similarly treated herpesvirus particles had increased carcinogenic potential. Thus there was the possibility that the photoinactivation therapy in humans might initiate skin cancer. To add to this uncertainty, a small number of patients who had been treated by this method developed Bowen's disease or intraepithelial carcinoma. Whether this was fortuitous or cause and effect has not undergone rigorous investigation. However, such information suggests that photo-dye therapy should, for the moment, be performed only in investigative situations where long-term follow-up is possible.

Part of the physician's role is to counsel patients with genital herpes infection, and this duty is both important and time-consuming. Patients are generally frightened, angry, and full of questions. Written material should be available for them to take home and read. Usually the patient is so upset that teaching in the initial interview is ineffective. Instructional pamphlets are available from the American Social Health Association, the National Institutes of Health, the Centers for Disease Control, and private organizations and universities. In the United States, the American Social Health Association sponsors a toll-free number where patients may have their questions answered and be referred for help. Women with herpes should be advised to have yearly Papanicolaou smears of the cervix. Patients with active lesions should avoid intercourse until epithelialization of the ulcers takes place. It is not known how infectious patients are between attacks. The condom and spermidical jellies may provide some protection, and their use should be encouraged. Patients should be cautioned that reinfections are possible from having intercourse with other herpes patients.

HERPES RESOURCES

In the United States:

Herpes Resource Center
American Social Health
  Association
HRC/ASHA
Post Office Box 100
Palo Alto, CA 94302

VD National Hotline (toll-free)
1-800-227-8922
In California
1-800-982-5883

Division of Venereal Disease
  Control
Center for Prevention Services
Center for Disease Control
Atlanta, GA 30333

In Canada:

REACH (Research, Education, and
  Assistance for Canadians with
  Herpes)
Post Office Box 649, Station P
Toronto, Ontario M5S 2Y4
416-961-2777

BIBLIOGRAPHY

Adam E, Kaufman RH, Melnick JL, et al. Seroepidemiologic studies of herpesvirus type 2 and carcinoma of the cervix. Amer J Epidemiol, 96:427-442, 1973.

Adam E, Kaufman RH, Mirkovic RR, et al. Persistance of virus shedding in asymptomatic women after recovery from herpes genitalis. Obstet Gynecol, 54:171-173, 1979.

Barton IG, Kinghorn GR, Najem S, Al-Omar LS, Potter CW. Incidence of herpes simplex virus types 1 and 2 isolated in patients with herpes genitalis in Sheffield. Br J Vener Dis, 58:44-47, 1982.

Belsey EM, Adler MW. Current approaches to the diagnosis of herpes genitalis. Br J Vener Dis, 54:115-120, 1978.

Berger RS, Papa CM. Photodye herpes therapy-Cassandra confirmed. J Amer Med Assoc, 238:133-134, 1977.

Brown ST, Jaffee HW, Zaidi A, et al. Sensitivity and specificity of diagnostic tests for genital infection with Herpes-virus hominis. Sex Transm Dis, 6:10-13, 1979.

Bryson YJ, Dillon M, Lovett M, et al. Treatment of first episodes of genital herpes simplex virus infection with oral acyclovir. N Eng J Med, 308:916-921, 1983.

Buchman TG, Roizman B, Nahmias AJ. Demonstration of exogenous genital reinfection with herpes simplex virus type 2 by restriction endonuclease fingerprinting of viral DNA. J Infect Dis, 140: 295-304, 1979.

Caplan LR, Kleeman FJ, Berg S. Urinary retention probably secondary to herpes genitalis. N Eng J Med, 297:920-921, 1977.

Corey L, Adams HG, Brown ZA, Holmes KK. Genital herpes simplex virus infections: Clinical manifestations, course, and complications. Ann Int Med, 98:958-972, 1983.

Corey L, Fife KH, Benedetti JK, et al. Intravenous acyclovir for the treatment of primary genital herpes. N Eng J Med, 98: 914-921, 1983.

Corey L, Holmes KK. Genital herpes simplex virus infections: Current concepts in diagnosis, therapy, and prevention. Ann Int Med, 98:973-983, 1983.

Crane LR, Gutterman PA, Chapel T, et al. Incubation of swab materials with herpes simplex virus. J Infect Dis, 141:531, 1980.

Deardourff SL, Deture FA, Drylie DM, et al. Association between herpes hominis type 2 and the male genitourinary tract. J Urol, 112:126-127, 1974.

Deture FA, Drylie DM, Kaufman AE, et al. Herpesvirus type 2: Study of semen in male subjects with recurrent infections. J Urol, 120:449-451, 1978.

Ekwo E, Wong YW, Meyers M. Asymptomatic cervicovaginal shedding of herpes simplex virus. Amer J Obstet Gynecol, 134: 102-103, 1979.

Felber TD, Smith EB, Knox JM, et al. Photodynamic inactivation of herpes simplex. J Amer Med Assoc, 223:289-292, 1973.

Fife KH, Schmidt O, Remington M, Corey L. Primary and recurrent concomitant genital infection with herpes simplex virus types 1 and 2. J Infect Dis, 147:163, 1983.

Glogau R, Hanna L, Jawetz E. Herpetic whitlow as part of genital virus infection. J Infect Dis, 136:689-692, 1977.

Goodell SE, Quinn TC, Mkrtichian E, Schuffler MD, Holmes KK, Corey L. Herpes simplex virus proctitis in homosexual men. Clinical, sigmoidoscopic, and histopathological features. N Eng J Med, 308:868-871, 1983.

Guinan ME, MacCalman J, Kern ER, Overall JC, Spruance SL. The course of untreated recurrent genital herpes simplex infection in 27 women. N Eng J Med, 304:759-763, 1981.

Hirsch MS, Schooley RT. Treatment of herpesvirus infections. N Eng J Med, 309:963-970, 1034-1039, 1983.

Jeansson S, Molin L. On the occurrence of genital herpes simplex virus infection. Acta Dermatol (Stockholm), 54:479-485, 1974.

Kalinyak JE, Fleagle G, Docherty JJ. Incidence and distribution of herpes simplex virus types 1 and 2 from genital lesions in college women. J Med Virol, 1:175-181, 1977.

Kaufman RH, Dreesman GR, Burek J, et al. Herpesvirus-induced antigens in squamous-cell carcinoma in situ of the vulva. N Eng J Med, 305:483-488, 1981.

Kaufman RH, Rawls WE. Herpes genitalis and its relationship to cervical cancer. Ca. A Cancer Journal for Clinicians, 24:258-265, 1974.

Kit S, Trkula D, Qavi H, et al. Sequential genital infections by herpes simplex viruses types 1 and 2: Restriction nuclease analysis of viruses from recurrent infections. Sex Transm Dis, 10:67-71, 1983.

Knox GE, Pass RF, Reynolds DW, et al. Comparative prevalence of subclinical cytomegalovirus and herpes simplex infections in the genital and urinary tracts of low-income urban women. J Infect Dis, 140:491-522, 1979.

Mindel A, Weller IVD, Faherty A, et al. Prophylactic oral acyclovir in recurrent genital herpes. Lancet, 2:57-59, 1984.

Myers MG, Oxymann MN, Clark JE, et al. Failure of neutral-red photodynamic inactivation in recurrent herpes simplex virus infections. N Eng J Med, 293:945-949, 1975.

Oates JK, Greenhouse PRDH. Retention of urine in anogenital herpetic infection. Lancet, 1:691-692, 1978.

Rattray MC, Corey L, Reeves WC, et al. Recurrent genital herpes among women symptomatic vs. asymptomatic viral shedding. Br J Vener Dis, 54:262-265, 1978.

Reeves WC, Corey L, Adams HG, et al. Risk of recurrence after first episodes of genital herpes. Relation to HSV type and antibody response. N Eng J Med, 305:315-319, 1981.

Reichman RC, Badger GJ, Guinan ME, et al. Topically administered acyclovir in the treatment of recurrent herpes simplex genitalis: A controlled trial. J Infect Dis, 147:336-340, 1983.

Reichman RC, Badger GJ, Mertz GJ, et al. Treatment of recurrent genital herpes simplex infections with oral acyclovir. A controlled trial. J Amer Med Assoc, 251:2103-2107, 1984.

Smith EF. Management of herpes simplex infections of the skin. J Amer Med Assoc, 235:1731-1733, 1976.

Sumaya CV, Marx J, Ullis K. Genital infections with herpes simplex virus in a university student population. Sex Transm Dis, 7:16-20, 1980.

Taylor PK, Doherty NR. Comparison of the treatment of herpes genitalis in men with proflavine photoinactivation, idoxuridine ointment and normal saline. Br J Vener Dis, 51:125-129, 1974.

Vesterinen E, Purola E, Saksela E, et al. Clinical and virological findings in patients with cytologically diagnosed gynecologic herpes simplex infections. Acta Cytol, 21:199-205, 1977.

Vontver LA, Hickok DE, Brown Z, Reid L, Corey L. Recurrent genital herpes simplex virus infection in pregnancy: Infant outcome and frequency of asymptomatic recurrences. Amer J Obstet Gyn, 143:75-84, 1982.

Waugh MA. Anorectal herpesvirus hominis infection in men.
J Amer Vener Dis Assoc, 3:68-70, 1976.

Wheeler CE. Pathogenesis of recurrent herpes simplex infections.
J Invest Dermatol, 65:341-346, 1975.

Whitney JE, Skinner GRB, Buchan A. Acquisition of type 1 herpes simplex vulvitis within a monogamous relationship. Br J Vener Dis, 54:121-123, 1978.

Willmott FE, Mair HJ. Genital herpes virus infection in women attending a venereal diseases clinic. Br J Vener Dis, 54:341-343, 1978.

Chapter 8

CONDYLOMA ACUMINATA (Genital Warts)

ETIOLOGIC AGENT

Condyloma acuminata are genital warts caused by infection
with the human wart virus. The human wart virus belongs to the papovavirus family, a group name taken from the names of the members of the family in the order that they were discovered: the papilloma, the polyoma, and the vacuolating viruses. The human wart
virus is a small DNA virus about 45–55 nm in diameter with an ico-
sahedral shape. The virus grows slowly in epithelial cell nuclei
and produces latent and chronic infections. For some time it was
believed that all human warts were caused by an identical virus
and that the different morphologic types of warts were the result of
environmental conditions associated with their location. Some
recent evidence indicates that a virus identified in condyloma acuminatum tissue differs antigenically from the virus isolated from
other human warts.
Human papillomaviruses (HPV) have been divided into at least
several different DNA types. Types 1, 2, 3, 4, and 7 have been
associated with benign skin warts. DNA sequences for HPV 6 DNA
have been found by DNA nucleic acid hybridization experiments in
approximately 90% of condyloma acuminata. The type 6 DNA also
has been found in Buschke-Loewenstein tumors. The HPV type 6
DNA does not seem to be associated with penile and cervical carcinoma, whereas HPV 11 DNA sequences have been identified in
atypical condyloma of the cervix. HPV 11 and HPV 16 DNA also
have been found in biopsies from some patients with cervical cancer. Whether these associations have any significance with respect
to some of the genital cancers remains to be seen. Crum believes
that the HPV 16 flat wart of the cervix is a precursor of invasive
cancer of the cervix.

EPIDEMIOLOGY

Warts are found on people in all parts of the world. In general, warts are uncommon in infancy and early childhood, and then they increase in frequency as individuals reach their mid-20s. Following this age, the incidence declines. From 1966 to 1981, the estimated number of consultations for condyloma acuminata with office-based, private physicians in the United States increased 459%. Genital warts are most commonly seen among sexually active people. Condyloma acuminata in children should alert the clinician to the possibility of sexual abuse.

Direct human and possibly fomite contact is presumed to be the mechanism of transmission, but there are a number of unexplained epidemiologic features. Some of these are as follows. Not all patients who are exposed to an infected individual will acquire warts. In homosexual men, warts are five to seven times more common around the anus than on the penis. Warts have been described in the oral cavity following oral-genital contact. Autoinoculation may take place from a genital to a nongenital site, but autoinoculation is uncommon from a nongenital to a genital site. Epidemiologic investigation of condyloma acuminata are difficult because of the long incubation period following exposure and the problem of tracing multiple sexual contacts.

CLINICAL MANIFESTATIONS

Condyloma acuminata occur in the genital and perianal areas. The incubation period following exposure is about 4 months, with a range of 1-20 months. Genital warts are found more frequently at certain sites. In men, they are found in decreasing order on the frenulum, the corona, the glans, the prepuce, the urinary meatus, the shaft of the penis, and the anus. They are infrequent on scrotum. As previously mentioned, they are more common around the anus than on the penis in homosexual men (see Figs. 8.1 and 8.2).

Anal warts in homosexual men are usually both perianal and intra-anal. Genital warts are more common in uncircumcised men, in whom they often first appear beneath the prepuce. In women, genital warts are found most frequently on the posterior part of the introitus, followed by the labia minora and clitoris, the labia majora, the perineum, the anus, the vagina, the urethra, and the cervix.

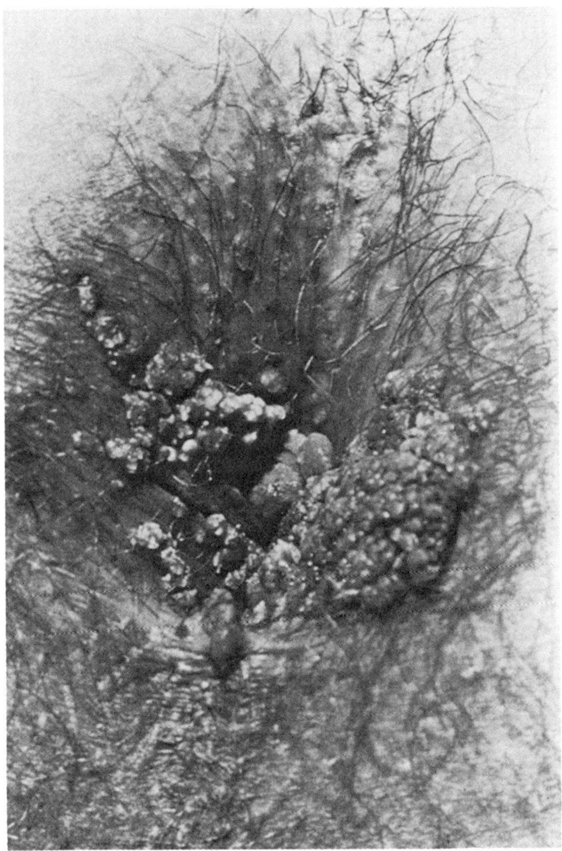

Figure 8.1   Condyloma acuminata or genital warts.   These in a perianal or intra-anal site may be a significant problem for homosexual men.   Anoscopy is required to demonstrate intra-anal condyloma.   Photograph courtesy of E. Stolz and J. van der Stek.*

It may be difficult to visually distinguish cervical intraepithelial neoplasia and cervical lesions caused by the papilloma virus. Walker et al. studied 50 women with vulval condylomata acuminata and found that 50% had evidence of cervical infection by papillomavirus and 36% had epithelial abnormalities consistent with cervical intraepithelial neoplasia.

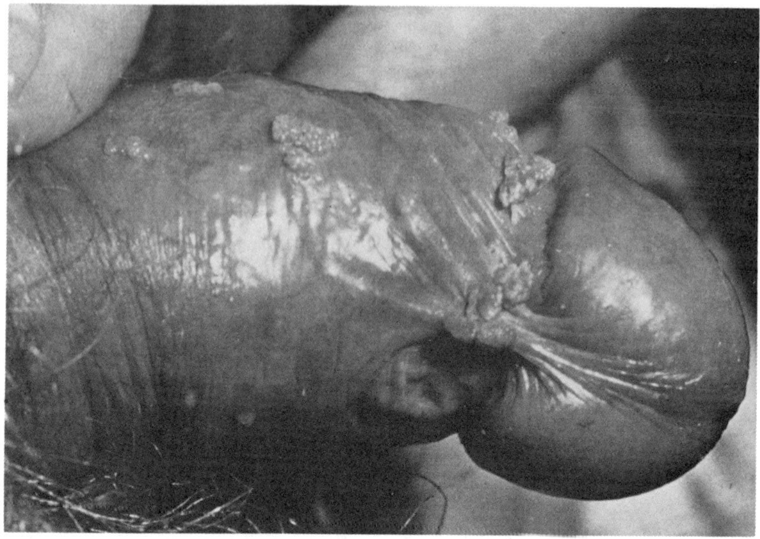

Figure 8.2   Condyloma acuminata on the penis, multiple lesions.
Photograph courtesy of E. Stolz and J. van der Stek.*

Condyloma acuminatum may be single or multiple. They
are characteristically soft and fleshy, and their morphology is
somewhat dependent on their location. Genital warts range in size
from 1 mm to large cauliflower masses several centimeters in
diameter. Fleshy, hyperplastic warts are most often seen in men
on the glans penis, beneath the prepuce, and in the urinary meatus.
Flattened warts are more common on the shaft of the penis. Genital warts resembling skin warts may be present but are uncommon.
Hyperplastic warts are more common in women. In pregnancy,
genital warts may become severe with enlargement, maceration,
and secondary infection. There is some evidence that infants born
to these women may be at higher risk for the development of laryngeal warts.

Buschke-Loewenstein giant condylomas are different from
ordinary condyloma acuminata. They have a malignant, fungating,
gross appearance, and they penetrate deeply into adjacent tissue.
Despite these characteristics, they are histologically benign, and
metastasis does not occur. However, Buschke-Loewenstein giant
condylomas do not respond to conventional therapy with topical
agents.

DIAGNOSIS

The diagnosis of genital warts is generally made on the gross appearance of the lesions. Where indicated, the lesions may be biopsied for histopathological examination. Typical histological features of genital warts include papillomatosis, hyperkeratosis, acanthosis, and parakeratosis. The basal layer is intact. In the upper part of the stratum spinosum, large vacuolated cells are present. Viral cultures are of no benefit in the diagnosis. A serologic test for syphilis and appropriate culture for Neisseria gonorrhoeae should be performed to rule out concurrent syphilis and gonorrhea. A Papanicolaou smear should be performed on women with cervical warts prior to therapy. Atypical or persistent warts should be biopsied.

TREATMENT

The treatment of genital warts ranges from physical destruction to suggestion. The detractors of wart "charming" say that this form of therapy yields results comparable to a placebo response in which a 35% cure rate is possible. The natural history of genital warts has not been completely studied. Skin warts are known to suddenly regress; however, both skin and genital warts can persist for years. Therapy is indicated in pregnant women, if the patient is experiencing discomfort or if the warts appear to be proliferating. In older patients, in patients complaining of pain, in patients with atypical appearing lesions, or in patients with a single lesion on the penis, excision and histologic examination are indicated to rule out malignancy.

Of the various topical therapies, 25% podophyllum in tincture of benzoin is the most popular. Podophyllum is an alcohol-soluble resin prepared from the dried rhizomes and roots of the mandrake or May apple plant. Podophyllum is by no means an ideal therapy. Because it is not a chemically defined compound, different lots may vary in activity. Large quantities of the agent should not be applied, as this material may cause local and systemic toxicity.

Podophyllum is frequently ineffective in eradicating anogenital warts. In one study of the therapy of penile warts, 10% podophyllum in benzotin was as effective as 25% podophyllum during a 3-month surveillance period. A purified active ingredient of podophyllum is podophyllotoxin. This material is available in some European countries and may be used in lower concentrations than the impure compound, and for that reason it may be less toxic than podophyllum.

Podophyllum is applied at weekly intervals until the lesions disappear. Adjacent skin around the warts should be protected with petrolatum prior to application of the podophyllum, and the podophyllum should be washed off 6 hr after application. If warts do not regress after 4 weeks of podophyllum therapy, another therapy should be substituted.

Other forms of therapy include curettage, scissor excision, electrocoagulation cryotherapy with nitrous oxide or liquid nitrogen, diathermy, or topical 5-fluorouracil. The 5-fluorouracil interferes with DNA synthesis, and the drug has been used to treat warts in the urinary meatus where podophyllum is inappropriate and where a destructive procedure may result in a urethral stricture. The 5-fluorouracil is available as a cream in a 25 g tube with a cone-shaped applicator. About 2 ml of the cream is instilled into the urinary meatus after each voiding and at bedtime. The cream should not touch uninvolved skin surfaces; for this reason, the patient should wear a scrotal support with a penile aperture. The treatment is continued for 1 week. Unfortunately, about one-half of the patients will experience erythema, itching, and burning, which may be followed by superficial painful erosions resulting in cessation of therapy. The erosions are said to heal without scarring. Autogenous wart vaccines are not significantly more effective than a placebo. Parenteral human fibroblast interferon shows promise as a therapy for genital warts.

Condyloma acuminata in pregnant women may make delivery difficult and may cause laryngeal warts in their infants. Consideration should be given to removal of the condyloma prior to delivery. Podophyllum is not recommended because of possible toxic effects in the mother and the fetus, and surgical excision may be hazardous because of excessive bleeding. Carbon dioxide laser therapy and electrocoagulation combined with curettage has been successfully used to remove the condyloma.

Patients with Buschke-Loewenstein giant condylomas should not be treated with topical therapy such as podophyllum, as this is not effective. Only surgical removal is of any value, and delay or inadequate local resection only serves to enhance patient morbidity.

BIBLIOGRAPHY

Alexander RM, Kaminsky DB. Giant condyloma acuminatum (Buschke-Loewenstein tumor) of the anus: Case report and review of the literature. Dis Col Rect, 22:561-565, 1979.

Almeida JD, Oriel JD, Stannard LM. Characterization of the
virus in human genital warts. Microbios, 3:225-232, 1969.

Ashiru JO, Ogunbanjo BO, Rotowa NA, Adeyemi-Doro FAB,
Osoba AO. Intraoral condylomata acuminata. A case report. Br
J Vener Dis, 59:325-326, 1983.

Baird PJ. Serological evidence for the association of papillomavirus and cervical neoplasia. Lancet, 2:17-18, 1983.

Burns TNC, Lauvetz RJ, Kerr ES, Ross G. Buschke-Loewenstein
giant condylomas: Pitfalls in management. Urology, 5:773-776,
1975.

Carr G, William DC. Anal warts in a population of gay men in
New York City. Sex Transm Dis, 4:56-57, 1977.

Clark GHV. The charming of warts. J Invest Dermatol, 45:15-21,
1965.

Crum CP, Ikenberg H, Richart RM, Grissman L. Human papillomavirus Type 16 and early cervical neoplasia. New Eng J Med,
310:880-883, 1984.

DeJong AR, Weiss JC, Brent RL. Condyloma acuminata in children. Amer J Dis Child, 136:704-706, 1982.

Dretler SP, Klein LA. The eradication of intraurethral condyloma
acuminata with 5 percent 5-fluorouracil cream. J Urol, 113:195-
198, 1975.

Ferenczy A. Treating genital condyloma during pregnancy with
the carbon dioxide laser. Amer J Obstet Gynecol, 148:9-12,
1984.

Friedman JM, Fialkow PJ. Viral "tumorigenesis" in man:
Cell markers in condylomata acuminata. Int J Cancer, 17:57-
61, 1976.

Gabriel G, Thin RNT. Treatment of anogenital warts. Comparison of trichloric acid and podophyllin versus podophyllin alone.
Br J Vener Dis, 59:124-126, 1983.

Ghosh AK. Cryosurgery of genital warts in cases in which podophyllin treatment failed or was contraindicated. Br J Vener Dis, 53:49-53, 1977.

Gissman L, deVilliers E-M, zur Hausen H. Analysis of human genital warts (condylomata acuminata) and other genital tumors for human papillomavirus type 6 DNA. Int J Cancer, 29:143-146, 1982.

Gissman L, Wolnik L, Ikenberg H, Koldovsky U, Schnurch HG, zur Hausen H. Human papillomavirus types 6 and 11 DNA sequences in genital and laryngeal papillomas and in some cervical cancers. Proc Natl Acad Sci, 80:560-563, 1983.

Gollock JM, Slatford K, Hunter JM. Scissor excision of anogenital warts. Br J Vener Dis, 58:400-401, 1982.

Harvey JM, Glen E, Watson GS. Buske-Loewenstein tumor of the penis. A case report. Br J Vener Dis, 59:273-276, 1983.

Judson FN. Condyloma acuminatum of the oral cavity: A case report. Sex Transm Dis, 8:218-219, 1981.

Krogh G von. 5-Fluorouracil cream in the successful treatment of therapeutically refractory condylomata acuminata of the urinary meatus. Acta Dermatovener (Stockholm), 56:297-301, 1976.

Krough G von. Penile condylomata acuminata: An experimental model for evaluation of topical self-treatment with 0.5-1.0% ethanolic preparations of podophyllotoxin for three days. Sex Transm Dis, 8:179-186, 1981.

Lee SH, McGregor DH, Kuziez MN. Malignant transformation of perianal condyloma acuminatum: A case report with review of the literature. Dis Colon Rectum, 24:462-467, 1981.

Lupulescu A, Mehregan AH, Rahbari H, Pinkus H, Birmingham DJ. Venereal warts vs. Bowen disease: A histologic and ultrastructure study of five cases. J Amer Med Assoc, 237:2520-2522, 1977.

Lutzner MA, Orth G, Dutronquay V, et al. Detection of human papillomavirus type 5 DNA in skin cancers of an immunosuppressed renal allograft recipient. Lancet, 2:422-424, 1983.

Malison MD, Morris R, Jones LW. Autogenous vaccine therapy for condyloma acuminatum. A double-blind controlled study. Br J Vener Dis, 58:62-65, 1982.

Mambo NC. Isoantigen status in condyloma acuminata of the uterine cervix: An immunoperoxidase study. Amer J Clin Path, 79:178-181, 1983.

Margolis D. Therapy for condyloma acuminatum: A review. Rev Infect Dis, 4(Suppl.):S829-S836, 1982.

New York City Department of Health. Condyloma acuminata— United States 1966-1981. City Hlth Info, 2:no. 24, 1983.

· Oriel JD. Anal warts and anal coitus. Br J Vener Dis, 47:373- 376, 1971.

Oriel JD. Natural history of genital warts. Br J Vener Dis, 47: 1-13, 1971.

Oriel JD. Genital warts. Review. Sex Transm Dis, 4:153-159, 1977.

Oriel JD, Almeida JD. Demonstration of virus particles in human genital warts. Br J Vener Dis, 46:37-42, 1970.

Partridge EE, Murad T, Shingleton HM, Austin JM, Hatch KD. Verrucous lesions of the female genitalia. I. Giant condylomata. Amer J Obstet Gynecol, 137:412-418, 1980.

Partridge EE, Shingleton HM, Austin JM, Hatch KD. Verrucous lesions of the female genitalia II. Verrucous carcinoma. Amer J Obstet Gynecol, 137:419-424, 1980.

Pettersson S, Hansson G, Blohme I. Condyloma acuminatum of the bladder. J Urol, 115:535-536, 1976.

Ray B. Condyloma acuminatum of the scrotum. J Urol, 117:739- 740, 1977.

Reid R, Laverty CR, Coppleson M, Isarangkul W, Hills E. Non-condylomatous cervical wart virus infection. Obstet Gynecol, 55: 476-483, 1980.

Rhatigan RM, Saffos RO. Condyloma acuminatum and squamous carcinoma of the vulva. South Med J, 70:591-594, 1977.

Schmauz R, Owor R. Epidemiology of malignant degeneration of condylomata acuminata in Uganda. Pathol Res Pract, 170:91-103, 1980.

Schonfeld A, Nitke S, Schattner A, et al. Intramuscular human interferon-β injections in treatment of condylomata acuminata. Lancet, 1:1038-1042, 1984.

Seidel J, Zonana J, Totten E. Condylomata as a sign of sexual abuse in children. J Ped, 95:553-554, 1979.

Simmons PD. Podophyllin 10% and 25% in the treatment of ano-genital warts. Br J Vener Dis, 57:208-209, 1981.

Simmons PD, Langlet F, Thin RNT. Cryotherapy versus electro-cautery in the treatment of genital warts. Br J Vener Dis, 57:273-274, 1981.

Swerdlow DB, Salvati EP. Condyloma acuminatum. Dis Col Rect, 14:226-231, 1971.

Walker PG, Colley NV, Grubb C, Tejerina A, Oriel JD. Abnor-malities of the uterine cervix in women with vulvar warts. A pre-liminary communication. Br J Vener Dis, 59:120-123, 1983.

Walker PG, Singer A, Dyson JL, Oriel JD. Natural history of cervical epithelial abnormalities in patients with vulval warts. A colposcopic study. Br J Vener Dis, 59:327-329, 1983.

Wallin J. 5-Fluorouracil in the treatment of penile and urethral condylomata acuminatum. Br J Vener Dis, 53:240-243, 1977.

Young RL, Acosta AA, Kaufman RH. The treatment of large con-dylomata acuminata complicating pregnancy. Obstet Gynecol, 41:65-73, 1973.

Zachow KR, Ostrow RS, Bender M, et al. Detection of human papillomavirus DNA in anogenital neoplasias. Nature, 300:771-773, 1982.

Chapter 9

MOLLUSCUM CONTAGIOSUM

ETIOLOGIC AGENT

Molluscum contagiosum is a superficial skin infection caused by a DNA virus of the pox virus family. The molluscum contagiosum virus is one of the largest pathogenic viruses in man ($300 \times 200 \times 100$ nm). It has a brick-shaped outer shell and a dumbbell-like inner core containing deoxyribonucleic acid. The virus is morphologically related to the variola, vaccinia, cowpox, orf, and other animal viruses; however, the exact antigenic relationship of this virus to the pox virus family is unclear.

EPIDEMIOLOGY

Molluscum contagiosum is found worldwide and most commonly affects children and sexually active adults. It is more common among boys than girls, and the lesions are generally located on the trunk, limbs, face, and eyelids. Patients attending venereal disease clinics usually have lesions located in the genital area. Molluscum contagiosum also has been reported in wrestlers, in infant-mother contacts, and in patrons of public baths and swimming pools.

CLINICAL MANIFESTATIONS

The incubation period following exposure to an infected individual varies from several days to 2 months. The lesions appear as shiny, smooth, firm, flesh-colored to pearly white papules

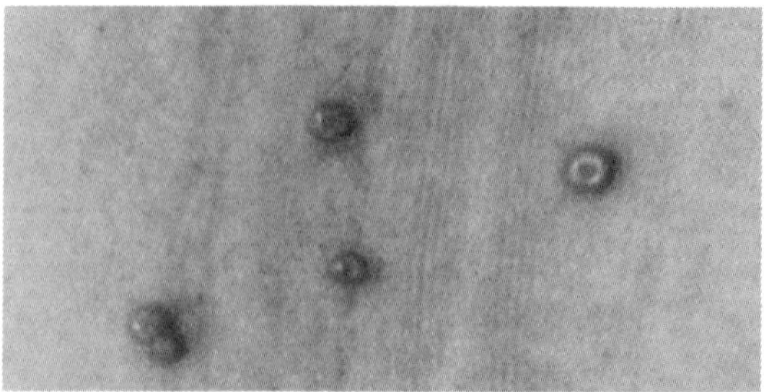

Figure 9.1   Molluscum contagiosum. Typical lesions are smooth papules with an umbilicated center, 1-5 mm in diameter. Patients may have 15-20 lesions located in the pubic area, on the genitalia, the upper inner aspects of the thighs, the perianal region, and the buttocks.

with an umbilicated center. They are painless and are confined to the skin and mucous membranes. Although the size of the lesions varies with their duration, they are usually 1-5 mm but may be as large as 1-2 cm. In patients with sexually transmitted disease, the lesions are located on the pubic area, genitalia, upper inner aspect of the thighs, perianal region, and buttocks. The lesions may be single, but more commonly a patient may have 15-20 lesions at the same time (see Fig. 9.1). Lesions are uncommon on the palms and soles.

DIAGNOSIS

The diagnosis is generally made by the typical appearance of the molluscum contagiosum lesions. From the umbilicated central pore of a papule, one may express a cheesy material. This may be smeared on a glass slide and stained with Giemsa stain. Microscopic examination of this material reveals cells containing basophilic inclusion bodies (molluscum bodies). Excisional biopsy is another method of diagnosis. Microscopic examination of hematoxylin- and eosin-stained tissue sections reveals a localized mass of hypertrophied, hyperplastic epidermis extending down to, but not below, the limiting basement membrane. Mature virus particles cannot be identified below the malpighian layer.

The virus-laden cells appear to migrate toward the surface of the epidermis. As the virus develops in the cytoplasm, the cell nucleus is pushed to one side of the cell. As the molluscum bodies move from the lower epidermis to the horny layer during their development, they become basophilic and Feulgen-positive. The core of the lesion is filled with large numbers of inclusion bodies, keratin, and cell debris. The virus of molluscum contagiosum has not been serially propagated in tissue culture, yet virus cytopathologic effects have been demonstrated in tissue cultures of material from freshly cultured lesions. Routine isolation attempts are not warranted. Virus-specific antibodies, mostly IgG, have been demonstrated in 69% of patients. However, there are no useful diagnostic serologic tests. The role of cellular and humoral immunity is unclear. The differential diagnosis includes basal cell epitheliomas, warts, nevi, adenomas, cysts, lichen planus, and furunculosis.

TREATMENT

The natural history of molluscum contagiosum is that the lesions eventually disappear over a period of a few years. Individual lesions may persist for about 2 months. Autoinoculation is possible, and for this reason removal by curettage may be advisable. Application of liquid nitrogen, podophyllin, 0.9% cantharidin solution, and other caustic liquids has been successfully employed. However, caution should be exercised in all treatments, as the natural history of the lesions is benign and infection does not result in scarring.

BIBLIOGRAPHY

Brown ST, Nalley JF, Kraus SJ. Molluscum contagiosum. Review. Sex Transm Dis, 8:227-234, 1981.

Brown ST, Weinberger J. Molluscum contagiosum: Sexually transmitted disease in 17 cases. J Amer Vener Dis Assoc, 1:35-36, 1974.

Cobbold RJC, MacDonald A. Molluscum contagiosum as a sexually transmitted disease. Practitioner, 204:416-422, 1970.

Hawley TG. The natural history of molluscum contagiosum in Fijian children. J Hyg (Camb), 68:631-632, 1970.

Jacobs PH. Molluscum contagiosum. Aerospace Med, 41:1196-1197, 1970.

Lutzner MA. Molluscum contagiosum, verruca and zoster viruses. Arch Dermatol, 87:436-444, 1963.

Lynch PJ, Minkin W. Molluscum contagiosum of the adult: Probably venereal transmission. Arch Dermatol, 98:141-143, 1968.

Mescon H, Gray M, Moretti G. Molluscum contagiosum: A histochemical study. J Invest Dermatol, 23:293-308, 1954.

Overfield JM, Brody JA. An epidemiologic study of molluscum contagiosum in Anchorage, Alaska. J Ped, 69:640-642, 1966.

Postlethwaite R. Molluscum contagiosum. A review. Arch Environ Hlth, 21:432-452, 1970.

Shand JH, Gibson P, Gregory DW, Cooper RJ, Keir HM, Postlethwaite R. Molluscum contagiosum: A defective poxvirus? J Gen Virol, 33:281-295, 1976.

Shirodaria PV, Mathews RS. Observations on the antibody responses in molluscum contagiosum. Br J Dermatol, 96:29-34, 1977.

Sutton JS, Burnett JW. Ultrastructural changes in dermal and epidermal cells of skin infected with molluscum contagiosum virus. J Ultrastruct Res, 26:177-196, 1969.

Wilkin JK. Molluscum contagiosum venereum in a women's outpatient clinic: A venereally transmitted disease. Amer J Obstet Gynecol, 128:531-535, 1977.

Chapter 10

SYPHILIS

ETIOLOGIC AGENT

The organism causing syphilis is the spirochete Treponema
pallidum. The spirochetes are a group of micro-organisms with a
distinct morphology. They have a slender, spiral shape that resembles a corkscrew. Pathogenic species are found among the
three genera Treponema, Borrelia, and Leptospira. The latter
are free-living spirochetes found in association with animals and
humans in surface waters and soil. The Leptospira species cause
leptospirosis or Weil's disease. The Borrelia spirochetes are
transmitted by lice or ticks and cause relapsing fever in humans.
The Treponema spirochetes are present in the mouth, intestinal
tract, and genital areas of humans and animals. Many are members of the normal microflora of the healthy human. Only T. pallidum (syphilis), T. pertenue (yaws), and T. carateum (pinta) are
pathogenic. The latter two diseases are endemic in populations
inhabiting certain tropical and subtropical climates.

Except for Borrelia, the spirochetes cannot be seen with the
light microscope unless special stains or dark-field illumination
is used. None of the pathogenic treponemes can be cultivated in
vitro. Their mechanism of locomotion is thought to be motion of
overlapping axial filaments wound around the length of the proto-
plasmic cylinder. The characteristic movement is helpful in dark-
field examinations of material from patients with syphilis.

EPIDEMIOLOGY

In recent years in the United States the number of reported
cases of syphilis has varied. A peak of 450 cases per 100,000

population per year occurred during 1943, and this was followed by a precipitous drop, presumably related to the availability of penicillin as well as the intensive treatment campaigns. Beginning in the late 1950s, the number of reported cases again rose.

By the mid-1960s there were approximately 10 cases per 100,000 population per year of primary and secondary syphilis. Since 1964 the number of reported cases per 100,000 population per year has remained approximately the same. Late syphilis has become increasingly infrequent, since the current cases reflect the incidence of the disease in this country 20 years ago. However, the Public Health Service estimates that approximately 50 million dollars is spent annually for the institutional care of the syphilitic insane and blind.

In 1981 syphilis followed gonorrhea and chickenpox as the third most frequently reported communicable disease in the United States. The ratio of gonorrhea to primary and secondary syphilis was 32:1. Syphilis is twice as frequent in men as in women. The chance of an uninfected sexual partner acquiring syphilis following sexual exposure is about 50-60%. Syphilis acquired from a blood transfusion is extremely rare. Syphilis is a hazard to the contacts of prostitutes and to homosexual and bisexual men and their partners. About one-half of the cases of early syphilis in the United States are in homosexual men. The largest reservoir of <u>T. pallidum</u> in Denmark is among homosexual men. In 1979 at least 48% and possibly as many as 71% of cases of early infectious syphilis were homosexually acquired. The city of Copenhagen accounted for 86% of the cases and, of the reinfections, 77% occurred in homosexual men. Syphilis in the United States is more common in large cities. In 1981, 61% of all cases of syphilis in the United States came from 63 cities with populations of ⩾200,000 comprising only 26% of this country's population.

CLINICAL MANIFESTATIONS

Of the sexually transmitted diseases, syphilis is one of the more difficult to recognize because of the many varieties of its presentation. The disease is characterized by having several clinical stages. The characteristic finding of the primary stage of syphilis is the chancre (Figs. 10.1 and 10.2).

Chancres of <u>primary syphilis</u> appear about 3 weeks (10-90 days) following exposure and usually are single in number. The chancre <u>may not be clinically apparent</u> if it is located in the mouth,

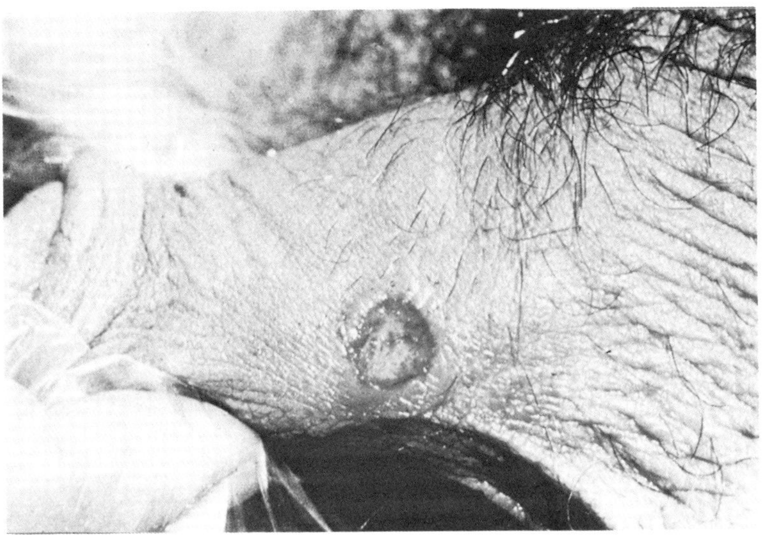

Figure 10.1   Chancre of syphilis on the shaft of the penis.   The
"classic" chancre of syphilis is painless, single, indurated, and
has a raised border.   Spirochetes may be demonstrated in the lesion by means of dark-field microscopy.   Photograph courtesy of
E. Stolz and J. van der Stek.*

vagina, or rectum.   When not secondarily infected, the chancre is
a painless, shallow, punched-out ulcer.   It is indurated and often
has a raised border.   Regional nodes may be enlarged, firm, and
painless.   Chancres vary in diameter from 3-4 mm to 1-2 cm.
Chancres may be ulcerated or covered with a thin crust which
overlays a firm, granular base.   Spirochetes may be demonstrated
in the lesion by means of dark-field microscopy and, if untreated,
the chancre may persist for 2-6 weeks.

A clinical study suggests that the "classic" chancre described
above may not be so common.   In the study, two or more lesions
were observed in 47% of the patients, nonindurated ulcers in 8% of
the patients, and irregular and undermined bordered ulcers in 8%
of the patients.   The chancres of heterosexual men are mostly
present on the prepuce, coronal sulcus, glans, or shaft of the
penis.   In women they may be unnoticed because of their location
on the vaginal wall, cervix, or posterior fourchette, but they may
also be visible on the labia or perineum.   In homosexual men,

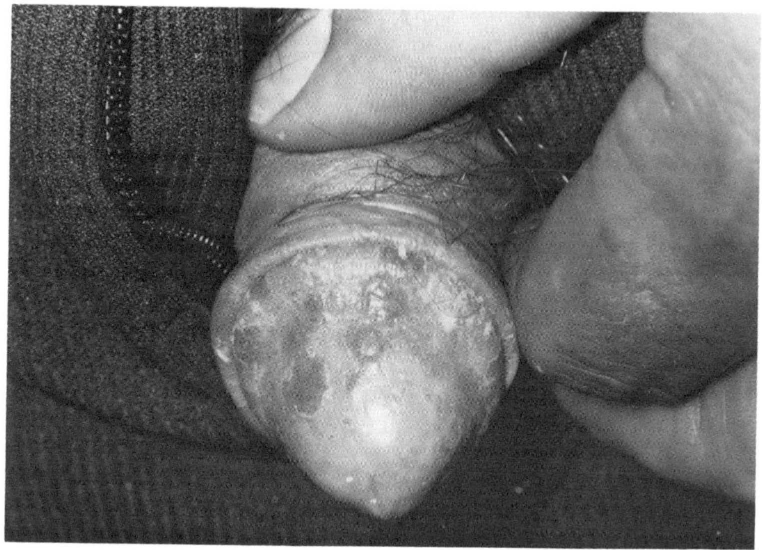

Figure 10.2   Thomas Chapel points out that the classic chancre may be the "atypical" lesion. In his study, two or more lesions were observed in 47% of the patients, nonindurated ulcers in 8%, and irregular and undermined bordered ulcers in 8% of the patients. The photograph demonstrates a nonclassic presentation of primary syphilis in a young man on the corona of the penis. We were surprised to find this lesion dark-field positive for spirochetes.

chancres may be found in the anal canal, on the rectal mucosa, or on the lips or on the oral mucosa or tonsil. Anorectal chancres sometimes may be painful and be accompanied by inguinal adenopathy. Rectal lesions may be easily confused with anal fissures, fistulas, idiopathic anal ulcers, traumatic lesions, rectal polyps, carcinoma, or other infectious diseases such as genital herpes or chancroid. Nongenital lesions also can be located on the fingers, nipples, and other sites.

A number of other diseases may produce lesions that resemble syphilis, and it is mandatory that syphilis be ruled out by the appropriate microscopic or serologic tests. Chancroid, lymphogranuloma venereum, and granuloma inguinale may produce genital lesions but are extremely uncommon in most of the United States. Trauma, drug eruptions, and Reiter's syndrome are more common but may be differentiated by the appropriate history and physical findings.

Secondary syphilis follows primary and usually occurs 6-8 weeks following the initial exposure (see Figs. 10.3-10.7). This form of syphilis has myriad manifestations and persists 2-6 weeks in the untreated patient. One-fourth of patients may have recurrences of secondary syphilis over a 2-year period.

In about one-third of patients, the manifestations of secondary syphilis begin while the chancre is still present (Fig. 10.3). Patients may have constitutional symptoms including low-grade fever, headache, malaise, weight loss, and anorexia. Aching in the long bones, muscles, and joints, sore throat, and lymphadenopathy may be disturbing to patients. Hair loss also may be a presenting complaint.

· The physical findings in secondary syphilis involve the skin in about three-fourths of patients, enlarged lymph nodes in about one-half, and oral or pharyngeal lesions in about one-third. Less

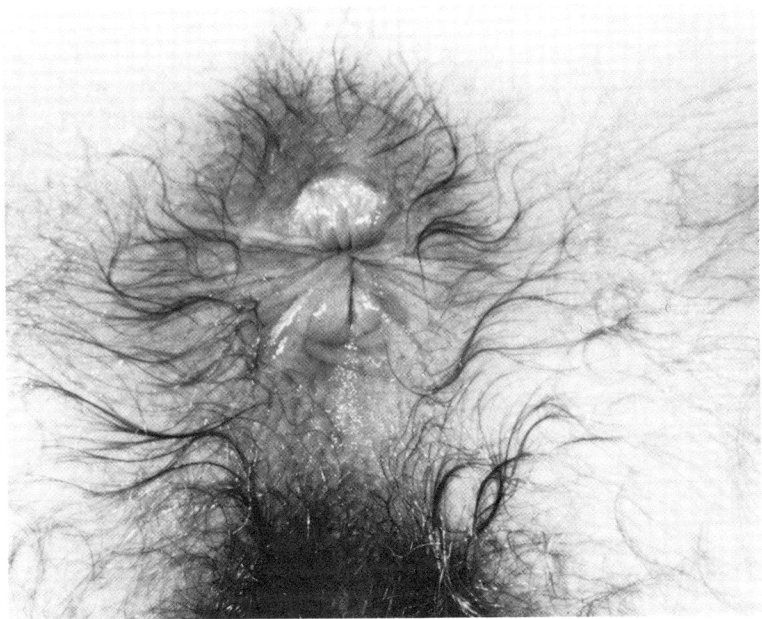

Figure 10.3   A 23-year-old homosexual man complained of a measles-like skin rash and a painful rectal fissure that had been unresponsive to topical lubricants. His "fissure" was a chancre, and his RPR card test was positive at a dilution of 1:32.

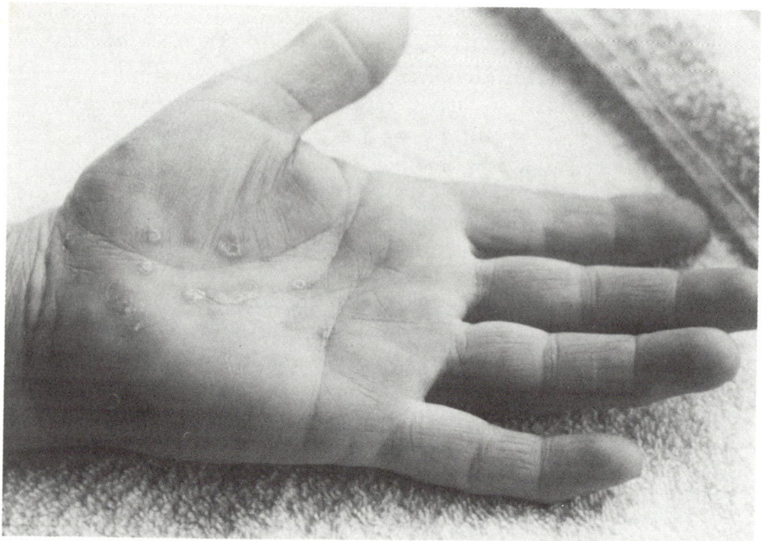

Figure 10.4   Skin lesions of secondary syphilis on the palm. A 38-year-old woman was referred to our oncology service because of the appearance of lymphadenopathy and fever. An alert intern saw the dry, nonpruritic lesions that were bilaterally present on her palms and ordered a VDRL.

than 10% have involvement of the eye, bone, and nervous system. Deafness and uveitis are two dreaded complications, but fortunately are rare. Hepatitis or at least liver function abnormalities are common. The skin lesions are generalized and variable, but they are not vesicular or bullous. The face, trunk, palms, and soles are frequently involved with the rash of secondary syphilis.

There are four major types of rash in patients with secondary syphilis: macular, papular, papulosquamous, and pustular. More than one type may be found on a patient at the same time. One characteristic finding in secondary syphilis is the appearance of a dry, bilaterally symmetrical rash associated with generalized non-tender lymphadenopathy. The rash is said to be generally non-pruritic. However, in a recent study of patients with secondary syphilis, 42% of the patients complained of pruritis. The macular rash is measles-like and consists of pink spots 0.5–1 cm in diameter on the trunk, and on flexor surface of the upper arms. The rash blanches with pressure from a glass slide.

The papular rash is the most common form of the rash and consists of dull-red papules less than 1 cm in diameter found on the palms, soles, arms, legs, face, genitals, and trunk. On warm, moist areas of the body, the rash forms moist papules called condyloma lata. These generally are found in the genital and anal areas, and frequently there is superficial erosion with oozing of serum loaded with T. pallidum. "Nickel and dime" lesions are small annular lesions 1.5-2.0 cm in diameter. Larger annular lesions have a dark border and a dry central clear area.

Other papular lesions are associated with hair follicles. (The hair comes out of the top of the papule.) If this rash is on the scalp there may be hair loss particularly at the sides and at the back of the head. The papulosquamous lesions are generally large, plaque-like, and covered with a scale. The lesions may be easily confused with psoriasis. Pustular lesions have an area of central necrosis. Lesions on mucous membranes (mouth, tongue, vaginal outlet, and cervix) are oval, shallow ulcers called mucous

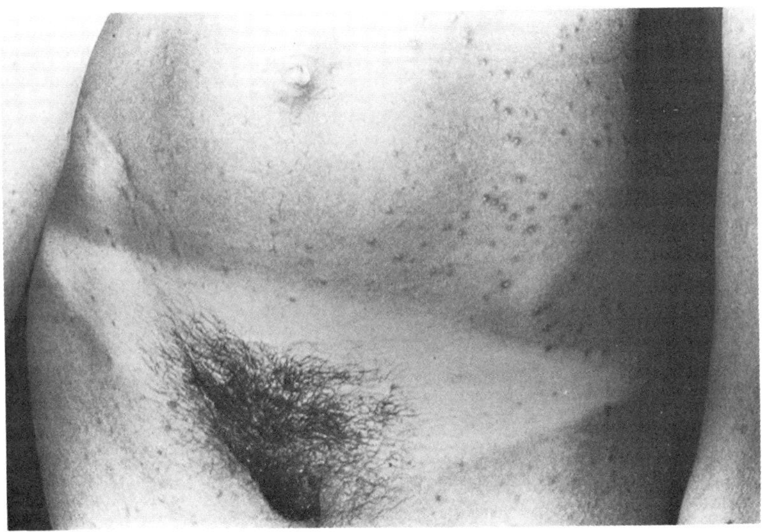

Figure 10.5 Skin lesions of secondary syphilis on the trunk. Apparently this young woman acquired syphilis during her summer at the beach. The lesions are papular in nature. Photograph courtesy of E. Stolz and J. van der Stek.[*]

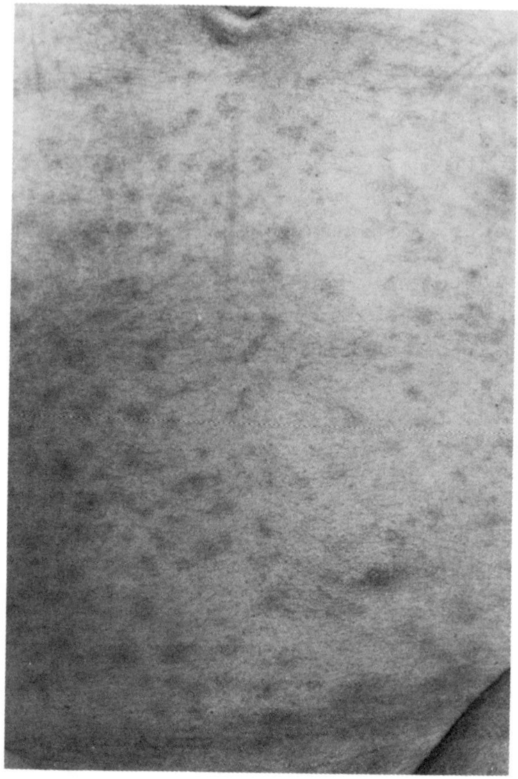

Figure 10.6   Skin lesions of secondary syphilis on the trunk. Secondary syphilis may mimic a number of dermatologic conditions. This macular rash is termed syphilitic roseola. Photograph courtesy of E. Stolz and J. van der Stek.*

patches. The gray-white color of the lesion is due to the presence of necrotic material in the shallow ulcer. Patients with pharyngeal mucous patches may complain of a sore throat.

The skin lesions of secondary syphilis are infectious and may be present at the same time as the primary chancre. Failure to demonstrate spirochetes in the lesions of secondary syphilis does not rule out the disease. In secondary syphilis, the serologic tests are more sensitive diagnostic ones. This is fortunate, because a large number of dermatologic conditions that may be confused with secondary syphilis may be eliminated in the presence of a reactive serologic test for syphilis. Secondary syphilis also can mimic lymphoma and other neoplastic diseases.

When the symptoms and signs of secondary syphilis disappear, the disease is said to be latent. Patients with latent syphilis have no clinical signs or symptoms of the disease. Just because the disease is latent does not mean that this form is not infectious to the patient's sexual partners or, in the case of women, to the fetus. However, after about 4 years in the latent state, syphilis is rarely

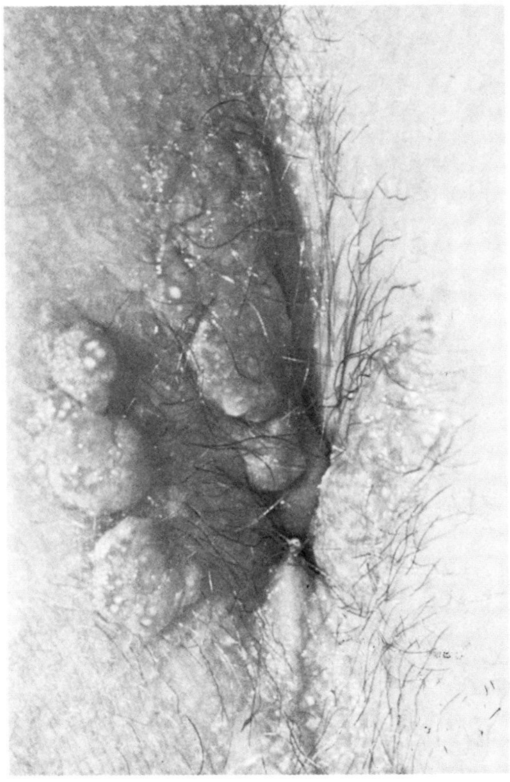

Figure 10.7 Condyloma lata on the anus. Condyloma lata are moist papules that are found on the anal or genital region. They are highly infectious and teem with spirochetes. The serologic tests will be uniformly positive in patients with secondary syphilis. Photograph courtesy of E. Stolz and J. van der Stek.*

transmitted, with the exception that the pregnant mother may transmit the disease to her unborn child. Also, not all patients with latent syphilis go on to more advanced stages of the disease. Only one-third of patients with latent disease develop late complications of syphilis. If the infection has persisted for 4 years, and the cerebrospinal fluid has not been involved, it is not likely to become involved. The spinal fluid examination may be normal in latent syphilis. In latent syphilis the serologic tests for syphilis are positive.

Late syphilis follows latent syphilis. Late syphilis may take several forms: benign, neurosyphilis, or cardiovascular syphilis. Those forms of syphilis occur in approximately one-third of all patients with untreated syphilis and may be found within 2-30 years after the original infection. Approximately 20% of patients develop neurosyphilis, 50% develop benign syphilis, and 30% develop cardiovascular syphilis. Some patients may have combined lesions.

The gumma is the lesion of the late benign syphilis. Benign refers to the fact that the lesions seldom reflect in death or physical incapacity. Gummas are found in the skin, mucous membranes, and subcutaneous tissue. In addition, they may be found in the bones, muscles, joints, and ligaments. Gummas may be the result of cell-mediated host defenses against the invading treponeme. When found in the skin, they may be single or multiple and are generally circular. They are chronic destructive lesions that heal centrally and extend peripherally. Localized gummas in mucous membranes are most commonly found in the tongue and oral cavity, the pharynx, the larynx, and the nasal system. The hard palate and the nasal septum may be perforated. Because of breakdown of surface structures, the gumma may present as an ulcer. In the abdominal cavity, gummas most commonly involve the liver. In bone, gummas are present most frequently in the cranial bones, the clavicle, and the tibia. In general the serologic tests for syphilis are positive in high titer, and material from biopsy may be examined pathologically.

Neurosyphilis is subdivided into three forms: asymptomatic, meningovascular, and parenchymatous. The latter presents as general paresis or tabes dorsalis. All patients with neurosyphilis have abnormal spinal fluid findings. A positive reagin test in the cerebrospinal fluid is indicative of neurosyphilis. The activity of neurosyphilis is indicated by the degree of abnormality of the spinal fluid protein value and the presence of cells in the spinal fluid. A cell count of greater than four lymphocytes is evidence of disease activity. Spinal fluid abnormalities may remain abnormal for extended periods following successful therapy and may not become normal for 1 year. The abnormalities generally return to normal or become nonreactive in the following order: cell count, protein and, finally, the serologic test. Colloidal gold tests on the spinal fluid are not diagnostically significant and should not be used to follow the activity of neurosyphilis.

The classification of neurosyphilis is somewhat arbitrary because the treponeme is unlikely to confine itself to the meninges or the parenchyma of the brain. Asymptomatic neurosyphilis patients have no clinical manifestations and only abnormalities in the cerebrospinal fluid. Patients with meningovascular involvement have a variety of signs and symptoms depending on where the area of damage lies. Headache, papilledema, cranial nerve palsies, seizures, hemiplagia, and loss of papillary response are some examples. Argyll Robertson pupils may be present. This sign indicates constricted, irregular pupils that have loss of light reflex but retention of accommodation reflex.

Parenchymous neurosyphilis includes the paretic and tabetic forms. General paresis patients may have personality changes ranging from mild to psychotic, and patients may undergo progressive changes of dementia. In addition to mental deterioration, the patient may suffer seizures, aphasia, or hemiplegia that may be transient in nature. Impairment of speech, handwriting, and pupillary changes are common. Gummas of the brain may produce symptoms as does any space-occupying lesions.

Tabes dorsalis is a form of neurosyphilis that appears 10-20 years after the original infection. In tabes dorsalis the posterior columns of the spinal cord are injured, and patients complain of sharp attacks of leg pains and ataxia. These attacks may be accompanied by paresthesias, impotence, distension of the bladder, and constipation due to loss of tone and sensory nerve supply. Patients may have an abdominal crisis with severe abdominal pain, nausea, and vomiting. The patient may have Argyll Robertson pupils, loss of reflexes in the legs, and loss or diminished sensation on various areas of the body and limbs. Vibratory loss is common in the lower extremities. The impairment of sensation may lead to injury to the joints (most commonly the knee). This form of osteoarthritis is called a Charcot's joint, and the joint may be severely deranged. Perforating ulcers may develop on the sole of the foot or toes as a result of pressure necrosis due to diminished sensation and, when the ulcers become secondarily infected, osteomyelitis is sure to follow. To add to this litany of horrors, deafness may occur, and patients may become blind as a result of syphilitic optic atrophy.

Cardiovascular syphilis generally involves the large vessels of the body 10-40 years after the initial infection. The ascending and transverse section of the aortic arch is the most frequently involved, and there is destruction of the elastic tissue and medial necrosis as a result of endarteritis obliterans of the vasa vasorum. The intimal surface of the vessel is damaged as well, and calcium in linear streaks may be deposited on the ascending aorta. Fibrosis resulting from damage to the intima may cause narrowing of the opening of the coronary arteries. The destruction of the elastic tissue of the proximal aorta results in dilatation of the aortic valve ring and aortic valve insufficiency.

The vessel weakness also results in aneurysm formation. Syphilitic aneurysms are more commonly present in the thoracic aorta, while atherosclerotic aneurysms are more commonly found in the abdominal aorta. It is rare today that they are discovered because of physical signs such as pulsations, hoarseness due to left recurrent laryngeal nerve damage, Horner's syndrome, or superior vena cava syndrome. More likely patients will complain of angina or symptoms secondary to aortic regurgitation, and the aneurysm will be first identified on a chest roentgenogram.

Cardiovascular syphilis is more common and occurs at an earlier age in men than in women and in blacks than in whites. Aortic regurgitation also is more common than aneurysm formation. Syphilis may be confused with atherosclerotic cardiovascular disease, hypertension, and rheumatic fever. In cardiovascular syphilis, the serologic tests for syphilis are usually positive.

Syphilis occurring in pregnancy and congenital syphilis remain a very real hazard. It was generally thought that prior to the eighteenth week of pregnancy treponemes did not cross the placenta to infect the fetus. This assumption is not correct and is of relatively little value, because frequently the physician has no idea when the infection occurred or the exact duration of the pregnancy. Women with latent syphilis may deliver infants who are infected yet do not have signs of syphilis. Therefore, the quantitative serologic tests for syphilis are a key in the management of pregnant patients.

In infants there is no primary stage of syphilis, since the infecting organisms are introduced via the maternal bloodstream. Early congenital syphilis appears before the age of 2 years. Shortly after birth, skin lesions of the bullous variety may occur. Later, however, papulosquamous lesions with symmetrical distribution are more typical. Condyloma lata may be present. A mucoid discharge may be present in the mucous membranes in the nose and pharynx. In the newborn period, a hemorrhagic nasal discharge may be present. These discharges are highly infectious, because they are teeming with spirochetes which may be demonstrated by dark-field examination. After the first month of life, osteochondritis of long bones may be seen by roentgenologic examination. Hepatosplenomegaly is present in two-thirds of the patients, and most have a self-limited hemolytic anemia. One-half of the infants will have an abnormal cerebrospinal fluid examination, although not all of them will have clinical manifestations of neurosyphilis.

Late congenital syphilis is defined as congenital syphilis that has persisted beyond 2 years of age. All will have a reactive serologic test for syphilis; however, one-third of the children will have other clinical manifestations. Late congenital syphilis is not infectious. Following is a list of some of the signs of late congenital syphilis. The dental lesions include mulberry molars, notched incisors, and abnormalities of the enamel. The skeletal changes include painless hydrathrosis (Clutton's joints), saber tibia, clavicular deformity, scaphoid scapula, saddle nose, short maxilla, frontal bossing of the skull, and high palatal arch. In the eye there may be uveitis, interstitial keratitis, and glaucoma. Skin lesions include cracks and fissures about the nose and mouth (rhagades) and gummas. Cardiovascular lesions are rare in congenital syphilis.

DIAGNOSIS

Serologic Tests for Syphilis

There are two basic types of serologic tests to diagnose syphilis: treponemal and nontreponemal tests. The tests measure two types of antibody. One is an antibody directed to components of the pathogenic treponeme. The other is an antibody that is formed to lipoidal antigens of the treponema and lipoidal antigens that are released as a result of the interaction of the spirochete and the host cells. The latter antibody also reacts with a substance extracted from beef heart called cardiolipin. This convenient cross-reaction is the basis for the nontreponemal tests. The standard antigen in the nontreponemal test contains cardiolipin, cholesterol, and lecithin. When this mixture reacts with antibody in patients with syphilis, a flocculation reaction takes place.

The standard antigen was devised by the Venereal Disease
Research Laboratories (VDRL), and this antigen is the basis for
all of the other nontreponemal tests currently in use: the VDRL,
the unheated serum reagin (USR) test, the automated reagin test
(ART), the rapid plasma reagin (RPR) card, and the reagin screen
test (RST). Another test, the toluidine red unheated serum test
(TRUST) currently is being investigated by the Centers for Disease
Control. The VDRL test is the only test that is recommended for
the evaluation of cerebrospinal fluid. The VDRL test in the United
States has become less popular in the past 15 years and has been
replaced by other nontreponemal tests because they are easier to
perform. The VDRL and the USR tests require a microscope to
perform, and the VDRL antigen must be made up daily. In addition, the patient's serum must be heated before performing the
VDRL test. The remainder of the tests are macroscopic tests,
and they are simpler to perform. With certain limitations, plasma may be used in the RPR card and the RST procedure. This is
especially convenient for blood that has been collected by blood
banks.

The specific treponemal antibody tests are generally performed only on those patients who have a positive nontreponemal
test. One of the earlier tests, the _T. pallidum_ immobilization
(TPI) test, is no longer routinely performed and has been sup-
planted by the fluorescent treponemal antibody absorption (FTA-
ABS) test. In that test the patient's serum is absorbed with the
nonpathogenic Reiter treponema, which removes antibodies that
cross-react with saprophytic treponemes and _T. pallidum_. The
serum is then layered over dead _T. pallidum_ (Nichols virulent
strain), which is fixed to a glass slide. If antibody is present in
the patient's serum, then the treponeme becomes coated with a
layer of antibody globulin. The presence of a positive reaction is
identified by then flooding the slide with fluorescein-labeled antibody to human gamma globulin. The excess labeled antibody is
removed, and the slide is examined under ultraviolet light with a
dark-field background. Under these conditions the antibody coated
spirochetes are easily identified. As noted later, the manner of
this fluorescence is important.

In addition to the FTA-ABS test, there are a number of other
specific treponemal antibody tests including the microhemagglutination assay for antibodies to _T. pallidum_ (MHA-TP), and the
hemagglutination treponemal test for syphilis (HATTS). Two other
tests are in the development stages, and they are the fluorescent
treponemal antibody absorption double staining (FTA-ABS DS) and

the syphilis bio-EnzaBead test. The two hemagglutination tests
are similar in design. T. pallidum antigens are broken up and
attached to the erythrocytes of sheep (MHA-TP) or turkey (HATTS).

Although not generally considered a serologic test, one should
not forget the direct fluorescent treponemal antibody test for
T. pallidum (DFA-TP). Here fluoresceine-labeled antibody is
reacted directly with a biopsy specimen or material taken from a
skin or mucous membrane lesion. This and dark-field microscopy are excellent tests when material is available from lesions of patients with primary or secondary syphilis. With dark-
field microscopy, the material has to be examined rapidly, but
with the DFA-TP, the specimen can be examined at any time since
the presence of living spirochetes is not required.

<u>Relative Value of the Serologic Tests for Syphilis</u>
<u>in the Different Stages of the Disease</u>

The physician needs to be selective in the test that is chosen
to assist in the diagnosis of syphilis. With few exceptions, it is
safer to use a nontreponemal test as the screening test. The performance of a test is in part dependent on the number of patients
with the disease in the population tested: the greater the number
of patients with the disease, the better the test performs. Even
a test with a very high sensitivity and specificity (see Tables 10.1
and 10.2) will give a large proportion of false positives when the
test is used in a population where the disease in question is rare.
Therefore, the predictive value of the treponemal tests is improved
when they are used only in those patients who have a positive nontreponemal test. Physicians should not be tempted to use the FTA-
ABS test as the only one in patients with primary syphilis despite
its greater sensitivity. Patients who may have late syphilis sometimes will have a negative nontreponemal test and a positive treponemal test. Patients with borderline FTA-ABS tests should have
them repeated.

The same nontreponemal test should be used to follow a patient
who is being treated for syphilis. There are up to fourfold differences in end points among the various nontreponemal tests.

The other thing to keep in mind when considering a serologic
test for syphilis is the test's performance in the particular patient's
stage of disease. Two measures of performance are the test's
sensitivity and specificity. The sensitivity of a test is its ability
to be positive in the presence of the disease. Sensitivity is expressed numerically as the percentage of true positives detected.

Table 10.1 Sensitivity and Specificity of the Nontreponemal Tests[a]

A. Percent Sensitivity by Stage of Untreated Syphilis

Stage	Primary	Secondary	Latent
Test			
VDRL	80 (74–87)[b]	100	96 (95–100)
RPR card	86 (81–100)	100	99 (95–100)
USR	80 (72–88)	100	95
TRUST	85 (77–86)	100	99 (97–100)

B. Percent Specificity

Test	Specificity	Range
VDRL	98	(96–99)
RPR card	98	(93–99)
USR	99	
TRUST	99	(98–99)

[a] From S. A. Larsen, Current status of laboratory tests for syphilis. Chapter V in J. H. Rippey and R. M. Nakamura, Diagnostic Immunology: Technology assessment and quality assurance CAP Conference/1983. College of American Pathologists, Skokie, Illinois, 1984.
[b] Range of sensitivity in CDC studies.

The specificity of a test is its ability to be negative in the absence of disease. Specificity is expressed numerically as the percentage of true negatives detected by the test. The available sensitivity and specificity of the nontreponemal and treponemal tests are presented in Tables 10.1 and 10.2.

Table 10.2   Percent Sensitivities and Specificities of the Treponemal Tests[a]

A.   Percent Sensitivity by Stage of Untreated Syphilis

Stage	Primary	Secondary	Latent	Late
Test				
FTA-ABS	98 (93-100)[b]	100	100	96
MHA-TP	82 (69-90)	100	100	94
HATTS	87	100	100	94

B.   Percent Specificity

Test	Specificity	Range
FTA-ABS	98	95-99
MHA-TP	99	98-100
HATTS	99	

[a] From S. A. Larsen, Current status of laboratory tests for syphilis. Chapter V in J. H. Rippey and R. M. Nakamura, Diagnoistic Immunology: Technology assessment and quality assurance CAP Conference/1983. College of American Pathologists, Skokie, Illinois, 1984.
[b] Range of sensitivity in CDC studies.

As seen in the tables, the FTA-ABS test and other treponemal tests, once positive, tend to remain positive. In this respect the treponemal test is inferior to the VDRL or other nontreponemal tests, which are more useful in following the course of successful therapy in syphilis. Successful therapy results in a more rapid fall in the VDRL than occurs in untreated patients. If treatment is given for early syphilis in appropriate dosage, up to 90% of patients may have a nonreactive VDRL after 12-15 months. However, the VDRL may remain positive for life if the patient has received therapy after having untreated syphilis for several years. A rising titer may indicate recent infection, reinfection, relapse, or biologic false positive.

Since the VDRL is often nonreactive in primary syphilis, the dark-field examination is extremely important in establishing the diagnosis. In patients with secondary syphilis, the VDRL antibody titers may be so high that the test appears to be negative due to the prozone phenomenon. This happens in less than 2% of sera from patients with secondary syphilis. In cases where secondary syphilis is suspected and the VDRL is negative, it would be wise to ask the laboratory to dilute the serum and retest it. At delivery, a positive VDRL on cord blood does not necessarily indicate that a baby has syphilis, as the antibody may be passively transferred from the mother. By 3 months the nontreponemal tests should no longer detect passively transferred antibodies. The FTA-ABS (IgM) test for neonatal congenital syphilis currently is thought to be unreliable for ruling out the presence of congenital syphilis. A false negative rate in this test may exceed 35%. A reactive VDRL test on a spinal fluid specimen indicates syphilis unless proven otherwise. The FTA-ABS test should not be performed on spinal fluid because its interpretation is unclear.

Despite adequate therapy, the VDRL may remain positive for life. Retreatment for syphilis is indicated when the VDRL or other nontreponemal test shows a fourfold rise in titer, i.e., 1:2 to 1:8. In congenital syphilis, however, titers may fluctuate in that degree for no apparent reason. In pregnant women, doubt about previous therapy should direct one toward retreatment.

False positive reactions to the VDRL and other nontreponemal tests are a source of concern both to the physician and the patient. False positives occur in 1-2% in the general population regardless of which test is used. Technical problems or errors in the laboratory may be the source, and this sometimes may be identified by simply repeating the test. When false positive reactions occur, the titers are usually less than 1:8. Twelve percent of false positive reactions are greater than or equal to 1:8. The treponemal diseases yaws and pinta will produce a reactive test. Some false positive reactions are acute and are associated with certain temporary conditions such as pregnancy, immunizations, certain antihypertensives, and infectious diseases such as malaria and mycoplasma pneumonia. Most of these false positive reactions disappear within 6 months. Chronic false positive reactions may be associated with aging, drug addiction, leprosy, and collagen-vascular disorders such as lupus erythematosus or Hashimoto's thyroiditis.

In heavy narcotics users, more than 10% of the sera may give
false positive results.

False positive reactions infrequently occur in the treponemal
tests as well. False positive FTA-ABS test results occur in 1-2%
of healthy persons for no apparent reason. A beaded fluorescence
reaction on the treponeme rarely may be seen in patients with lupus
erythematosus, rheumatoid arthiritis, scleroderma, mixed connective tissue disorders, and malignancy. Homogenous fluorescence has been reported in lupus, discoid lupus, drug-induced
lupus, rheumatoid arthritis, autoimmune hemolytic anemia, alcoholic cirrhosis, and lymphosarcoma. False positive FTA-ABS
reactions also have been reported in patients with vaccinations,
viral infections, and pregnancy.

METHOD OF LABORATORY APPROACH IN THE
DIAGNOSIS OF SYPHILIS

Primary Syphilis

In primary syphilis it is necessary to perform a dark-field
examination on exudate from the ulcerative lesion whenever possible.
Alternatively, material from the lesion should be stained by the
direct fluorescent antibody method (DFA-TP). Early in syphilis
the serologic tests are not positive. However, the FTA-ABS becomes positive slightly more rapidly than the nontreponemal tests.
If laboratory facilities are not available for the dark-field examination, then the physician should draw the appropriate serologic test
(in this case the VDRL or RPR as well as the FTA-ABS) prior to
therapy. The microhemagglutination tests are less sensitive than
the FTA-ABS in patients with primary syphilis.

A patient with typical lesions and a reactive test should be
treated even in the absence of a positive dark-field test. It is
worthwhile, in the face of a negative test, to repeat the serologic
test at 1 week, at 1 month, and at 3 months to see if the test will
become positive or if a different diagnosis is established. Nonreactive tests during the 3-month period excludes the diagnosis of
syphilis. It is again emphasized that in the diagnosis of primary
syphilis, the dark-field examination is most important. If a genital lesion is healing, a presumptive diagnosis can be made without
a confirmatory dark-field examination in the presence of lymphadenopathy, a reactive serologic test, and a history of sexual
exposure to an infected patient.

Table 10.3   Criteria for the Diagnosis of Early Congenital Syphilis (Patient Younger Than 2 Years)[a]

<u>Diagnosis Should Be Made When</u>

1. The absolute criterion is met
2. The patient meets one major criterion and one major or minor criterion in another category
3. The patient meets at least one minor criterion in each of the three categories

<u>Clinical Criteria</u>

Absolute:

1. Specimen from lesions showing <u>Treponema pallidum</u> on dark-field or histologic examination

Major:

2. Positive reagin test of cerebrospinal fluid
3. Condyloma lata
4. Osteochondritis, periostitis
5. Snuffles, hemorrhagic rhinitis
6. Bullous lesions, palmar/plantar rash

Minor:

7. Mucous patches
8. Hepatomegaly, splenomegaly
9. Generalized lymphadenopathy
10. Central nervous system signs
11. Hemolytic anemia, diffuse intravascular coagulation
12. Elevated cell count or protein in cerebrospinal fluid
13. Pneumonitis
14. Edema, ascites
15. Placental villitis or vasculitis
16. Intrauterine growth retardation

Table 10.3   (Cont'd.)

Serologic Criteria

Major:

1. Fourfold rise in reagin titer and positive treponemal antibody test
2. Development of a positive treponemal antibody test after birth

Minor:

3. Positive reagin test after 4 months of age
4. Positive treponemal antibody test after 1 year of age

Epidemiologic Criteria

Major:

1. Untreated early syphilis in the mother within 4 weeks of delivery

Minor:

2. Untreated late latent syphilis in the mother
3. Early syphilis in the mother within 3 months of child's birth
4. Mother an untreated contact to lesion syphilis during pregnancy
5. Mother treated for syphilis during pregnancy with a drug other than penicillin
6. Mother treated for syphilis during pregnancy and not followed to delivery

---

[a] From K. C. Rathbun. Congenital syphilis: A proposal for improved surveillance, diagnosis, and treatment. Sex Transm Dis, 10:102–107, 1983.

Secondary Syphilis

In secondary syphilis the dark-field examination or DFA-TP
may be performed on material aspirated from lymph nodes or taken
from moist lesions, such as condyloma lata. However, in this
stage of the disease the serologic tests are uniformly reactive.
Thus one needs only to have the clinical suspicion plus the positive
VDRL or other nontreponemal test. Generally the nontreponemal
titers are greater than 1:16 dilution. Only a rare prozone reaction (see above) may cause confusion. In this form of the disease
the FTA-ABS is rarely required except when a false positive reaction is suspected. Abnormal cerebral spinal fluid findings have
been reported in 5-32% of patients with primary and secondary
syphilis. However, CSF examinations are not generally indicated
because patients who are treated with the standard penicillin therapy generally respond and the CSF findings return to normal. The
VDRL is the only test that is currently recommended for testing of
the cerebrospinal fluid.

Latent Syphilis

Patients with latent syphilis have reactive reagin and treponemal serologic tests in the absence of clinical findings. A
cerebrospinal fluid examination is indicated in patients with
syphilis of greater than 1 year's duration to exclude asymptomatic
neurosyphilis. Approximately 20% of patients with late latent
syphilis will have nonreactive nontreponemal test results.

Tertiary Syphilis

In this form of the disease the treponemal tests are the most
sensitive; thus the diagnostic evaluation should include an FTA-
ABS serologic test. In addition, a lumbar puncture should be performed in order to rule out neurosyphilis. The VDRL (quantitative)
is performed on the spinal fluid.

Congenital Syphilis

Katharine C. Rathbun, Texas public health officer, points
out that congenital syphilis is difficult to diagnose. She suggests
sets of diagnoistic criteria for patients younger than and older than
2 years of age. These are outlined in Tables 10.3 and 10.4.

Table 10.4 Criteria for the Diagnoisis of Late Congenital Syphilis (Patient Older Than 2 Years)[a]

Diagnosis Should Be Made When

1. An absolute criterion is met
2. The patient meets criteria in at least two categories

Absolute Criteria

1. Mulberry molars
2. Notched incisors

Epidemiologic Criteria

1. Untreated syphilis in the mother
2. Positive treponemal antibody test in mother
3. Sibling with congenital syphilis

Serologic Criteria

1. Positive reagin test[b]
2. Positive treponemal antibody test[b]

Clinical Criteria

1. Rhagades
2. Clutton's joints
3. Interstitial keratitis, uveitis
4. Delayed mental development, seizures, hydrocephalus[c]
5. Saddle nose, saber tibia
6. High palatal arch, palatal perforation
7. Cardiovascular defects
8. Eighth-nerve deafness[b]
9. Gummas[b]
10. Paresis, paralysis[b]

[a] From K. C. Rathbun. Congenital syphilis: A proposal for improved surveillance, diagnosis, and treatment. Sex Transm Dis, 10:102-107, 1983.
[b] These criteria should be considered only when it is unlikely that they could be caused by acquired syphilis.
[c] These criteria should be considered only when other diagnoses have been excluded.

Many times the first thought that syphilis might be present comes when the physician finds that the patient has a positive VDRL. Lee and Sparling have provided an algorithm to systematically approach the evaluation of a patient with a positive VDRL. The algorithm has three main branches: suspicious lesions (Fig. 10.8), keys within the history (Fig. 10.9), and pregnancy (Fig. 10.10).

SEROLOGIC TESTS TO ASSESS THE
RESPONSE TO THERAPY

The quantitative VDRL test is the one to use to follow the course of therapy. In patients with primary or secondary syphilis who are treated with the appropriate therapy, the VDRL titer generally will fall by at least two dilutions in a 2-year period.

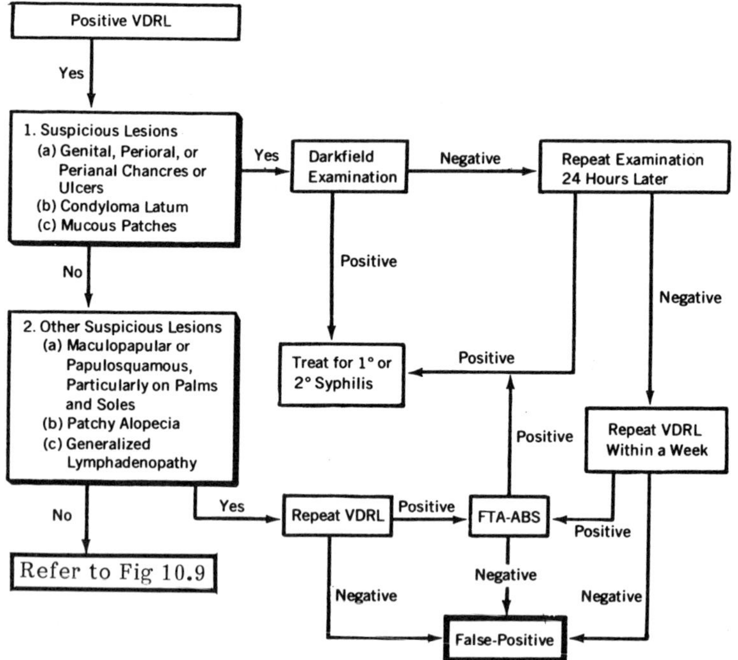

Figure 10.8   Suspicious lesions (positive VDRL). From T. J. Lee and P. F. Sparling, Syphilis. An algorithm. J Amer Med Assoc, 242:1187-1189, 1979.

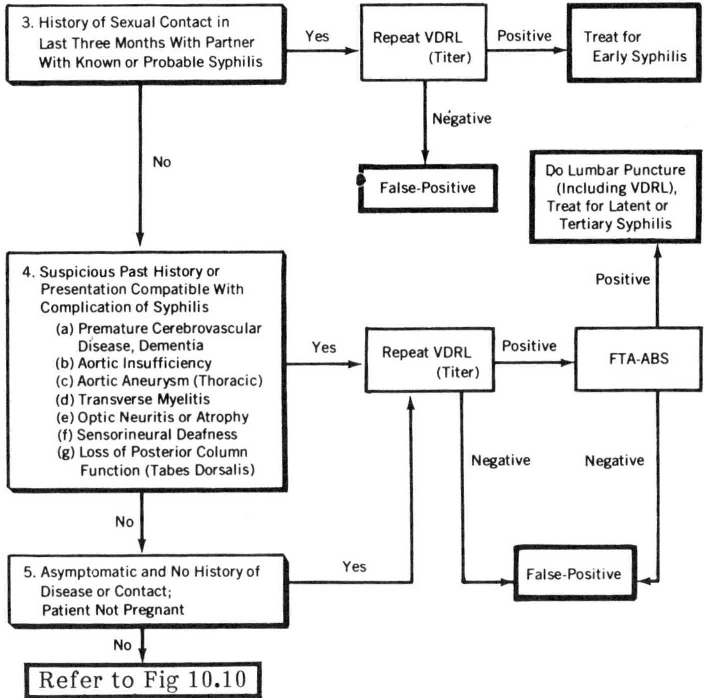

Figure 10.9   Keys in history (positive VDRL). From T. J. Lee and P. F. Sparling, Syphilis. An algorithm. J Amer Med Assoc, 242:1187–1189, 1979.

Two years after the appropriate therapy, the VDRL titer will fall to negative in 97% of patients with seropositive primary syphilis and in 76% of patients with secondary syphilis.

SPECIMEN COLLECTION FOR
DARK-FIELD MICROSCOPY

Surface Lesions

The surface of the lesion should be wiped clean of crusts, pus, or epithelial cells, and then the lesion should be gently abraded to the point of bleeding. Pressure should be applied to produce a serous exudate. A glass slide is placed on the lesion to

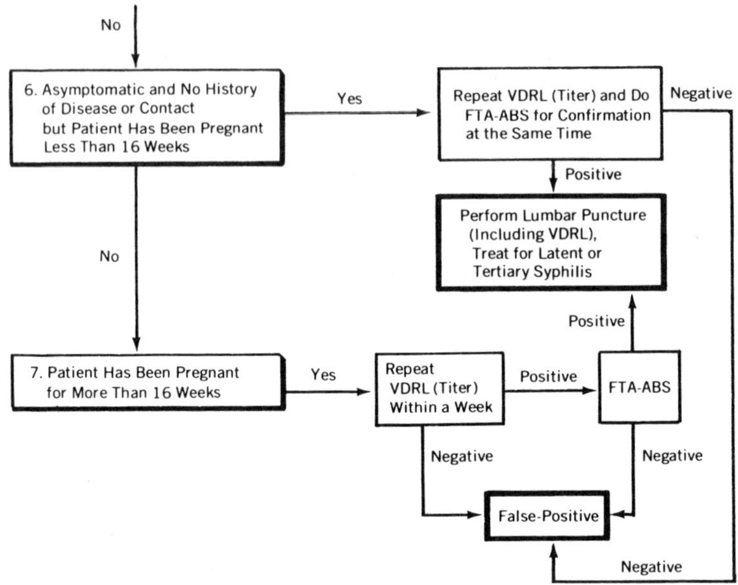

Figure 10.10   Pregnancy (positive VDRL).   From T. J. Lee and
P. F. Sparling, Syphilis.   An algorithm.   J Amer Med Assoc,
242:1187-1189, 1979.

collect the exudate.   The exudate should be quickly covered with
a glass coverslip and taken directly to the dark-field microscope.
Treatment of the lesion with 5% acyclovir ointment does not interfere with detection of T. pallidum by dark-field microscopy.
Mucous patches or chancres in the mouth may be examined after
thorough cleansing; however, the presence of nonpathogenic oral
spirochetes may be confused with T. pallidum.   It is worth attempting direct fluorescent antibody (DFA-TP) examination on material
from the lesion or a biopsy of the lesion.

The dark-field examination may be useful for perianal and
anal lesions.   However, the presence of nontreponemal spirochetes
in the rectum may cause confusion.   Intrarectal lesions should be
biopsied and stained with the Warthin-Starry silver stain or with
the direct immunofluorescent antibody stain (DFA-TP) for T. pallidum.

<u>Lymph Nodes</u>

Diagnostic material may be aspirated from enlarged regional lymph nodes. The overlying skin is cleaned and prepared with an antiseptic solution. When the solution has dried, a 20-gauge needle is inserted into the node and a small amount (0.1 ml) of normal sterile saline without preservative is injected. The needle tip is manipulated in order to free some of the lymph node tissue, and the material is aspirated in order to look for the presence of spirochetes.

RECOMMENDED TREATMENT SCHEDULES FOR PATIENTS WITH SYPHILIS[1]

EARLY SYPHILIS

Recommended Regimen

Early syphilis (primary, secondary, latent syphilis is less than 1 year's duration) should be treated with:
   Benzathine penicillin G: 2.4 million units total, IM, at a single session

Penicillin-Allergic Patients

Patients who are allergic to penicillin should be treated with:
   Tetracycline HCl: 500 mg, by mouth, four times a day for 15 days
   Tetracycline appears to be effective but has been evaluated less extensively than penicillin. Patient compliance with this regimen may be difficult, so care should be taken to encourage optimal compliance.
   Penicillin-allergic patients who cannot tolerate tetracycline should have their allergy confirmed. For these patients there are two options:

---

[1] From Centers for Disease Control, Sexually Transmitted Diseases Treatment Guidelines, 1982. Morbid Mortal Weekly Rept, 31:33S-60S, 1982.

1. If compliance and serologic follow-up can be as-
    sured, administer erythromycin 500 mg by
    mouth four times a day for 15 days.
2. If compliance and serologic follow-up cannot be
    assured, the patient should be managed in consul-
    tation with an expert.

SYPHILIS OF MORE THAN ONE YEAR'S DURATION

Recommended Regimen

Syphilis of more than 1 year's duration, except neurosyphilis (latent syphilis of indeterminate or more than 1
year's duration, cardiovascular, or late benign syphilis)
should be treated with:

Benzathine penicillin G: 2.4 million units, IM, once
a week for 3 successive weeks (7.2 million units total).

The optimal treatment schedules for syphilis of
greater than 1 year's duration have been less well established than schedules for early syphilis. In general,
syphilis of longer duration requires more prolonged
therapy.

Therapy is recommended for established cardiovascular syphilis. Antibiotics may not reverse the pathology associated with this disease, however,

Penicillin-Allergic Patients

There are no published clinical data that adequately
document the efficacy of drugs other than penicillin for
syphilis of more than 1 year's duration. Cerebrospinal
fluid examinations should be performed before therapy
with these regimens.

Patients who are allergic to penicillin should be
treated with:

Tetracycline HCl: 500 mg, by mouth, four times a
day for 30 days. Patient compliance with this regimen
may be difficult, so care should be taken to encourage
optimal compliance.

Penicillin-allergic patients who cannot tolerate tetracycline should have their allergy confirmed. For these
patients there are two options:

1. If compliance and serologic follow-up can be as-
    sured, administer erythromycin 500 mg by mouth,
    four times a day for 30 days.
2. If compliance and serologic follow-up cannot be
    assured, the patient should be hospitalized and
    managed in consultation with an expert.

Cerebrospinal Fluid Examination

Cerebrospinal fluid (CSF) examination should be done for
patients with clinical symptoms or signs consistent with
neurosyphilis. This examination also is desirable for
other patients with syphilis of greater than 1 year's duration to exclude asymptomatic neurosyphilis.

NEUROSYPHILIS

Published studies show that a total of 6.0-9.0 million
units of penicillin G over a 3-4-week period results in a
satisfactory clinical response in approximately 90% of
patients with neurosyphilis. This information must be
considered along with the observation that regimens em-
ploying benzathine penicillin or procaine penicillin in
doses under 2.4 million units daily do not consistently
provide treponemicidal levels of penicillin in CSF and
with the knowledge that several case reports show the
failure of such regimens to cure neurosyphilis.

Drug Regimens

Potentially effective regimens, none of which have been
adequately studied, include:
    Aqueous crystalline penicillin G: 12-24 million units,
IV, per day (2-4 million units every 4 hours) for 10 days,
followed by benzathine penicillin G 2.4 million units, IM,
weekly for three doses
                    OR
    Aqueous procaine penicillin G: 2.4 million units, IM,
daily plus probenecid 500 mg, by mouth, four times a day,
both for 10 days, followed by benzathine penicillin G 2.4
million units, IM, weekly for three doses
                    OR
    Benzathine penicillin G: 2.4 million units, IM, week-
ly for three doses

Penicillin-Allergic Patients

Patients with histories of allergy to penicillin should
have their allergy confirmed and managed in consultation
with an expert.

SYPHILIS IN PREGNANCY

Evaluation of Pregnant Women

All pregnant women should have a nontreponemal serologic test for syphilis, such as the VDRL or RPR test, at
the time of the first prenatal visit. The treponemal tests
such as the FTA-ABS test should not be used for routine
screening. For women suspected of being at high risk
for syphilis, a second nontreponemal test should be done
during the third trimester, and the cord blood should be
tested for syphilis antibody.

Seroactive patients should be expeditiously evaluated.
This evaluation should include a history and physical
examination, as well as a quantitative nontreponemal
test and a confirmatory treponemal test.

If the FTA-ABS test is nonreactive and there is no
clinical evidence of syphilis, treatment may be withheld.
Both the quantitative nontreponemal test and the confirmatory test should be repeated within 4 weeks. If there is
clinical or serologic evidence of syphilis or if the diagnosis of syphilis cannot be excluded with reasonable certainty, the patient should be treated as outlined below.

Patients for whom there is documentation of adequate
treatment for syphilis in the past need not be treated
again unless there is clinical or serologic evidence of
reinfection such as dark-field positive lesions or a four-
fold rise in titer when a quantitative nontreponemal test
is used.

Recommended Regimens

For patients at all stages of pregnancy who are not allergic to penicillin, it should be used in dosage schedules
appropriate for the stage of syphilis as recommended for
the treatment of nonpregnant patients.

Penicillin-Alergic Patients

For patients at all stages of pregnancy who have documented allergy to penicillin:
1. If compliance and serologic follow-up can be assured, administer erythromycin in dosage schedules appropriate for the stage of syphilis as recommended for the treatment of nonpregnant patients. [Erythromycin therapy may not be successful and newer antibiotics are currently being studied.] Infants born to mothers treated during pregnancy with erythromycin for early syphilis <u>should</u> be treated with penicillin.
2. If compliance and serologic follow-up cannot be assured, the patient should be hospitalized and managed in consultation with an expert.

Tetracycline is not recommended in pregnant women because of potential adverse effects on the fetus.

Follow-Up

Pregnant women who have been treated for syphilis should have monthly quantitative nontreponemal serologic tests for the remainder of the current pregnancy. Women who show a four-fold rise in titer should be treated again. After delivery, follow-up is as outlined for nonpregnant patients.

CONGENITAL SYPHILIS

Congenital syphilis may occur if the mother has syphilis during pregnancy. If the mother has received adequate penicillin treatment during pregnancy, the risk to the infant is minimal. However, all infants should be examined carefully at birth and at frequent intervals thereafter until nontreponemal serologic tests are negative.

Infected infants are frequently asymptomatic at birth and may be sero-negative if the maternal infection occurred late in gestation. Infants should be treated at birth if maternal treatment was inadequate, unknown, or with drugs other than penicillin or if adequate follow-up of the infant cannot be ensured.

Infants with congenital syphilis should have a CSF examination before treatment.

Symptomatic Infants or Asymptomatic Infants
with Abnormal Cerebrospinal Fluid

Aqueous crystalline penicillin G: 50,000 units/kg, IM
or IV, daily in two divided doses for a minimum of 10
days

OR

Aqueous procaine penicillin G: 50,000 units/kg, IM,
daily for a minimum of 10 days

Asymptomatic Infants with Normal
Cerebrospinal Fluid

Benzathine penicillin G: 50,000 units/kg, IM, in a single dose

Although benzathine penicillin has been previously
recommended and widely used, published clinical data on
its efficacy in congenital neurosyphilis are lacking. If
neurosyphilis cannot be excluded, the aqueous crystalline
or procaine penicillin regimen is recommended. Only
penicillin regimens are recommended for neonatal congenital syphilis.

After the neonatal period, penicillin therapy for
congenital syphilis should be with the same dosages used
for neonatal congenital syphilis. For larger children
the total dose of penicillin need not exceed the dosage
used in adult syphilis or more than 1 year's duration.
After the neonatal period, the dosage of tetracycline for
congenital syphilis in patients who are allergic to penicillin should be individualized but need not exceed dosages used in adult syphilis of more than 1 year's duration.
Tetracycline should not be given to children less than 8
years of age.

SYPHILIS CAUSING COCHLEOVESTIBULAR
DYSFUNCTION (not included in the CDC guidelines)

Cochleovestibular dysfunction and sensorineural hearing
loss may result from either congenital or acquired syphilis. The cerebrospinal fluid may be normal in patients
with syphilitic hearing loss. Most clinicians agree that
steroids such as prednisone and prolonged penicillin therapy are indicated. Agreement as to how much and how
long has not been reached. One suggestion is to treat

patients with intramuscular benzathine penicillin G, 2.4 million units weekly for 3 months, along with prednisone, 80 mg orally every other day. The prednisone is discontinued after 1 month if no clinical improvement has been demonstrated. Other clinicians have suggested that prednisone should be given in a daily dose of 30–60 mg by mouth for 2 weeks. If symptomatic improvement takes place, the dose is then tapered to a level that will maintain this improvement.

EPIDEMIOLOGIC TREATMENT

Persons who have been exposed to infectious syphilis within the preceding 3 months and other persons who on epidemiologic grounds are at high risk for early syphilis should be treated as for early syphilis. Every effort should be made to determine if such persons have syphilis.

FOLLOW-UP AFTER TREATMENT AND RETREATMENT

All patients with early syphilis and congenital syphilis should be encouraged to return for repeat quantitative nontreponemal tests at least 3, 6, and 12 months after treatment. For these patients quantitative nontreponemal tests will decline to nonreactive or to reactive with a low titer within a year following successful treatment with benzathine penicillin G. Titers decline more slowly with serologic tests for patients treated for disease of longer duration. Patients with syphilis of more than 1 year's duration also should have a repeat serologic test 24 months after treatment. Careful follow-up serologic testing is particularly important in patients treated with antibiotics other than penicillin. Examination of CSF should be planned as part of the last follow-up visit after treatment with alternative antibiotics.

All patients with neurosyphilis must be carefully followed with periodic serologic testing, clinical evaluation at 6-month intervals, and repeat CSF examinations for at least 3 years.

The possibility of reinfection always should be considered when patients with early syphilis need to be treated a second time. A CSF examination should be performed

before retreatment unless reinfection and a diagnosis of
early syphilis can be established.

Retreatment should be considered when

1. clinical signs or symptoms of syphilis persist or recur
2. there is a four-fold increase in titer with a nontreponemal test
3. a nontreponemal test showing a high titer initially fails to
   show four-fold decrease within a year

Patients should be retreated according to the schedules recommended for syphilis of more than 1 year's duration. In general a patient should be retreated only once,
since patients may maintain stable, low titers when nontreponemal tests are used or may have irreversible ana-
tomical damage. Table 10.5 is advice given by Rathburn
for posttherapy follow-up of patients with congenital
syphilis.

COMPLICATIONS OF THERAPY

The Jarisch-Herxheimer reaction may follow antibiotic therapy for syphilis. It is thought to be due to the rapid release of
treponemal products from organisms whose cells have been dis-
rupted by the drugs used in the therapy. The systemic effects do
not always occur, and they are variable in their severity. The
onset is generally within 2 hr after treatment with a peak at 4-8 hr.
There may be generalized aches and pains with the appearance of
burning discomfort in the local lesions. Vasodilation and hypotension also may occur. The local lesions may intensify in their coloration and may become edematous. Most patients with the reaction experience a rise in temperature of approximately $1.5°C$, but
this may vary widely. The leukocyte count rises at the height of
the reaction with a predominance of neutrophiles and lymphocyto-
penia. Following the reaction, the leukocyte count returns to
normal.

Most reactions occur within 12 hr of treatment and are most
common in primary and secondary syphilis. The overwhelming
majority of the reactions are benign. There has been some concern that the local reaction may adversely affect patients with cardiovascular syphilis; however, such events must be rare. Patients
should be informed of the possibility of the reaction and that it may
be treated symptomatically with analgesic and antipyretic agents.

Table 10.5   Schedule of Follow-Up After Treatment or
Prophylaxis for Congenital Syphilis[a]

For patients diagnosed as having congenital syphilis:

1. Reagin testing every 3 months for the first 15 months, then
   every 6 months until negative or stable at low titer
2. Treponemal antibody test after 15 months of age
3. Repeat cerebrospinal fluid evaluation 2 years after treatment if the patient was treated for or showed any signs of
   central nervous system disease
4. Careful developmental evaluation, vision testing, and hearing testing before 3 years of age or at the time of diagnosis

For patients treated in utero or at birth because of maternal
syphilis[b]:

1. Reagin testing at birth and then every 3 months until at
   least 6 months of age and test is negative
2. Treponemal antibody test after 15 months of age

For women treated for syphilis during pregnancy:

1. Reagin testing monthly until delivery, then every 3 months
   until negative
2. Retreatment anytime there is a fourfold rise in reagin
   titer

---

[a] From K. C. Rathburn, Sex Transm Dis, 10:102–107, 1983.
[b] Anytime the patient meets the criteria for diagnosis of congenital
syphilis, follow-up should be that indicated for a diagnosed case.

BIBLIOGRAPHY

Adams DA, Kerr AG, Smyth GDL, Cinnamond MJ. Congenital
syphilitic deafness—a further review. J Laryngol Otol, 97:399–
404, 1983.

Bauer TJ, Price EV, Cutler JC. Spinal fluid examinations among patients with primary or secondary syphilis. Amer J Syph Gonn Vener Dis, 36:309-318, 1952.

Baum EW, Bernhardt M, Sams M, Alexander WJ, McLean GL. Secondary syphilis. Still the great imitator. J Amer Med Assoc, 249:3069-3070, 1983.

Becker GD. Late syphilitic hearing loss: A diagnostic and therapeutic dilemma. Laryngoscope, 89:1273-1288, 1979.

Belin MW, Baltch AL, Hay PB. Secondary syphilitic uveitis. Amer J Ophthal, 92:210-214, 1981.

Bergstrom JF, Navin JJ. Luetic lymphadenitis: Lymphographic manifestations simulating lymphoma. Radiology, 106:287-288, 1973.

Brown ST. Update on recommendations for treatment of syphilis. Rev Infect Dis, 4(Suppl.):S837-S841, 1982.

Center for Disease Control: Criteria and Techniques for the Diagnosis of Early Syphilis, Publ. No. 98-376, March 1976.

Chapel TA. The variability of syphilitic chancres. Sex Transm Dis, 5:68-70, 1978.

Chapel TA. The signs and symptoms of secondary syphilis. Sex Transm Dis, 7:161-164, 1981.

Cole GW, Amon RB, Russell PS. Secondary syphilis presenting as a pruritic dermatitis. Arch Derm, 113:489-490, 1977.

Dobbin JM, Perkins JH. Otosyphilis and hearing loss: Response to penicillin and steroid therapy. Laryngoscope, 93:1540-1543, 1983.

Drusin LM, Singer C, Valenti AJ, et al. Infectious syphilis mimicking neoplastic disease. Arch Int Med, 137:156-160, 1977.

Ducas J, Robson HG. Cerebrospinal fluid penicillin levels during therapy for latent syphilis. J Amer Med Assoc, 246:2583-2584, 1981.

Felman YM. Syphilis serology today. Arch Dermatol, 118:84-89, 1980.

Fiumara NJ. Serologic responses to treatment of 128 patients with late latent syphilis. Sex Transm Dis, 6:243-246, 1979.

Fiumara NJ. Treatment of primary and secondary syphilis. Serologic response. J Amer Med Assoc, 243:2500-2502, 1980.

Fiumara NJ, Lessell S. The stigmata of late congenital syphilis: An analysis of 100 patients. Sex Transm Dis, 10:126-129, 1983.

Friendly G, Zartarian MW, Wood JC, et al. Hemagglutination treponemal test for syphilis. J Clin Microbiol, 18:775-778, 1983.

Greene BM, Miller NR, Bynum TE. Failure of penicillin G benzathine in the treatment of neurosyphilis. Arch Int Med, 140:1117-1118, 1980.

Hambie EA, Larsen SA, Perryman MW, Pettit DE, Feeley JC. Heated versus unheated sera in the hemagglutination treponemal test for syphilis. J Clin Microbiol, 15:337-337, 1982.

Hardy PH. Death knell for the Treponema pallidum immobilization test. Sex Transm Dis, 7:145-148.

Harter CA, Benischke K. Fetal syphilis in the first trimester. Amer J Obstet Gynecol, 124:705-711, 1976.

Haskisaki P, Wertzberger GG, Conrad GL, Nicholas CR. Erythromycin failure in the treatment of syphilis in a pregnant woman. Sex Transm Dis, 10:36-38, 1983.

Huber TW, Storms S, Young P, et al. Reactivity of microhemagglutination, fluorescent treponemal antibody absorption, venereal disease research laboratory, and rapid plasma reagin tests in primary syphilis. J Clin Microbiol, 17:405-409, 1983.

Hungerbühler JP, Regli F. Cochleovestibular involvement as the first sign of syphilis. J Neurol, 219:199-204, 1978.

Idsoe O, Guthe T, Wilcox RR. Penicillin in the treatment of syphilis. The experience of three decades. Bull World Hlth Org (Suppl.), 47:1-68, 1972.

Jaffe HW. The laboratory diagnosis of syphilis: New concepts.
Ann Int Med, 83:846-850, 1975.

Jaffe HW, Kabins SA. Examination of the cerebrospinal fluid in
patients with syphilis. Rev Infect Dis, 4(Suppl.):S842-S847, 1982.

Kaufman RE, Olansley DC, Wiesner PJ. The FTA-ABS (IgM)
test for neonatal syphilis: A critical review. J Amer Vener Dis
Assoc, 1:79-84, 1974.

King A, Nichol C. Venereal Diseases 3rd ed. Williams and Wilkins, Baltimore, 1975.

Larsen SA. Current status of laboratory tests for syphilis.
Chapter V in J. H. Rippey and R. M. Nakamura, Diagnostic
immunology: Technology assessment and quality assurance.
CAP Conference/1983. College of American Pathologists, Skokie,
Illinois, 1984.

Larsen SA, Hambie EA, Pettit DE, Perryman MW, Kraus SJ.
Specificity, sensitivity, and reproducibility among the fluorescent
treponemal antibody-absorption test, the microhemagglutination
assay for Treponema pallidum antibodies, and the hemagglutination
treponemal test for syphilis. J Clin Microbiol, 14:441-445, 1981.

Larsen SA, Pettit DE, Perryman MW, Hambie EA, Mullally R,
Whittington W. EDTA-treated plasma in the rapid plasma card
test and the toluidine red unheated serum test for serodiagnosis of
syphilis. J Clin Microbiol, 17:341-345, 1983.

Lee TJ, Sparling PF. Syphilis. An Algorithm. J Amer Med
Assoc, 242:1187-1189, 1979.

Luger A, Schmidt BL, Spendlingwimmer I, Steyrer K. Specificity
of the Treponema pallidum haemagglutination test. Analysis of
results. Br J Vener Dis, 57:178-180, 1981.

Luger A, Schmidt BL, Steyrer K, Schonwald E. Diagnosis of
neurosyphilis by examination of the cerebrospinal fluid. Br J
Vener Dis, 57:232-237, 1981.

McNulty JS, Fassett RL. Syphilis: An otolaryngologic perspective. Laryngoscope, 91:889-903, 1981.

Mohr JA, Griffiths W, Jackson R, et al. Neurosyphilis and penicillin levels in cerebrospinal fluid. J Amer Med Assoc, 236:2208-2209, 1976.

National Communicable Disease Center. Syphilis. A synopsis. Public Health Service Publ. No. 1660, January 1968.

Peterson CS, Pedersen NS. The profile of early infectious syphilis in Denmark. Danish Med Bull, 30:49-51, 1983.

Pettit DE, Larsen SA, Harbee PS, et al. Toluidine red unheated serum test, a nontreponemal test for syphilis. J Clin Microbiol, 18:1141-1145, 1983.

Pettit DE, Larsen SA, Pope V, Perryman MW, Adams MR. Unheated serum reagin test as a quantitation test for syphilis. J Clin Microbiol, 15:238-242, 1982.

Polnikorn N, Witoonpanich R, Vorachit M, et al. Penicillin concentrations in cerebrospinal fluid after different treatment regimens for syphilis. Br J Vener Dis, 56:363-367, 1980.

Quinn TC. Anorectal syphilis. Brief guide to office counseling. Med Aspects Human Sex, 17:21-28, 1983.

Rathbun KC. Congenital syphilis. Sex Transm Dis, 10:93-99, 1983.

Rathbun KC. Congenital syphilis: A proposal for improved surveillance, diagnosis, and treatment. Sex Transm Dis, 10:102-107, 1983.

Rein MF, Banks GW, Logan LC, et al. Failure of _Treponema pallidum_ immobilization test to provide additional diagnostic information about contemporary problem sera. Sex Transm Dis, 7:101-105, 1980.

Risseeuw-Appel IM, Kothe FC. Transfusion syphilis: A case report. Sex Transm Dis, 10:200-201, 1983.

Roddy R, Lukehart SA, Hansfield HH. Acyclovir ointment does not affect the dark-field examination in primary syphilis. Sex Transm Dis, 10:198-199, 1983.

Rudolph AH. The microhemagglutination assay for _Treponema pallidum_ antibodies (MHA-TP). A new treponemal test for syphilis: Where does it fit? J Amer Vener Dis Assoc, 3:3-8, 1976.

Schober PC, Gabriel G, White P, Felton WF, Thin RN. How infectious is syphilis? Br J Vener Dis, 59:217-219, 1983.

Schoreter AL, Lucas JB, Price EV, et al. Treatment for early syphilis and reactivity of serologic tests. J Amer Med Assoc, 221: 471-476, 1972.

Tait IA. Uveitis due to secondary syphilis. Br J Vener Dis, 59: 397-401, 1983.

Tramont EC. Persistence of _Treponema pallidum_ following penicillin therapy. J Amer Med Assoc, 236:2206-2207, 1976.

Warrell DA, Perine PL, Bryceson ADM, et al. Physiologic changes during the Jarisch-Herxheimer reaction in early syphilis. Amer J Med, 51:176-185, 1971.

Wiet RJ, Milko DA. Isolation of the spirochetes in the perilymph despite prior antisyphilitic therapy. Arch Otolaryng, 101:104-106, 1975.

Yoder, FW. Penicillin treatment of neurosyphilis. Are the recommended dosages sufficient? J Amer Med Assoc, 232:270-271, 1975.

Zoller M, Wilson WR, Nadol JB. Treatment of syphilitic hearing loss. Combined penicillin and steroid therapy in 29 patients. Ann Otol, 88:160-165, 1979.

Chapter 11

SHIGELLOSIS, AMEBIASIS, GIARDIASIS, VIRAL HEPATITIS,
AND OTHER SPECIAL PROBLEMS FOR HOMOSEXUAL MEN

INTRODUCTION

Homosexual men as a group are likely to suffer from a large
number of sexually transmitted diseases. For the purpose of this
brief discussion, a homosexual male is defined as a man who has
oral-genital, penile-anal or oral-anal sexual contact with another
man. This definition includes bisexuals. In reality, when venere-
ologists talk about homosexuals, their data are probably derived
from a subpopulation of homosexual men who are sexually active
with a large number of anonymous partners. As with heterosexu-
als, the greater the number of partners, the greater the chance of
acquiring a sexually transmitted disease. It is probable that homosexuals as a group have a larger number of sexual partners than
their heterosexual male counterparts. When these partners are
anonymous and the health care system is not well oriented to homosexual behavior and the pathogens adapted to transmission by homosexual contact, then all of the elements are in place for a venereal
disease problem in the homosexual community.

Homosexual patients may be reluctant to identify their sexual
preference because they fear adverse social consequences. On the
other hand, physicians may neglect to ask about sexual preference
because of embarrassment or because they assume the patient is
heterosexual. The characterization of the homosexual male as the
effeminate, prancing, bent-wrist dandy is not useful in identifying
the majority of homosexuals. The presence of anal warts or re-
laxed anal sphincter tone in a young man has been suggested as an
indicator of homosexuality. However, only the patient can disclose
his sexual preference. The physician should ask for and respond

to this information in a nonjudgmental way. Failure of the physician to perform an appropriate rectal or pharyngeal culture may
result in therapeutic mismanagement.

In many larger cities, public health departments have responded specifically to the problem of sexually transmitted diseases in
homosexuals. There, public health personnel have participated in
establishing clinics which serve predominantly homosexual men,
and special screening programs have been organized in gay bath-
houses and bars. These screening methods are cost-effective in
detecting cases of gonorrhea. However, the methods do not appear
to lower the prevalence of infection. The term "gay" is preferred
by many homosexual men to describe their sexual orientation.

It may be that rectal intercourse itself in addition to multiple
partners may make the homosexual more susceptible to certain
venereal diseases. Rectal warts are more common than penile
warts in homosexual men. Syphilis and gonorrhea may be more
easily transmitted by rectal infections because of their often
asymptomatic nature. _Chlamydia_ urethritis is less common in
homosexual than heterosexual men. Yet _Chlamydia_ as well as
gonococci cause proctitis in homosexual men. Hepatitis B seems
to be an infection perfectly matched for the homosexual life-style,
and cytomegalovirus is almost ubiquitous in this group. This combination of pathogens and behavior patterns along with the appearance of the acquired immune deficiency syndrome, AIDS, will be a
challenge to the very best efforts of the venereal disease control
physicians. Although very little is known about sexually transmitted
diseases in lesbians, as a group, they do not appear to be a significant reservoir of sexually transmitted diseases. Lesbians appear
to have fewer sexual partners than homosexual men. Generaliza-
tions for either group, however, do not apply to individuals. The
acquired immune deficiency syndrome with Kaposi's sarcoma,
Pneumocystis carinii pneumonia and other opportunistic infections
appearing among previously healthy homosexual men has been recently reported by the U.S. Center for Disease Control. The
appearance of these patients in increasing numbers warrants concern among all physicians and public health officials. AIDS will be
discussed in more detail in a later chapter.

ENTERIC DISEASES IN HOMOSEXUAL MEN

Homosexuals infected with one enteric pathogen frequently
may harbor more than one. Patients have been reported with

simultaneous giardiasis, amebiasis, and shigellosis infections.
The diseases covered in this chapter are some of those more recently discussed in relation to the homosexual. They are by no
means an exhaustive list. Any bacteria or parasite not requiring
an intermediate host may be transmitted by the oral-genital-anal
routes. Since, however, these diseases are not generally sexually
transmitted, they will not be treated in detail.

The homosexual man may present in a number of ways to the
physician. Table 11.1 is derived from Quinn's study and shows
some of the pathogens associated with three clinical syndromes:
proctitis, proctocolitis, and enteritis. Enteric pathogens were
found in 80% of 119 consecutive homosexual men in Seattle with
anorectal or intestinal symptoms and in almost 40% of 75 randomly
selected homosexual men. In a New York City venereal disease
clinic, Phillips found Entamoeba histolytica or Giardia lamblia
(or both) in 22% of homosexual men, in 6% of bisexual men, and in
0% of heterosexual men. Figure 11.1 presents an algorithm
for the management of anorectal or intestinal infection in homosexually active men.

Anoscopy or sigmoidoscopy is necessary to adequately visualize the involved area as well as to collect specimens in all of
the following enteric diseases. To repeat, remember that more
than one pathogen may be present even in asymptomatic patients.

<u>Proctitis</u>

Proctitis in homosexual men frequently is caused by N. gonorrhoeae, C. trachomatis, herpes simplex virus and T. pallidum.
In some patients no identifiable etiology is identified. Patients
may be asymptomatically infected with any of these pathogens, or
they may have anorectal pain, tenesmus, and rectal discharge.

Non-LGV immunotypes may be seen in men with mild proctitis or men with no symptoms. McMillan cultured the urethra,
pharynx, and rectum of 150 homosexual men consecutively attending a sexually transmitted disease clinic in Glasgow. The isolation
rates for Chlamydia trachomatis were 6.7% from the urethra, 4%
from the rectum, and 1.3% from the pharynx.

In the United States studies, C. trachomatis of the nonlympho-
granuloma venereum serotypes has been the more common infecting agent and responsible for a milder form of proctitis than that
caused by the lymphogranuloma venereum serotypes of C. trachomatis. The LGV strains may produce a severe infection that
resembles Crohn's disease of the rectum. The infection by both

Table 11.1   Pathogens Associated with Intestinal Infections in Homosexual Men[a]

Type of Infection[b]	Symptoms
Proctitis	Anorectal pain or burning
Neisseria gonorrhoeae	Anorectal discharge
Herpes simplex virus	Tenesmus, constipation
Chlamydia trachomatis	
(lymphogranuloma venereum and non–LGV serotypes)	
Treponema pallidum	
Proctocolitis	Symptoms as above and/or bloating, abdominal pain, abdominal cramps
Campylobacter jejuni	Diarrhea with blood
Shigella flexneri	
Chlamydia trachomatis	
(lymphogranuloma venereum serotypes)	
Entamoeba histolytica	
Enteritis	Abdominal pain, cramps, bloating
Gardia lamblia	Nausea, diarrhea without blood
Cryptosporidium	

[a] Adapted from T. C. Quinn et al. New Engl J Med, 309:576–582, 1983.

[b] Multiple pathogens are frequent. Pathogens may be associated with more than one syndrome.

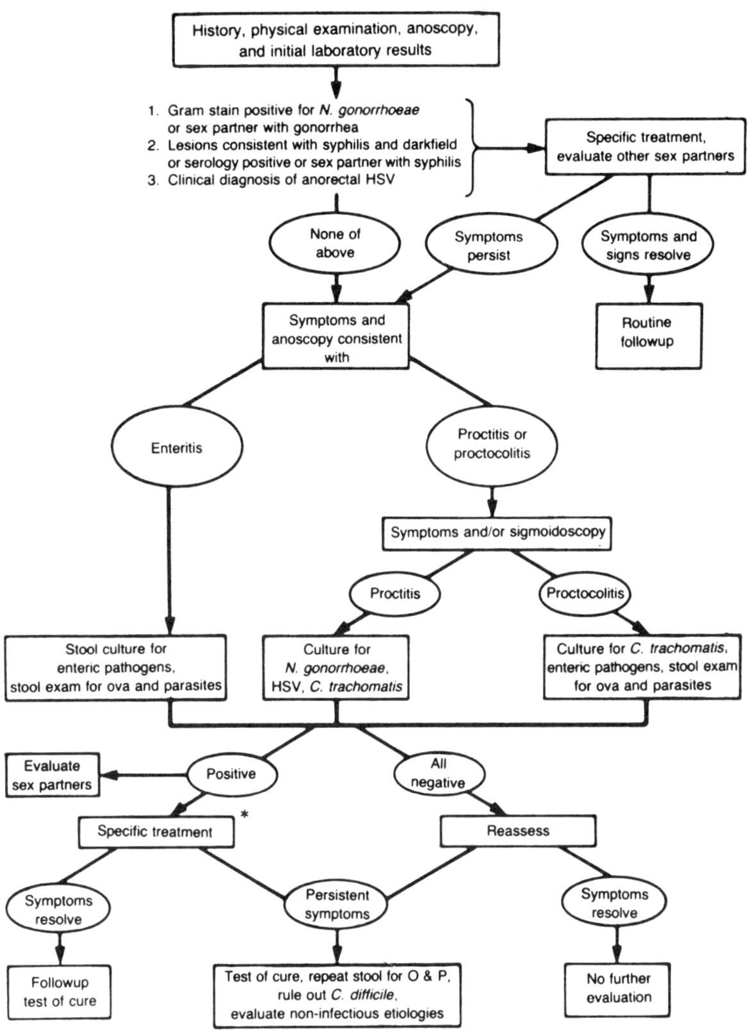

Figure 11.1   Algorithm for management of anorectal or intestinal symptoms or both in homosexually active men.   Anoscopy, culture for <u>N. gonorrhoeae</u>, and a serologic test for syphilis should be performed in all cases.   The asterisk indicates that specific antiviral therapy for herpes simplex virus proctitis is currently under study.   Empirical therapy for enteritis and proctitis can be given pending results of microbiologic studies as discussed in the text. HSV denotes herpes simplex virus, and O and P denotes ova and parasites.   Printed by permission of N Engl J Med, 309:576–582, 1983.

serotypes also can take place in women. Both sexes have anorectal pain, tenesmus and a bloody mucopurulent discharge from the anus. Therapy for enteric chlamydial infections is tetracycline 800 mg four times a day for 2-3 weeks.

Proctocolitis

The etiologic agents of proctocolitis are shown in Table 11.1, and the pathogens are discussed in more detail in this chapter. Patients complain of abdominal pain and diarrhea. The diarrhea may be bloody and contain large numbers of leukocytes. Sigmoidoscopy should be performed on these patients to adequately visualize the involved anatomy and to properly collect specimens.

Campylobacter infection

It is unknown if sexual contact is an important route of transmission of Campylobacter infections in homosexual men. Nevertheless, Campylobacter jejuni (originally called Vibrio fetus) has been recognized as a leading cause of enteritis in the world. Specifically in Europe and North America, C. jejuni is isolated from patients with diarrhea at least as often as Salmonella or Shigella species. Its recognition is due to the discovery of practical laboratory techniques to isolate the pathogen from human feces. Like the other enteric infectious diseases, C. jejuni often causes illness in small children. However, the peak isolation rate for C. jejuni in the United States is in people age 10-29 years, and in Sweden, age 20-34 years. In adults, the illness produces a wide range of symptoms. It may resemble the 24-hour "stomach flu" or mild gastroenteritis, or it may cause more severe disease with diarrhea, abdominal pain, fever, malaise, nausea, and vomiting. Grossly bloody stools are common. Some patients may have severe enterocolitis resembling acute ulcerative colitis. Peritoneal signs are rare, and most patients recover in a week.

The diagnosis usually is confirmed with a positive stool culture or occasionally with a positive blood culture. The fecal specimen may be examined by dark-field or phase-contrast microscopy in patients with acute diarrhea. In addition to leukocytes and red blood cells, C. jejuni occasionally may be seen with their characteristic darting movements. If the stool is gram stained, C. jejuni appears in the shape of a "seagull" or "equivalent sign" ($\sim$) approximately 1.5-3.5 μm in length and 0.2-0.4 μm in width.

Most patients do not require therapy. However, if there are
prolonged symptoms, high fever, or frequent or bloody diarrhea,
antibiotic therapy is indicated. Erythromycin is the drug of
choice. (Erythromycin base, ethylsuccinate, or sterate is preferred.) Erythromycin is administered in a dosage of 500 mg four
times daily for seven days.

Campylobacter fetus subspecies fetus

This causes a much less common and more severe illness
not generally associated with diarrhea. Patients may have fatal
systemic illnesses with bacteremia, meningitis, vascular infection, or abscesses.

Shigellosis

Shigellosis is an enteric infection caused by a bacillus of the
species Shigella. Shigella species are gram-negative rods and
members of the Enterobacteriaceae. In the United States, Shigella
sonnei (group D) now accounts for approximately 70% of the Shigella
isolates reported. Shigellosis is most common in children ages
1-4, and man is the principal vector. Infection occurs by fecal-
oral transmission, and convalescent or asymptomatic carriers
are the reservoir. Shigellosis is most commonly recognized in
outbreaks, and these are common when crowding or substandard
hygiene occurs. Populations at risk for shigellosis include those
at mental institutions, boarding schools, prisons, or refugee
camps and travelers in endemic areas.
   Homosexuals recently have been recognized as a population
at risk for shigellosis. The bacillus is probably acquired by oral-
anal or oral-genital contact. Oral infestion of as few as 200 virulent Shigella can produce illness in one-quarter of individuals thus
challenged. In the mid-1970s in Seattle, homosexual men accounted for 30% of all reported cases of shigellosis. Around the same
time, a retrospective hospital chart review in metropolitan New
York examined men with shigellosis between the ages of 19 and 61,
and 45% were homosexuals.
   The incubation period following exposure is two to three days.
The bacilli invade the intestinal epithelium and migrate into the
submucosa and muscularis of the large intestine. The invasion of
polymorphonuclear leukocytes into these areas causes microab-
scesses. Bleeding may occur from superficial ulcerations. The

patient experiences fever, crampy abdominal pain, and watery diarrhea that may develop into dysentery containing blood and mucus. Sigmoidoscopic examination of the colon reveals the mucosa to be friable and hyperemic. Multiple, shallow ulcers 3-7 mm in diameter may be present.

The diagnosis of shigellosis is made by the presence of a positive stool culture. Blood cultures are not generally positive. Rectal swabs or stool specimens should be transported without delay to the diagnostic laboratory to prevent loss of viability of the <u>Shigella</u>. Polymorphonuclear leukocytes may be demonstrated microscopically in the stool specimen by mixing a few drops of methylene blue solution. Clumps of leukocytes, macrophages, and erythrocytes are characteristic of the stool in shigellosis, and these cells are not generally present in toxin-induced diarrheas caused by viruses or food poisoning.

Treatment of shigellosis in healthy adults may not be necessary. Patients usually become afebrile within three days, and the dysentery usually stops within a week. Patients who have recovered may continue to excrete the bacillus in the stool for several weeks. Positive stool cultures are rare beyond 3 months. Contacts of such individuals should take precautions to prevent infection until at least two weekly stool cultures are negative.

Antibiotic therapy may reduce the duration of illness and is definitely indicated in all patients with severe disease. Ampicillin, 500 mg orally every 6 hr for five to seven days, is generally effective. Antibiotic sensitivity studies must be performed on the isolate because in certain locations antibiotic resistance is a problem. In such patients, alternative drugs include trimethoprim-sulfamethoxazole or tetracycline. Antidiarrheal agents which inhibit intestinal peristalsis and prolong the fever and excretion of the bacillus and should be avoided. Fluid and electrolyte replacement are important factors in therapy because dehydration may be present.

Amebiasis

Amebiasis results from infection with the protozoan parasite <u>Entamoeba histolytica.</u> This parasite is distinguished morphologically from two other nonpathogenic ameba inhabiting humans, <u>Entamoeba coli</u> and <u>Entamoeba hartmanni.</u> Ameba generally inhabit the gut, and infections are present in approximately 5% of the population in the temperate zones. The parasite exists in two forms: a trophozoite, 12-50 μm in diameter, and a cyst, 10-20 μm

in diameter. The trophozoite is the active form generally found
in the stool of patients without diarrhea. The cysts are more resistant than the trophozoites to environmental changes. Amebic
cysts resist gastric acid and are important in the epidemiology of
the disease. Ameba are spread by ingestion of cyst-contaminated
food and drink, by oral-anal contact, and by contamination of
improperly cleaned enema apparatus. The latter form of spread
has been reported in patients attending a chiropractic clinic.
Physicians should be aware that enema apparatus may be a vector
of enteric disease in homosexual man. Man is the only reservoir
for amebiasis.

The clinical features of amebic infection are varied. Not
everyone who is infected becomes symptomatic, and only 2-8% of
infected patients develop invasive disease. The reason for this
variation in the expression of amebiasis is unknown. Intestinal
amebiasis is characterized by the gradual onset of colicky abdominal pain, tenesmus, and frequent bowel movements stained with
blood and mucus. The sigmoidoscopic examination in one-quarter
of patients demonstrates typical lesions. These are shallow ulcers
a few millimeters to 2 cm in diameter with raised and undermined
edges. Fever is present in about 40% of patients. Peritonitis
occurs in about 3% of patients. Genital lesions are extremely
rare, but infections have been described on the penis of uncircumcised men and on the cervix, vagina, and clitoris of women. The
mortality of uncomplicated amebic dysentery is 0.5%. If it is
complicated by peritonitis, the mortality rate rises to 40%.

Invasive amebiasis most commonly involves the right lobe of
the liver in the form of a liver abscess. The abscess is solitary in
about 90% of patients. More than half of patients with amebic liver
abscesses do not have diarrhea, but 75% have fewer. The liver is
enlarged and tender in about 80% of patients. Patients with an
uncomplicated liver abscess have a mortality of about 1%. In 10%
of patients with liver abscess, the abscess may be complicated by
extension into the chest, the pericardium or the peritoneal cavity,
with a resulting mortality ranging from 2 to 30%. Amebic meningitis is almost universally fatal and occurs in individuals swimming
in warm, freshwater ponds.

The diagnosis of intestinal amebiasis is made by identifying
the trophozoites or cysts in stool specimens or material scraped
from the wall of an ulcer. These specimens must be examined
within 1/2 hr of collection, since the mobility of the trophozoites
is rapidly lost, making their identification often impossible. If
trained laboratory personnel are not available, the stool specimen

may be preserved in three times its volume of polyvinyl alcohol fixative. This preparation is suitable for deferred morphologic examination. Ameba may cling to cotton swabs; therefore, ulcers should be scraped with a nonabsorbent instrument. Stools may be stained by the Trichrome method, which demonstrates both the trophozoites and cysts.

When examining stool specimens for cysts, it is better to employ concentration methods and to collect several specimens, because the appearance of cysts may be intermittent. If nonpathogenic ameba or other protozoa are found in the patient's stool specimen, it is wise to continue looking with several repeat specimens, because pathogenic ameba may be found in the later specimens. Administration of the following substances may interfere with the stool examination: tetracyclines, sulfonamides, antiprotozoal agents, laxatives, enemas, radiologic contrast medium, and antidiarrheal preparations containing bismuth or kaolin. Rectal biopsy also is an excellent technique for identifying ameba, even when stool examinations are negative. Direct fluorescent antibody or periodic acid Schiff staining may be used on ethanol-fixed tissue sections.

An indirect hemagglutination serologic test is available through state health department laboratories. This may be positive in 80-90% of patients with active intestinal infection. It is not as useful in the asymptomatic patient who is only passing cysts.

The diagnosis of amebic liver abscess is made by the combination of a positive serology and the demonstration of a liver defect by means of a contrast study. Indirect hemagglutination titers of $\geq$1:128 are reported in almost all patients with amebic liver abscess. Liver abscesses may be identified by means of scans, using radioactivity labeled substances that are concentrated in the liver. Ultrasound techniques and advanced computerized body tomography scanning techniques also are beneficial in identifying liver abscesses. Needle aspiration of a liver abscess can be used to obtain material for examination. It is not known if aspiration will prevent rupture of an abscess.

There is some controversy as to the therapy of amebic infections. Luminal amebicides should be used for patients who are asymptomatic cyst passers. Luminal amebicides include diloxanide furoate and iodoquinol (formally called diiodohydroxyquin). Metronidazole plus a luminal amebicide are required for patients passing trophozoites as a result of mild to moderate intestinal disease. In some of these patients, paromomycin may be used as a single drug. Metronidazole or dehydroemetine and a luminal amebicide are necessary for treating patients with severe intestinal amebiasis. Patients with amebic liver abscess generally are treated with metronidazole.

Diloxanide furoate and dehydroemetine must be obtained in the United States from the Parasitic Disease Drug Service, Centers for Disease Control, Atlanta, Georgia. Iodoquinol is difficult to obtain in the United States. The most up-to-date sources of iodoquinol and paramomycin may be requested from the Centers for Disease Control. Nitroimidazole derivatives other than metronidazole (tinidazole, ornidazole, and nimorazole) also have been used successfully to treat both giardiasis and amebiasis; however, these drugs are not commercially available in the United States.

The dose of iodoquinol is 650 mg three times a day for 3 weeks. Diloxanide furoate is given in a dosage of 500 mg three times a day for ten days. Metronidazole is given in a dose of 750 mg three times a day after meals for five to ten days. Dehydroemetine is given in a dosage of 1-1.5 mg/kg per day (maximum, 90 mg per day) intramuscularly for five days.

One of the disadvantages of the therapies of amebic infection is that many of the drugs have unpleasant side effects and toxicities. Iodoquinol may cause furunculosis, diarrhea, chills, fever, and drug rash. The 8-hydroxyquinolines are contraindicated in patients with iodine allergies and liver damage. Diloxaine furoate causes flatulence. Metronidazole often causes gastrointestinal upset and a metallic taste in the mouth. A disulfiram-like reaction may take place after coincidental alcohol ingestion. Dehydroemetine is thought to be less cardiotoxic than emetine, but it should be used cautiously in patients with existing cardiovascular, muscular or neurological diseases.

In patients with sexually transmitted amebiasis, careful examination of the sexual contacts should be undertaken.

<u>Enteritis</u>

Patients with enteritis complain of diarrhea, abdominal pain, cramps, nausea, and bloating. The sigmoidoscopic examination is usually normal. <u>Giardia lamblia</u> is the most common pathogen. <u>Cryptosporidium</u> is also a cause of enteritis, and this parasite is most troublesome in the immunocompromised AIDS patients.

Giardiasis

Giardiasis is caused by a pear-shaped flagellated protozoan that resides in the human duodenum and jejunum. Under the microscope, the trophozoite (10-25 μm in length) resembles the face of a cartoon character, with the two nuclei as eyes and the flagella as tufts of hair. Giardia trophozoites are motile and feed by attaching a ventral sucker to the intestinal wall. Cysts (8-12 μm in diameter) develop as the parasite traverses the colon. The cysts are the infective form and are transmitted by the fecal-oral route. In homosexual men, giardiasis is probably sexually transmitted through oral-anal contact.

Infections are common in children and travelers to endemic areas. Endemic areas include Southeast and South Asia, West and Central Africa, Mexico, Korea, South America, and the Soviet Union. In the latter country, travelers to Leningrad have been infected via tap water. Similar infections also have occurred following exposure to the water of lakes, mountain streams, and tap water in parts of the United States, including Colorado, Utah, Oregon, Washington, New Hampshire, and New York State. Acquired immunity to giardiasis infestation may be present in residents of endemic areas.

Patients with hypogammaglobulinemia may be more prone to infection. Available epidemiologic data suggest, but do not prove, that G. lamblia infection is transmitted by sexual contact in homosexual men.

The incubation period of giardiasis ranges from 1 to 3 weeks. Patients may be asymptomatic or may experience watery, foul-smelling diarrhea associated with abdominal cramps, distention, flatulence, nausea, and anorexia. In chronic cases, patients may have asymptomatic periods. The illness may be confused with hiatal hernia, peptic ulcer, or gallbladder disease.

The diagnosis generally is made by detecting cysts in the stool. In contrast to amebiasis, polymorphonuclear leukocytes and erythrocytes are not present, and trophozoites are rarely seen, except in patients with active diarrhea. Cysts may be detected by means of a direct smear or a formol-ether concentration of three separate stool specimens. Stool specimens that cannot be examined immediately may be preserved in polyvinyl alcohol.

Parasites may be more difficult to find in patients who have received antibiotics, antacids, barium, antidiarrheal agents, certain oily laxatives, and enema preparations. If cysts cannot be demonstrated in the stool, trophozoites may be identified in a sample of duodenal fluid or a biopsy specimen from the duodeno-jejunal junction stained with Giemsa stain.

An indirect immunofluorescence test with G. lamblia trophozoites as antigen has been used to detect anti-G. lamblia antibodies in serum. Counterimmunoelectrophoresis also can be used to detect G. lamblia antigen in stool specimens. Although not commercially available, these types of tests may be useful in the future for identifying patients with symptomatic disease.

Treatment is recommended for all infected patients. Three drugs are effective. Quinacrine is licensed in the United States for the treatment of giardiasis and has a cure rate of 80-95%. Quinacrine is given in a dose of 100 mg orally, three times per day after meals for ten days. Side effects of quinacrine include nausea, vomiting, stomach cramps, and the appearance of toxic psychosis in 1.5% of patients. Metronidazole is available in the United States but is unlicensed for the treatment of giardiasis. It is better tolerated than quinacrine and is frequently prescribed in a dose of 250 mg orally, three times per day for ten days. A third drug, tinidazole, closely related to metronidazole and not available in the United States, is effective for giardiasis in a single oral dose of 2 g. Alcohol should be avoided when patients are taking either drug since both may cause the "antabuse syndrome." Furazolidone, an antiprotozoal agent, is an alternative drug for treating giardia infections. It is given orally 100 mg four times a day for seven days. None of the drugs is safe for pregnant women.

Cryptosporidiosis

Cryptosporidium is a coccidian parasite normally of importance to veterinary medicine as it causes a diarrheal illness in animals including guinea pigs, calves, lambs, turkeys, and chickens. The parasite may also be transmitted to mice, cats, dogs, and goats. The parasite occasionally infects humans, and the type of disease produced depends on the immunocompetence of the patient. Cryptosporidial oocysts have been identified in one to two percent of patients with diarrhea in the United Kingdom, Australia, the United States, and Finland. The disease probably occurs worldwide.

The parasite has both sexual and asexual reproduction and is spread by fecal-oral transmission. The villi of the large and small intestine are usually infected although the parasites have been identified in the respiratory tract, gallbladder, bile, and pancreatic ducts. After exposure to infected calves, the incubation period in humans is usually five to fourteen days.

The illness in the normal host is usually a self-limited gastroenteritis with watery diarrhea, abdominal pain, nausea, and fever. In most respects, the illness is distinguishable from giardiasis.

Without any therapy, the diarrhea resolves within three to ten days. In immunocompromised individuals such as the AIDS patients, the illness is much more severe and protracted. Patients may have up to several liters of watery diarrhea in a day. Mucous and blood are not present, but patients have crampy abdominal pain, nausea and vomiting and severe weight loss. Fever and lymphadenopathy may also be present. The diarrhea usually persists without remission until the patient succumbs to some other infectious or neoplastic complication resulting from their immunocompromised status.

The diagnosis of cryptosporidiosis is based on the demonstration of the parasite in the stool (oocysts) or in a biopsy specimen from the intestinal mucosa. The oocysts are round and 4 μm in diameter. They are identified in stool specimens by flotation and concentration techniques, and their detection may be aided by phase contrast microscopy or special stains including the Giemsa and the modified Ziehl-Neelsen method. When stained sections of biopsy material are examined from the rectum or small or large intestine, the cryptosporidium organisms are seen as 2 or 5 μm spherical bodies adhering to the microvillous border. The organisms are best seen with hematoxylin-eosin, Giemsa, and the methylene blue counterstain of the modified Kinyoun stain. Electron microscopy can be used to distinguish the stages of the parasite; trophoozoite, schizont, and macrogametocyte. Villous atrophy is commonly found in small bowel biopsies of patients with cryptosporidiosis. There is no diagnostic serologic test.

Treatment of cryptosporidiosis in the normal host is not necessary since the disease is self-limiting. In the immunosuppressed patients, particularly the AIDS patients, the disease appears unremitting and no successful therapy has been identified. Patients are generally supported with parenteral nutrition. The status of the following drug therapies is unclear: spiromycin, the combination of quinine and clindamycin, and furazolidone.

VIRAL HEPATITIS

General

Epidemiologic and laboratory data indicate that most viral hepatitis is caused by two distinct viruses, hepatitis A virus (HAV or infectious hepatitis) and hepatitis B (HBV or serum hepatitis). Another clinically similar disease, designated non-A/non-B

Table 11.2   Causes of Acute Hepatitis in Homosexual Men

Disease	Diagnostic Tests
Hepatitis B	HBsAg, anti-HBc, anti-HBs
Hepatitis A	Anti-HAV IgM
Non-A/Non-B hepatitis	By exclusion of other etiologies
Infectious mononucleosis	EBV serology
Cytomegalovirus mononucleosis	CMV isolation and serology
Syphilis	VDRL or other syphilis serology
Drug induced hepatitis	By exclusion and history
Cholangitis	Clinical signs and symptoms and laboratory findings

hepatitis, may be caused by at least two agents and is diagnosed
only by exclusion. Non-A/non-B hepatitis is the most important
cause of hepatitis following blood transfusions. Hepatitis A virus
is spread primarily by the fecal-oral route among individuals exposed to the same infected material or among those with intimate
contacts. The differential diagnosis of acute hepatitis in homosexual men is shown in Table 11.2.

Hepatitis A

Hepatitis A infection in homosexual men is most likely the
result of oral-anal contact. Until relatively recently the diagnosis
of hepatitis A was made only by excluding hepatitis B by serologic
methods. However, the availability of a test to detect antibody to
hepatitis A virus (anti-HAV) has indicated that hepatitis A in addition to hepatitis B may be a problem in homosexual men. In New
York City the prevalence of anti-HAV among homosexual men was
similar to the prevalence in middle-class white men. However,
in Seattle, Washington, the prevalence of anti-HAV was 30% in

homosexual men and 12% in heterosexual men. The annual incidence of hepatitis A in seattle was higher in homosexual men. Also, a large outbreak of hepatitis A was reported in homosexual men in Stockholm in the winter of 1980.

Clinical illness

Patients with hepatitis A virus infection become ill 15-50 days (usually 1 month) after exposure to the virus, usually through close contact with an infected patient or ingestion of fecally contaminated water or food. Transmission by blood products or transfusion is rare. Virus excretion is present late in the incubation phase and diminishes rapidly within several days after the patient becomes jaundiced. The patient is most likely to transmit the disease in the 2 weeks before he is jaundiced at a time when he may be feeling well. The illness varies in severity depending on age. Infants and young children may be asymptomatic, while adults usually have clinical illness. Chronic carriage of the hepatitis A virus does not happen, and death is rare. Patients usually experience malaise, anorexia, nausea, fever, abdominal discomfort and, finally, the diagnosis is considered with the appearance of jaundice.

Diagnosis

The diagnosis of hepatitis A has been greatly simplified by the availability of serologic tests to distinguish hepatitis A from hepatitis B. Patients with acute hepatitis A infection will have a IgM antibody to the virus (anti-HAV-IgM). The IgM antibody will be replaced by IgG antibody during convalescence. In the United States more than half of the population over 40 years of age has serologic evidence of past hepatitis A infection (anti-HAV-IgG).

Prophylaxis

There is no specific therapy for hepatitis A. Immune globulin ("gamma globulin") given shortly after exposure is protective—the sooner, the better. If the exposure interval is greater than 2 weeks, immune globulin should not be given. Sexual contacts (homosexual and heterosexual) as well as household contacts of a patient with hepatitis A should be given a single intramuscular dose of 0.02 ml/kg of body weight. School or office contact does not warrant immune globulin administration. Because of the expense and time wasted, routine testing for anti-HAV before prophylaxis with immune globulin is inadvisable. A vaccine to hepatitis A is currently under development.

Hepatitis B

Hepatitis B infection appears to be a common problem with homosexual men. Among venereal disease clinic patients, about 50-75% of homosexual men show serologic evidence of prior or current hepatitis B infection.

In one large study of 3785 homosexual men from United States venereal disease clinics, 6% had detectable HBsAg, 52% were positive for anti-HBs, and 3% were positive for anti-HBc. In surface antigen-positive specimens (HBsAg), 91% also were positive for 3 e antigen or antibody, indicating that these individuals pose a considerable risk of infection to their sexual partners. (There is a correlation between e antigen, virus-specific DNA polymerase activity, and circulating Dane particles indicating ongoing viral replication.)

Among homosexual men, evidence of infection with hepatitis B virus is more frequent in patients who engaged in anal-genital intercourse, oral-anal intercourse, and rectal douching before or after intercourse. The common feature to these practices appears to be trauma to the rectal mucosa and probable loss of small quantities of blood asymptomatically. HBsAg has been found in swabbed specimens of rectal and anal canal mucosa and in feces of homosexual men who had active hepatitis B virus infection. Infection is also more common in homosexual men with longer durations of homosexual activity and in homosexual men who have frequent intercourse with large numbers of nonsteady partners.

The risk of infection for hepatitis B among heterosexual sexual contacts is unknown. Some evidence is available from Japan indicating that women who carry HBsAg can transmit hepatitis to their husbands. HBsAg was not detected in the specimens of their sputum or cervical mucus. However, the antigen was found in some of the women in their vaginal discharge during days 1-6 of their menstrual cycle. The precise risk of sexual transmission in the contacts of chronic HBsAg carriers is also unknown. Thus, the epidemiology in regard to the sexual transmission of HBV is incomplete.

Exposure to hepatitis B virus may take place in a number of other ways. Direct innoculation of infected blood or blood products can take place through transfusion, sharing of contaminated needles (drug addicts) or puncture wounds (hospital workers, persons being tatooed or having their ears pierced). Infection may be due to exposure to infected secretions such as might take place in a laboratory accident or sexual encounter.

Clinical illness

Clinical illness with hepatitis B virus begins after an incubation period of 45-160 days (average 2-3 months) and is not as abrupt as with hepatitis A. The signs and symptoms are similar: malaise, anorexia, nausea, vomiting, abdominal pain, and jaundice. Asymptomatic illness may occur. In about 10% of patients with hepatitis B, an immune complex-mediated syndrome develops which results in petechial skin rashes, urticaria, arthralgias, and arthritis. This is uncommon in hepatitis A or hepatitis non-A/non-B. Fatality rates for hospitalized patients are around 1%. About 5-10% of patients with acute type B hepatitis develop a chronic infection with HBsAg present in the blood. The persistence of high levels of HBeAg during the early part of the illness suggests the development of the chronic carrier state. The complications of chronic hepatitis B include cirrhosis, hepatic failure, immune complex disorders, and hepatocellular carcinoma.

Diagnosis

Dark urine and light-colored stools generally precede the development of jaundice. When jaundice appears, the liver may become enlarged and tender. The diagnosis is generally made by the clinical syndrome coupled with the following abnormal laboratory values: elevated serum transaminases (SGOT and SGPT) and bilirubin. The alkaline phosphatase also may be mildly elevated. The diagnosis of HBV hepatitis is established by the presence of HBsAg or antibody to hepatitis B core antigen (anti-HBc). Anti-HBc is present in the early acute phase of the illness and may remain measurable for many years. The presence of anti-HBsAg appears later and indicates immunity. Table 11.3 attempts to make some sense out of the interpretation of the serologic tests.

Prophylaxis

There is no specific medical therapy for viral hepatitis other than supportive. Immunoprophylaxis with either immune serum globulin or hepatitis B immune globulin may be of some benefit in preventing hepatitis in sexual contacts of patients with HBV

Table 11.3   Interpreting Serologic Results in Patients
with Type B Viral Hepatitis

Test Result			Interpretation
HBsAg	anti-HB$_S$	anti-HBc	
−	−	−	No past or present HBV infection
+	−	−	Early hepatitis B
+	−	+	Acute or chronic hepatitis B
+	+	+	Late acute or chronic hepatitis B
−	+	+	Recovery from hepatitis B
−	−	+	Late in recovery phase, or possibly carrier state with low level of antigen present
−	+	−	Late in recovery phase or post-hepatitis B vaccine

infections. The maximum benefit occurs if the globulin is given
within 48 hr after exposure. However, recommendations for passive immunization to prevent hepatitis B, presumably acquired by
sexual contact, are not currently available from the U.S. Public
Health Service. However, many physicians would recommend both
passive immunization with hepatitis immune globulin and active
immunization with hepatitis B vaccine in nonimmune individuals
with a sexual exposure to a patient with hepatitis B.

A major event in the control of hepatitis B infection has been
the recent development of a hepatitis B vaccine. The efficacy of
the vaccine was demonstrated in a control clinical trial in homosexual men in New York City. The vaccine appears to be safe and
free from major side effects. The commercial production of this
product is welcomed by homosexual men as well as health workers
who are at risk for HBV infection.

The hepatitis B vaccine definitely should be administered to homosexual men regardless of their age or homosexual practices. Because of the high incidence of asymptomatic hepatitis B in homosexual men, it is advisable to check for serological markers of previous hepatitis B infection before administering the vaccine, which is expensive. Such tests include HBsAg, anti-HBs, and anti-HBc. If these tests are negative, then the vaccine should be administered. The primary adult vaccination consists of three intramuscular injections. The second dose is given at 1 month, and the third dose is given 6 months after the initial dose. Protection from subsequent HBV infection is not complete, and antibody is induced in 85% of the recipients. The duration of protection is unknown. Hepatitis B immune globulin should be given within 14 days of sexual contacts with persons (homosexual or heterosexual) with acute hepatitis B virus infection.

OTHER DISEASES

Neisseria meningitidis

Neisseria meningitidis is normally found in the nasopharynx. However, genital and anal infection has been identified in both men and women. In homosexual men, anal infection is thought to be the result of oral-anal contact. Although many data are not available, the routine antibiotic therapies for gonococcal infection are probably adequate for genital or anal meningococcal infection. A warning is in order. On rare occasions the microbiology laboratory can inadvertently misdiagnose a meningococcus and call it a gonococcus because of aberrant sugar reactions. This small point is worth remembering because of the possible legal implications of a misdiagnosis of gonorrhea.

Anal Warts

Anal warts are more common in homosexual men (see Chapter 8).

Trauma

Trauma is a result of anal intercourse or insertion of objects into the rectum and may result in pathology in homosexual men. Fecal incontinence does not appear to be common among men practicing anal intercourse. However, nonspecific proctitis, anal fissures, anal fistulas, rectal ulcers, rectal tears, and perirectal abscesses may occasionally be seen. Cases of peritonitis have resulted from rectosigmoid tears after insertion of a fist or forearm for sexual gratification. <u>Chlamydia trachomatis</u> proctitis may be confused with trauma in men who practice anal intercourse.

<u>Cancer</u>

There are suggestions that anal intercourse may be a risk factor for anal cancer.

TOLL-FREE TELEPHONE NUMBER FOR HOMOSEXUAL MEN IN THE UNITED STATES

The National Gay Task Force has a toll-free telephone number for homosexual men who have questions about social and medical problems relating to homosexuality. The crisis line also provides up-to-date information about sexually transmitted diseases and particularly acquired immunodeficiency syndrome. The line sends information to health care professionals and local groups and provides referral to treatment centers, support groups, and research facilities. The line is open weekdays from 3 to 9 p.m. The nationwide toll-free number is 1-800-221-7044 and, from New York, Alaska, and Hawaii, 212-807-6016

BIBLIOGRAPHY

<u>Homosexual Men</u>

Barker RW, Peppercorn MA. Gastrointestinal ailments of homosexual men. Medicine, 61:390-405, 1982.

Bath R, Sketchley J. Homosexuality. Treating patients in general practice. Br Med J, 283:827-829, 1981.

Dritz SK, Ainsworth TE, Back A, et al. Patterns of sexually transmitted enteric diseases in a city. Lancet 2, 3-4, 1977.

Felman YM, Morrison JM. Examining the homosexual male for sexually transmitted diseases. J Amer Med Assoc, 238:2046-2047, 1977.

Merino HI, Richards JB. An innovative program of veneral disease case-finding, treatment and education for a population of gay men. Sex Transm Dis, 4:50-52, 1977.

Mildvan D, Gelb AM, William D. Venereal transmission of enteric pathogens in male homosexuals. Two case reports. J Amer Med Assoc, 238:1387-1389, 1977.

Ostrow DG, Altman NL. Sexually transmitted diseases and homosexuality. Sex Transm Dis, 10:208-215, 1983.

Ostrow DG, Sandholzer TA, Felman YM. Sexually transmitted diseases in homosexual men. Diagnosis, treatment, research. Plenum Publishing, New York, 1983.

Owen WF. The clinical approach to the homosexual patient. Ann Int Med, 93:90-92, 1980.

Phillips SC, Mildvan D, William DC, Gelb AM, White MC. Sexual transmission of enteric protozoa and helminths in a venereal-disease-clinic population. N Eng J Med, 305:603-606, 1981.

Quinn TC, Corey L, Chaffee RG, Schuffler MD, Brancato FP, Holmes KK. The etiology of anorectal infections in homosexual men. Amer J Med, 71:395-406, 1981.

Quinn TC, Stamm WE, Goodell SE, et al. The polymicrobial origin of intestinal infections in homosexual men. N Eng J Med, 309, 576-582, 1983.

Washington AE, Schultz MG, Cohen ML, Juranek DD, Owen RL. Treatment of sexually transmitted bacterial and protozoal enteric infections. Rev Infect Dis, 4(Suppl.):S864-S876, 1982.

William DC, Feldman YM, Marr JS, et al. Sexually transmitted enteric pathogens in male homosexual population. NY State J Med, 77:2050-2052, 1977.

William DC. Sexually transmitted diseases in gay men: An insider's view. Sex. Transm Dis, 6:278-280, 1979.

Wolf FC, Judson FN. Intensive screening for gonorrhea, syphilis and hepatitis B in a gay bathhouse does not lower the prevalence of infection. Sex Transm Dis, 7:49-52, 1980.

Proctitis Caused by Chlamydia

Boland RK, Sands M, Schachter J, Miner RC, Drew WL. Lymphogranuloma venereum and acute ulcerative proctitis. Amer J Med, 72:703-706, 1982.

Klotz SA, Drutz DJ, Tam MR, Reed KH. Hemorrhagic proctitis due to lymphogranuloma venereum serogroup L2. Diagnosis by fluorescent monoclonal antibody. N Eng J Med, 308:1563-1565, 1983.

Munday PE, Taylor-Robinson DT. Chlamydial infection in proctitis and Crohn's disease. Br Med Bull, 39:155-158, 1983.

Quinn TC, Corey L, Chaffee RC, et al. The etiology of anorectal infections in homosexual men. Amer J Med, 71:395-406, 1981.

Quinn TC, Corey L, Chaffee RG, et al. Campylobacter proctitis in a homosexual man. Ann Int Med, 93:458-459, 1980.

Quinn TC, Goodell SE, Mkrtichian E, et al. Chlamydia trachomatis proctitis. N Eng J Med, 305:195-200, 1981.

Sohn N, Robilotti JG. The gay bowel syndrome. A review of colonic and rectal conditions in 260 male homosexuals. Amer J Gastroenterol, 67:478-484, 1977.

Campylobacter Enteritis

Blazer MJ, Reller LB. Campylobacter enteritis. N Eng J Med, 305:1444-1452, 1981.

Blazer MJ, Wells JG, Feldman RA, et al. Campylobacter enteritis in the United States. A multicenter study. Ann Int Med, 98: 360-365, 1983.

Ho DD, Ault MJ, Ault MA, Murata GH. Campylobacter enteritis. Early diagnosis with Gram's stain. Arch Int Med, 143:1858-1860, 1982.

Svedhem Å, Kaijser B. Campylobacter fetus subspecies jejuni: A common cause of diarrhea in Sweden. J Infect Dis, 142:353-359, 1980.

Shigellosis

Bader M, Pedersen AHB, Williams R, et al. Venereal transmission of shigellosis in Seattle—King County. Sex Transm Dis, 4:89-91, 1977.

Blaser MJ, Pollard RA, Feldman YM. Shigella infections in the United States, 1974-1980. J Infect Dis, 147:771-775, 1983.

Butler T, Mahmoud AAF, Warren KS. Algorithms in the diagnosis and management of exotic diseases. XXVII. Shigellosis. J Infect Dis, 136:465-468, 1977.

Dritz SK, Back AF. Shigella enteritis venereally transmitted. N Eng J Med, 291:1194, 1974.

Drusin LM, Genvert G, Topf-Olstein B, et al. Shigellosis, another sexually transmitted disease? Br J Vener Dis, 52:348-350, 1976.

DuPont HL, Hornick RB. Adverse effect of lomotil therapy in shigellosis. J Amer Med Assoc, 226:1525-1528, 1973.

Amebiasis

Adams EB, MacLeod IN. Invasive amebiasis. I. Amebic dysentery and its complications. Medicine, 52:315-323, 1977.

Adams EB, MacLeod IN. Invasive amebiasis. II. Amebic liver abscess and its complications. Medicine, 46, 325-334, 1977.

Cooke RA, Rodrigue RB. Amoebic balanitis. Med J Austral, 1: 114-116, 1964.

Gilman R, Islam M, Paschi S, et al. Comparison of conventional and immunofluorescent techniques for the detection of Entamoeba histolytica in rectal biopsies. Gastroenterology, 78:435-439, 1980.

Istre GR, Kreiss K, Hopkins RS, et al. An outbreak of amebiasis spread by colonic irrigation at a chiropractic clinic. N Eng J Med, 307:339-342, 1982.

Kean BH. Venereal amebiasis. NY State J Med, 76:930-931, 1976.

Krogstad DJ, Spencer HC, Healy GR. Current concepts of parasitology. Amebiasis. N Eng J Med, 298:262-266, 1978.

Krogstad DJ, Spencer HC, Healy HR, et al. Amebiasis: Epidemiologic studies in the United States, 1971-1974. Ann Int Med, 88:89-97, 1978.

Mahmond AAF, Warren KS. Algorithms in the diagnosis and management of exotic diseases, XVII. Amebiasis. J Infect Dis, 134: 639-643, 1976.

Majmudar B, Chaiken ML, Lee KU. Amebiasis of clitoris mimicking carcinoma. J Amer Med Assoc, 236:1145-1146, 1976.

Mulas H, Rodrigue RB. Amoebic infestation of the female genitalia. Med J Austral, 2:179-180, 1964.

Patterson M, Healy GR, Shabot JM. Serologic testing for amoebiasis. Gastroenterology, 78:136-141, 1980.

Phillips SC, Mildvan D, William DC, et al. Sexual transmission of enteric protozoa and helminths in a venereal-disease-clinic population. New Eng J Med, 305:603-606, 1981.

Schmerin MJ, Gelston A, Jones TC. Amebiasis, an increasing problem among homosexuals in New York City. J Amer Med Assoc, 238:1386-1387, 1977.

Giardiasis

Craft JC, Nelson JD. Diagnosis of giardiasis by counterimmunoelectrophoresis of feces. J Infect Dis, 145:499-504, 1982.

Jokipii L, Jokippi AMM. Single-dose metronidazole and tinidazole as therapy for giardiasis: Success rates, side effects, and drug absorption and elimination. J Infect Dis, 140:984-988, 1979.

Mahmond AAF, Warren KS. Algorithms in the diagnosis and management of exotic diseases, II. Giardiasis. J Infect Dis, 131:621-624, 1975.

Meyers JD, Kuharic HA, Holmes KK. Giardia lamblia infection in homosexual men. Br J Vener Dis, 53:54-55, 1977.

Schmerin JJ, Jones TC, Klein H. Giardiasis: Association with homosexuality. Ann Int Med, 88:801-803, 1978.

Visvesvara GS, Smith PD, Healy GR, et al. An immunofluorescence test to detect serum antibodies to Giardia lamblia. Ann Int Med, 93:802-805, 1980.

Wolfe MS. Current concepts in parasitology. Giardiasis. N Eng J Med, 293:319-321, 1978.

Cryptosporidiosis

Centers for Disease Control. Update: Treatment of Cryptosporidiosis in patients with Acquired Immunodeficiency Syndrome (AIDS). Morbid Mortal Weekly Rep, 33:117-119, 1984.

Current WL, Rees NC, Ernst JV, Bailey WS, Heyman MB, Weinstein WM. Human cryptosporidiosis in immunocompetent and immunodeficient persons. N Eng J Med, 308:1252-1257, 1983.

Jokiph L, Pohjola S, Jokiph AMM. Cryptosporidium: A frequent finding in patients with gastrointestinal symptoms. Lancet, 2:358-361, 1983.

Soave R, Danner RL, Honig CL, et al. Cryptosporidiosis in homosexual men. Ann Int Med, 100:504-511, 1984.

Viral Hepatitis

Berris B, Wrobel DM, Sinclair JC, et al. Hepatitis B antigen in families of blood donors. Ann Int Med, 79:690-693, 1973.

Blecker A, Coutinho RA, Bakker-Kok J, Tio D, deKoning GAJ. Prevalence of syphilis and hepatitis B among homosexual men in two saunas in Amsterdam. Br J Vener Dis, 57:196-199, 1981.

Catterall RD. Some observations on the epidemiology and transmission of hepatitis B. Br J Vener Dis, 54:335-340, 1978.

Christenson B, Brostrom CH, Bottinger M, et al. An epidemic outbreak of hepatitis A among homosexual men in Stockholm. Amer J Epidemiol, 116:599-607, 1982.

Coleman JC, Waugh W, Dayton R. Hepatitis B antigen and antibody in a male homosexual population. Br J Vener Dis, 53:132-134, 1977.

Corey L, Holmes KK. Sexual transmission of hepatitis A in homosexual men: Incidence and mechanism. New Eng J Med, 302:435-438, 1980.

Coutinho RA, Schut BJT, Albrecht-van Lent A, Reerink-Brongers EE, Jesdijk LS. Hepatitis B among homosexual men in the Netherlands. Sex Transm Dis, 8:333-335, 1981.

Dietzman DE, Harnisch JP, Ray G et al. Hepatitis B surface antigen ($HB_S Ag$) and antibody to $HB_S Ag$. Prevalence in homosexual and heterosexual men. J Amer Med Assoc, 238:2625-2626, 1977.

Feinman SV, Berris B, Rebane A, et al. Failure to detect hepatitis B surface antigen ($HB_S Ag$) in feces of $HB_S Ag$-positive persons. J Infect Dis, 140:407-410, 1979.

Francis DP, Hadler SC, Thompson SE, et al. The prevention of hepatitis B with vaccine. Report of the Centers for Disease Control multi-center efficacy trial among homosexual men. Ann Int Med, 97:362-366, 1982.

Immunization Practices Advisory Committee. Inactivated hepatitis B virus vaccine. Morbid Mortal Weekly Rep, 31:317-328, 1982.

Immunization Practice Advisory Committee. Immune globulins for protection against viral hepatitis. Morbid Mortal Weekly Rep, 30:423-435, 1981.

Immunization Practices Advisory Committee. Postexposure prophylaxis of hepatitis B. Morbid Mortal Weekly Rep, 33:285-290, 1984.

Inaba N, Ohkawa R, Matsurra A, et al. Sexual transmission of hepatitis B surface antigen. Infection of husbands by $HB_S Ag$ carrier-state wives. Br J Vener Dis, 55:366-368, 1979.

Murphy BL, Schreeder MT, Maynard JE, Hadler SC, Sheller MJ. Serological testing for hepatitis B in male homosexuals:

Special emphasis on hepatitis B e antigen and antibody by radioimmunoassay. J Clin Microbiol, 11:301-303, 1980.

Papaevangelou G, Trichopoulos D, Papoutsakis G, et al. Hepatitis B antigen in prostitutes. Br J Vener Dis, 50:228-231, 1974.

Parker HW, Varma RR, Rothwell DJ, et al. Venereal transmission of hepatitis B virus. The possible role of vaginal secretions. Obstet Gynecol, 48:410-412, 1976.

Peters CJ, Purcell RH, Lander JJ, et al. Radioimmunoassay for antibody to hepatitis B surface antigen shows transmission of hepatitis B virus among household contacts. J Infect Dis, 134:218-223, 1976.

Reiner NE, Judson FN, Bond WW, Francis DP, Peterson NJ. Asymptomatic rectal mucosal lesions and hepatitis B surface antigen at sites of sexual contact in homosexual men with persistent hepatitis B virus infection. Ann Int Med, 96:170-173, 1982.

Robinson WS, Lutwick LI. The virus of hepatitis, type B. N Eng J Med, 295:1168-1175, 1232-1236, 1976.

Schreeder MT. Thompson SE, Hadler SC, et al. Hepatitis B in homosexual men: Prevalence of infection and factors related to transmission. J Infect Dis, 146:7-15, 1982.

Scott RM, Snitbhan R, Bancroft WH, et al. Experimental transmission of hepatitis B virus by semen and saliva. J Infect Dis, 124:64-71, 1980.

Szmuness W, Dienstag JD, Purcell RH, et al. Distribution of antibody to hepatitis A antigen in urban adult populations. N Eng J Med, 295:755-759, 1976.

Szmuness W, Much MI, Prince AM, et al. On the role of sexual behavior in the spread of hepatitis B infection. Ann Int Med, 83: 489-495, 1975.

Szumness W, Stevens CE, Harley EJ, et al. Hepatitis B vaccine. Demonstration of efficacy in a controlled trial in a high-risk population in the United States. N Eng M Med, 303:833-841, 1980.

Wright RA. Hepatitis B and HB$_S$Ag carrier. An outbreak related to sexual contact. J Amer Med Assoc, 232:717-721, 1975.

Other Diseases

Bigger RJ, Andersen HK, Ebbesen P, et al. Seminal fluid excretion of cytomegalovirus related to immunosuppression in homosexual men. Br Med J, 286:2010-2012, 1983.

Carlson BL, Fiumara NJ, Kelly JR, et al. Isolation of <u>Neisseria meningitidis</u> from anogenital specimens from homosexual men. Sex Transm Dis, 7:71-73, 1980.

Cooper HS, Patchefsky AS, Marks G. Cloacogenic carcinoma of the anorectum in homosexual men: An observation of four cases. Dis Col Rect, 22:557-558, 1979.

Dahling JR, Weiss NS, Klopfenstein LL, Cochran LE, Chow WH, Daifuku R. Correlates of homosexual behavior and the incidence of anal cancer. J Amer Med Assoc, 247:1988-1990, 1982.

Drew WL, Mintz L, Miner RC, et al. Prevalence of cytomegalovirus infection in homosexual men. J Infect Dis, 143:188-192, 1981.

Dritz SK, Braff EH. Sexually transmitted typhoid fever (letter). N Eng J Med, 296:1359-1360, 1977.

Goldmeier D. Proctitis and herpes simplex virus in homosexual men. Br J Vener Dis, 56:111-114, 1980.

Judson FN, Ehret JM, Eickhoff TC. Anogenital infection with <u>Neisseria meningitidis</u> in homosexual men. J Infect Dis, 137:458-463, 1978.

Judson FN, Penley KA, Robinson ME, et al. Comparative prevalence rates of sexually transmitted diseases in heterosexual and homosexual men. Amer J Epidemiol, 112:836-843, 1980.

Marino AW. Proctologic lesions observed in male homosexuals. Dis Col Rect, 7:121-128, 1964.

McMillan A, Sommerville RG, McKie PMK. Chlamydial infection in homosexual men. Frequency of isolation of <u>Chlamydia trachomatis</u> from the urethra, ano-rectum, and pharynx. Br J Vener Dis, 57:47-49, 1981.

Mintz L, Drew WL, Miner RC, Braff EH. Cytomegalovirus infections in homosexual men. Ann Int Med, 99:326-329, 1983.

Noble RC, Cooper RM. Meningococcal colonization misdiagnosed as gonococcal pharyngeal infection. Br J Vener Dis, 55:336-339, 1979.

Owen WF. Sexually transmitted diseases and traumatic problems in a homosexual man. Ann Int Med, 92:805-808, 1980.

Chapter 12

LICE

ETIOLOGIC AGENT

The head, body, and pubic lice infesting humans are small,
wingless insects and are members of the order Anoplura or sucking lice. These are to be distinguished from the biting lice that
parasitize birds and other mammals. Fortunately, the lice of
humans and animals are distinct and highly selective in their feeding habits. Human lice have no animal vector. It is said that fleas
and lice are humanity's worst insect enemies in the temperate
zone, comparable to the mosquito in the tropics. Strictly speaking,
lice are not a sexually transmitted parasite; they are transmitted
by close contact. However, sexual intercourse is a frequent mode
of transmission for the crab louse.

The pathogenic lice in humans are _Pediculus humanis_ variety
capitis (the head louse), _Pediculus humanis_ variety _corporis_ (the
body louse), and _Phthirus pubis_ (the pubic or crab louse). Their
morphology and life cycles will be discussed together because of
their basic similarities (Table 12.1). Lice are small (0.8–3.0
mm), are flattened dorsoventrally, and possess five-jointed anten-
nae and three pairs of legs with distal clawlike structures for
grasping hairs or clothing fibers. The morphologic differences
between the head and body lice are slight, and distinction of these
varieties is of little practical importance.

Body and head lice can be bred to have fertile offspring. Lice
have gripping appendages on a tubelike mouth, and in feeding they
inject two cutting stylettes through the skin. Saliva is injected,
and a mixture of blood and saliva is withdrawn by means of a power-
ful sucking pharynx. The saliva is an irritant and in the case of
the body louse also may be a vector of disease. Body lice transmit
typhus (_Rickettsia prowazekii_), relapsing fever (_Borrelia recurrentis_),

Table 12.1 Characteristics of Lice Parasitic on Man[a]

	Body Louse	Head Louse	Crab Louse
Size of adults:			
Male	2.0–3.0 mm	1.0–1.5 mm	0.8–1.0 mm
Female	2.0–4.0 mm	1.8–2.0 mm	1.0–1.2 mm
Abdomen	Elongate without hairy lateral processes	Elongate without hairy lateral processes	Short with hairy processes
Legs	Approximately equal	Approximately equal	First pair smaller and more slender than second and third pairs
Color	Grayish white	Grayish white with dark margins	Grayish white

[a] Adapted from H. D. Pratt and K. S. Littig, Lice of Public Health Importance and Their Control: Training Guide, USPHS Publication No. 772, Insect Control Service, Part VIII, 1961.

and trench fever (<u>Rickettsia quintana</u>). Head and body lice are
more active than the relatively sedentary crab louse. Lice placed
onto the center of the back of a man's undershirt were observed to
wander an average of 30.5-35.5 cm within 2 hr.

Lice mate frequently, and egg laying occurs one to two days
later. The eggs or "nits" are attached to head hairs (head lice),
pubic hairs (crab lice), or clothing (body lice). Body lice can lay
9-10 eggs per day with a lifetime production of 270-300 eggs.
Head lice lay about 4 eggs per day with a lifetime total of 90-140.
The crab louse has been less studied, but the egg production is
probably less than that of the head louse, and about 50 per lifetime.

Lice eggs are operculated, i.e., they have a cap on the top.
This allows air into the developing organism. At the time they are
laid, the eggs are cemented firmly to hairs or fibers. The cement
resists solubilization by almost anything that is harmless to the
human skin. The crab louse egg is smaller than those of the other
two varieties. Depending on environmental conditions, the eggs
hatch in roughly 1 week. The hatching takes place when the eggs
are warmed to 21-36°C but may be delayed by lower temperatures.
The nymphs pop through the operculum and begin feeding. In
another 8-14 days the newly hatched lice go through three nymphal
stages to reach adulthood. The adult life span is approximately 1
month. The average life cycle of the body or head louse is 18 days
and that of the crab louse is 15 days.

Lice are dependent on their human hosts for blood as a source
of nutrition. When lice feed, they pass dark red feces which may
transfer rickettsial or spirochetal diseases. Individuals who wear
clothes intermittently are at less risk from lice. Clothing stored
for 1 month should become free of lice, as all eggs would hatch
and the nymphs would starve.

EPIDEMIOLOGY

Lice thrive in conditions of social disruption: poverty, famine,
and war. Head and body lice are acquired by personal contact or
by wearing infected clothes. Head lice also may be acquired by
sharing combs or brushes or from coming into contact with temporarily infested upholstered headrests. Modern air travelers probably do not appreciate the cloth or paper towels on the headrests
of the airplane seat. Lice may temporarily infest beds occupied
by parasitized individuals. Head lice are still prevalent in children,
mostly girls who have otherwise good personal hygiene. Lice have

been observed to leave feverish patients. At 40°C they are unable
to feed. Crab lice are much more sluggish than the head and body
lice and are spread predominantly by intimate contact. Sexual
intercourse is a common mechanism, but contacts with infested
beds, bath towels, and toilet seats also may result in infestation.
Small children may acquire crab lice from an infected mother or
nurse. Crab lice are thought to be able to survive only a day or
so away from their hosts. Crab lice are not significant vectors of
disease. Hospitalized patients infested with lice should be isolated
appropriately until treatment is instituted.

CLINICAL MANIFESTATIONS

The life cycle of the body lice is carried out on the clothes
and body of the host. The eggs are laid along the seams of underclothing, and the adults go onto the body for feeding. Body lice
feed on the waist, shoulder, and interscapular regions.

The clinical manifestations are initially caused by a reaction
to the saliva injected during the feeding process. A small red
macule appears, followed by a papule which may become wheal-
like. Microscopically, this appears as edema in the dermis with
lymphocytic infiltration and extravasated erythrocytes. The lesions
produces intense itching and the scratching results in excoriations
of the skin and crust formation. The presence of parallel interscapular excoriations suggest lice infestation. Patients with long-
standing infestations may have chronic skin changes, including
postinflammatory hyperpigmentation. Head lice infestations are
more common in girls and women. Patients may complain of
severe itching, and secondary infection is common. Cervical
adenopathy may be present.

The crab louse spends its entire life cycle on humans. These
lice remain attached to the same site for many days. The bites
resulting from feeding may produce varying skin reactions. Secondary infection in excoriated areas is found, although some patients may be asymptomatic. Itching is a common symptom. Patients
may develop characteristic blue spots, 2-20 mm in diameter
(maculae caeruleae). The lesions are a reaction to the saliva of
the crab louse and are occasionally seen on the skin of the thighs,
abdomen, thorax, and eyebrows of the patients. The latter location
was said to be used by quarantine physicians in examining immigrants coming into the United States. Crab lice commonly feed on
hairs in the pubic region, but they have been observed on the thorax

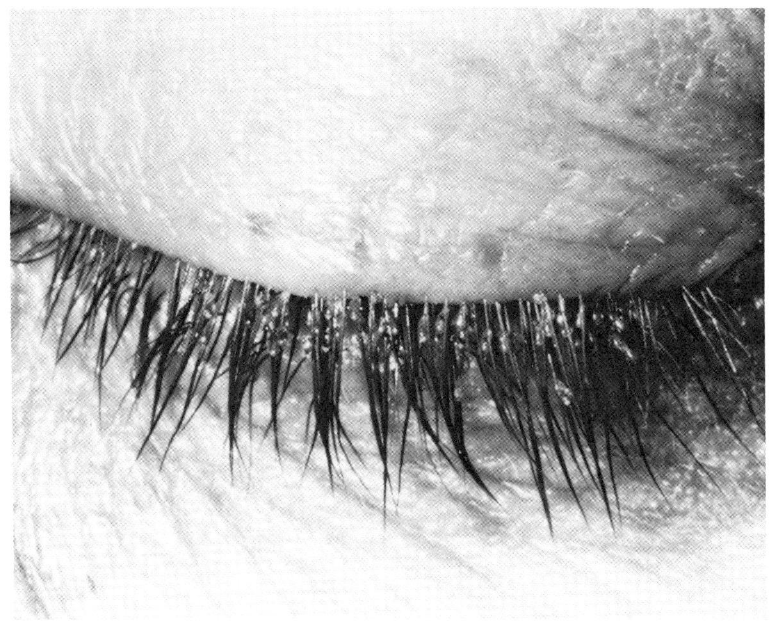

Figure 12.1   Crab louse infestation of the eyelashes.   Crab lice may infest the eyebrows and eyelashes.   This is a heavy infestation with many nits.

and axillae.   Eyebrow and eyelash infestations also should be looked for in all patients, especially small children.   Infestation of the eyelashes with secondary infection may result in phlyctenular conjunctivitis, keratitis, or blepharitis (Fig. 12.1).

DIAGNOSIS

The diagnosis of lice infestation frequently is made by the patient.   Confirmation of this is accomplished by identification of the adult form or the egg in an appropriate location.   Crab lice have a rather distinctive shape, looking somewhat like an oblong turtle with large, lobster-like claws present on the second and third pairs of appendages.   The eggs are found deposited on the pubic hair near the base of the shaft (Fig. 12.2).   The adults and nymphs of the head lice are found on the scalp, with heaviest

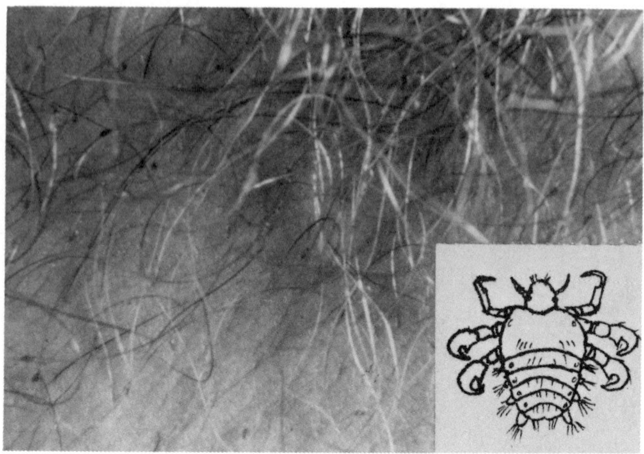

Figure 12.2   Crab lice. <u>Phthirus pubis</u> is commonly transmitted by sexual encounters. Left: The nits are present in the pubic hair. The adults are sluggish and may be located with the aid of a hand lens. Their appearance under low-power microscopy is not to be forgotten. Inset: Drawing of a crab louse.

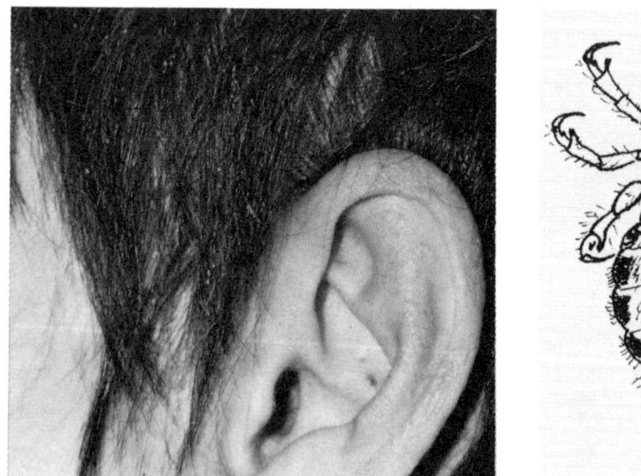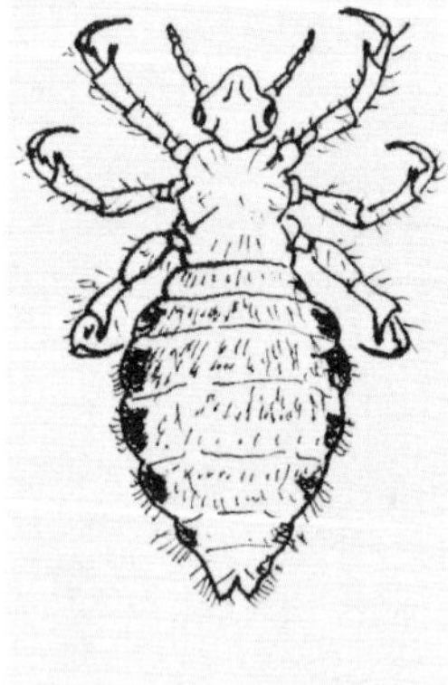

Figure 12.3   Head lice. <u>Pediculus humanis</u> variety <u>capitis</u> is seen more commonly in patients with poor hygiene and in outbreaks among schoolchildren than in patients attending sexually transmitted disease clinics. Left: The nits appear as small white flecks on the hair shaft. Right: The adults are 1-3 mm in length and rarely seen. The eggs or nits are shown in Fig. 12.4.

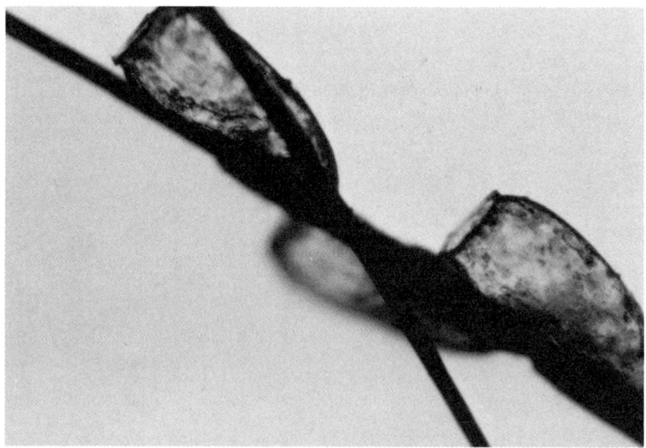

Figure 12.4 Lice eggs attached to a hair shaft (original magnification 18×). The eggs are empty and the operculum, or egg cap, is missing, indicating successful therapy. A fine-tooth comb is the only effective way of removing the eggs.

concentrations behind the ears and on the back of the neck (Fig. 12.3). They are not found on the eyelashes or eyebrows, as are crab lice. The eggs or nits are found in the same location as the adults and are attached to the base of the hair shafts. Not uncommonly, the adult forms of the head and body lice are difficult to find.

Body lice generally reside on the underclothes next to the skin. Females congregate on the seams of the clothing, where they lay their eggs. About 70% of the eggs are laid on clothing and the remainder on body hair. Although large numbers may be present on certain individuals, a dozen lice is a more typical infestation. The diagnosis may be made by finding the eggs along the seams of the underclothing. Wool is preferred by body lice to other clothing materials.

The nits or eggs are best examined under a low-power microscope at magnifications of less than 40× (Fig. 12.4). The eggs look like a tapered barrel that is cemented to a hair shaft. However, following successful therapy, most eggs will be empty and without an operculum. Head and body lice or crab lice, if captured, also can be more clearly seen under a microscope at low magnifications. The sight of an active, greatly enlarged louse is not to be forgotten.

A definitive diagnosis by direct examination of eggs or nits is warranted because of the possible adverse physiologic or psychologic consequences of misdiagnosis. Hair casts or pseudonits may confuse the physician. Hair casts are 2-7 mm long, discrete, firm, shiny, white, freely movable tubular accretions that encircle the hair shafts of the scalp. The casts may result from the persistence of the inner root sheath of the hair, and this condition requires no treatment. To the casual observer, the hair casts are indistinguishable from nits. However, microscopic examination of hair samples under low power will differentiate the two conditions.

TREATMENT

Lice may be treated effectively with a number of different insecticides. The foundation of all therapy is good personal hygiene and the availability of changes of clean clothing. It is worthwhile to treat sexual partners of the infested patient and examine other household contacts for evidence of infestation. Shaving of the hair is unnecessary. Lice resistant to insecticides such as gamma benzene hexachloride (lindane), malathione, or chlorphenothane (DDT) have not been a serious problem in the United States.

After all of the following lice treatments, the patients should put on clean clothing and dry-clean or machine wash and automatically dry (hot cycle in both) all clothing, hats, towels, bed linens, etc. Where this is not possible, boiling clothing or bedding items will kill the developing larvae. Brushes, combs, hair clips, etc. may be discarded, boiled, or washed with 1% gamma benzene hexachloride shampoo. The hair of family and sexual contacts should be thoroughly checked for nits.

Many patients expect that all therapy for lice infection will remove the nits as well. These generally must be removed with a fine-tooth comb that may be included in some commercially available treatment kits. The nits or egg cases are firmly cemented to the hair shaft, and examination under a low-power microscope (30×) can easily assess the viability of the ovum. An ovum is viable if it is yellow or creamy white and has an intact operculum (lid). Nonviable ovum are dark in color and have shrunken shells. Empty or hatched eggs are translucent and have the operculum popped open or absent.

HEAD LICE

Head lice are effectively treated with 1% gamma benzene hexachloride in shampoo form. Approximately 2 tablespoonfuls, or 1 oz, is rubbed into the scalp and adjacent hairy areas. The hair is wetted with small amounts of warm water to make a lather. The lather is then thoroughly massaged into hair for at least 4 min. The hair is rinsed with water and dried. The nit shells are removed with a fine-tooth comb. The shampoo should be repeated in 1 week. Hypersensitivity to gamma benzene hexachloride has been reported, and there is a theoretical possibility of central nervous system toxicity in infants and children.

A second pediculicide is a combination of pyrethrins 0.3%, piperonylbutoxide technical 3.0% equivalent to 2.4% (butylcarbityl) 6-propylpiperonyl ether and petroleum distillate. Slightly different proportions of the ingredients are present in various brands of this agent. The patient wets the hair and scalp thoroughly with the preparation and allows it to remain for 10 min only. The hair is then shampooed, and the dead lice and nits are combed out. The treatment may be repeated in 1 week.

Malathion is the third insecticide effective in killing both adult lice and their eggs. Malathion, an organophosphate cholinesterase inhibitor, is prepared in a 0.5% lotion in isopropyl alcohol for treatment of head lice. The preparation is effective in killing lice resistant to DDT and lindane. Laboratory colonies of body lice have not developed resistance to malathion despite repeated exposure. The lotion is applied to the scalp in a quantity sufficient to wet the hair. The patients should protect their eyes from the alcohol in the preparation by holding a folded towel to their foreheads. The hair is allowed to dry naturally, and 12 hr later the patients may wash the preparation out of their hair with a shampoo. Since at seven days about 5% of treated patients have live lice remaining in the hair, the treatment should be repeated at 1 week. If patients have excoriated areas or pyoderma of the scalp, the alcoholic vehicle in the lotion is likely to cause stinging. Otherwise there are no known major side effects. The medicine is flammable, and patients should be warned about the possibility of fire.

A fourth method of treating head lice is with benzyl benzoate emulsion. The hair is shampooed and dried in the normal manner. The eyes are covered with a towel. A 25% benzyl benzoate emulsion is generously applied to the hair and scalp with a brush. The

emulsion is massaged into the hair and scalp, and the hair is
combed in the normal manner. Twenty-four hours later the hair
is shampooed for a second time. The hair is dried and then combed
with a fine-tooth comb to remove the empty nits.

A fifth pediculicide is copper oleate in a mixture of Tetralin
(tetrahydronaphthalene), acetone, and mineral oil. Three or four
tablespoons of the mixture is gently massaged into the scalp or
other affected areas and allowed to remain for 15 min. Then the
hair is shampooed thoroughly with soap and water. The dead lice
and nits are removed with a fine-tooth comb. The treatment is
repeated in 1 week. The copper oleate is contraindicated in the
presence of infection or skin irritation.

BODY LICE

The treatment of body lice starts with bathing the patient and
separating the patient from the louse- and nit-infested clothes.
The clothing and bedding should be handled as previously described.
One percent gamma benzene hexachloride lotion or cream may be
used if eggs are identified on body hair. In situations where
laundry facilities are not available, or under conditions where
fresh clothing changes are absent, insecticide in powder form may
be applied to the inner garments and to the shirt and trousers,
particularly along the seams.   Examples of these powder preparations are 10% DDT in pyrophyllite, 1% gamma benzene hexachloride,
and 1% malathion containing 0.2% pyrethrin or 0.3% allethrin synergized with pyperonyl butoxide (1:10). These topical powders are
not readily available.

CRAB LICE

Crab lice are treated similarly to head lice. One percent
gamma benzene hexachloride in the form of a cream or lotion is
a convenient therapy. Patients should bathe and dry themselves
prior to application of the insecticide. A thin layer of gamma
benzene hexachloride lotion or cream is applied to the skin and
hairs of the perineum and the perianal areas. In certain hairy
patients other areas must be treated. Although unusual in occurrence, crab lice may infest the body hairs and the beard. The
medication is left on for 12-24 hr, and then the patient should
bathe. Treatment should be repeated in 1 week. Sexual partners

should be treated simultaneously. Treatment is not necessary for
members of the same household unless infestation is present. Alternate therapies include DDT powder, benzyl benzoate, pyrethrins,
and copper oleate, as described in preceding sections.

Crab louse infestations of the eyebrow or eyelids require
special care. Application of 0.25% physostigmine ointment or yellow oxide of mercury is effective. The lice then should be carefully removed with forceps. Another therapy is to apply ophthalmic petrolatum twice daily for eight days, accompanied and followed
by mechanical removal of the lice and nits. In eye infestations it
is prudent to treat the scalp concomitantly with 1% gamma benzene
hexachloride shampoo.

BIBLIOGRAPHY

Ackermann A. Crabs: The resurgence of Phthirus pubis. N Eng
J Med, 278:950-951, 1968.

Bloomers L, van Leenep M, van der Koay HJ. Gammaxane and
malathion in the treatment of pediculosis capitis. Ned Tijdschr
Geneeskd, 122:664-668, 1978.

Chapel TA, Katla T, Kuszmar T, DeGiusti D. Pediculosis pubis
in a clinic for treatment of sexually transmitted diseases. Sex
Transm Dis, 6:257-260, 1979.

Frisch Karl von. Ten Little Housemates. Pergamon Press, London, 1960.

Gordon RM, Lavoipierre MMJ. Entomology for Students of
Medicine, Blackwell Scientific Publications, Oxford, 1962.

Greaves WL, Juranek DD, Washington EA. Treatment of scabies
and pediculosis pubis. Rev Infect Dis, 4(Suppl.):S857-S863, 1982.

Juranek DD. Epidemiological investigations of Pediculosis capitis
in school children. In Orkin M, Maibach HI, Parish LC, Schwartz-
man MB (eds). Scabies and Pediculosis, Lippincott, Philadelphia,
1977, p. 203.

Kohn SR. Hair casts or pseudonits. J Amer Med Assoc, 238:
2058-2059, 1977.

Kraus SJ, Glassman LH. The crab louse—Review of physiology and study of anatomy as seen by the scanning electron microscope. J Amer Vener Dis Assoc, 2:12-18, 1976.

Newsome JH, Fiore, JL, Hackett E. Treatment of infestation with Phthirus pubis: Comparative efficacies of synergized pyrethrins and gamma-benzene hexachloride. Sex Transm Dis, 6:203-205, 1979.

Orkin M, Epstein E, Mailbach HI. Treatment of today's scabies and pediculosis. J Amer Med Assoc, 236:1136-1139, 1976.

Pratt HD, Littig KS. Lice of public health importance and their control: Training guide, USPHS Publication No. 772, Insect Control Series, Part VIII, 1961.

Proceedings of the International Symposium of the Control of Lice and Louse-born Diseases, Washington, DC, Pan American Health Organization, Scientific Publication No. 263, 1973.

Robinson DH, Shepherd DA. Control of head lice in school children. Curr Ther Res, 27:1-6, 1980.

Scott MJ, Scott MJ, Sr. Nits or not? Pseudonits: Simple office diagnosis. J Amer Med Assoc, 243:2325-2326, 1980.

Smith DE, Walsh J. Treatment of pubic lice infestations. Cutis, 26:618-619, 1980.

Taplin D, Castillero PM, Spiegel J, et al. Malathion for treatment of Pediculus humanus var capitis infestation. J Amer Med Assoc, 247:3103-3105, 1982.

Chapter 13

SCABIES

ETIOLOGIC AGENT

Sarcoptes scabiei causes scabies in humans. This mite
belongs to a family of itch and mange mites of the genus Sarcoptes
that infest mammals by burrowing into the skin. S. scabiei is the
species most frequently infecting humans. Animal species infrequently cause human disease. The animal mites do not differ morphologically from the human mites, but they are thought to differ
biologically.

S. scabiei is a small, oval mite, just visible to the naked eye,
with a flat underside and a convex dorsum covered with numerous
bristles (Figs. 13.1-13.4). The female (330-450 μm) is larger
than the male (200-250 μm). The adult mite has eight short, squat
legs. In the female, the two anterior pairs end in long tubular
processes, each with a bell-shaped sucker and claws. The two
posterior pairs end in long bristles. In the male, the posterior
pair of legs also possess suckers.

The female mite burrows into the stratum corneum or superficial portion of the skin (see Fig. 13.1). The burrows parallel the
skin surface and do not extend below the stratum corneum. The
female lives about 1 month and lays about 40-50 eggs. When egg
laying is complete, the female mites die at the end of the burrow.
In 3-10 days the eggs hatch, and six-legged larvae emerge and
burrow just below the surface of the skin, where maturation stages
take place. This "maturation chamber" forms a papule in the
outermost epidermis. The larva becomes an eight-legged nymph
by molting and, following several molts, an adult.

The life cycle is complete in about 2 weeks. Fortunately,
less than 10% of the eggs become adult mites. The female can

205

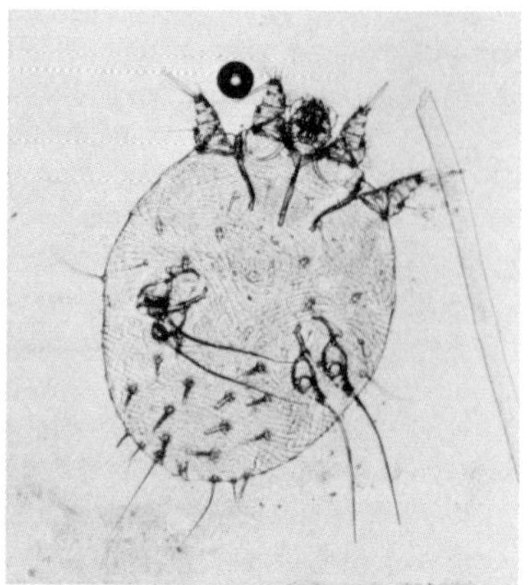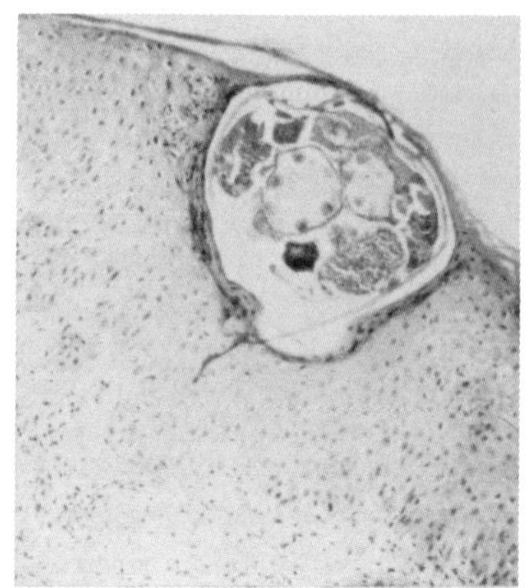

Figure 13.1   Left: <u>Sarcoptes scabiei</u> (original magnification 240×) is a mite causing scabies. Scabies appears to be increasing in frequency in the United States. Right: The female burrows into the stratum corneum of the skin, where the eggs are laid. The diagnosis is made by the identification of the mite, the eggs, or the mite scybala (inspissated excrement).

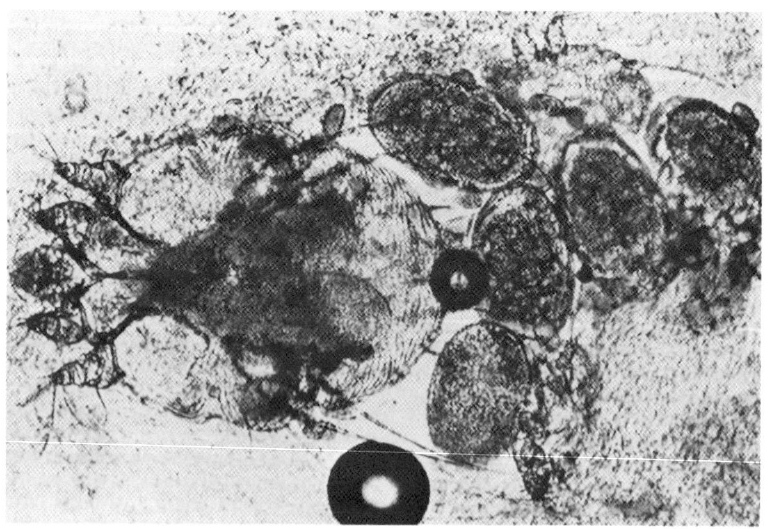

Figure 13.2   Mite as seen in skin scrapings and observed by magnification. Several mite eggs are present in the right side of the photograph. Photograph courtesy of E. Stolz and J. van der Stek.[*]

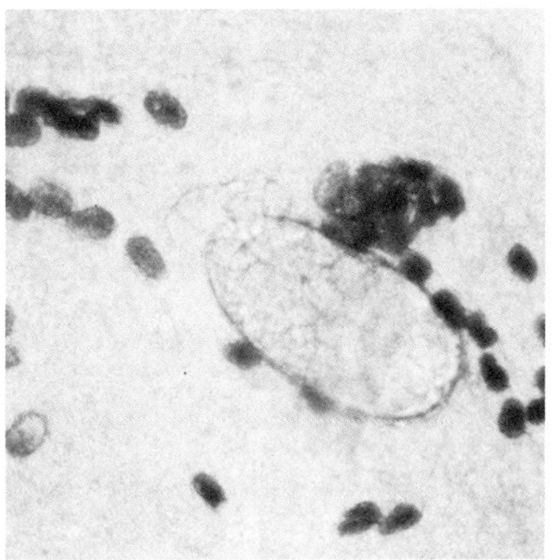

Figure 13.3   Egg and scybala from skin scrapings of a patient with scabies (original magnification 240×).

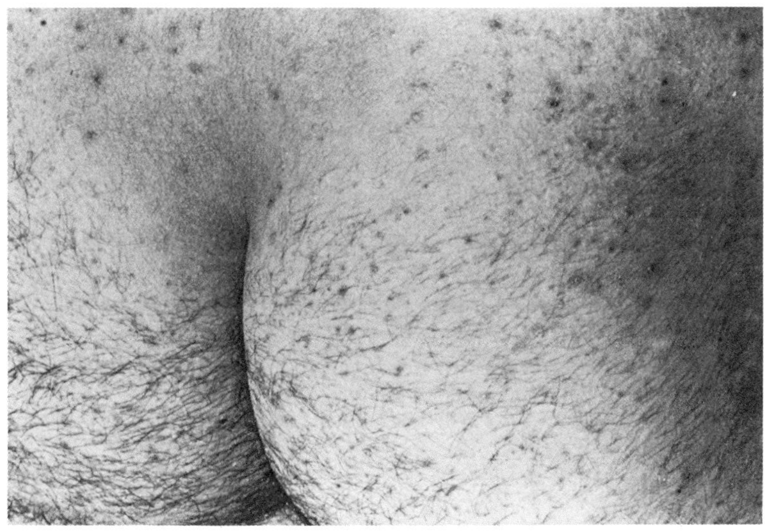

Figure 13.4   Buttocks of a man with scabies.   Patients in general complain of intense itching, worse at night.   Photograph courtesy of E. Stolz and J. van der Stek.[*]

survive away from the host for about two to three days. It is
thought that the male mite lives on the skin surface and enters the
shallow burrows only intermittently. The female mite remains
below the skin surface during her life cycle. The mites produce
small fecal compactions (scybala) that remain in the burrows.
They are of diagnostic value and are present in burrows in a ratio
to living organisms of 30:1 to 50:1.

EPIDEMIOLOGY

Scabies is not exclusively a sexually transmitted disease;
rather it is a disease of social contact. Traditionally scabies was
a disease of the unwashed poor; currently, however, scabies does
not respect traditional social, economic, or geographic boundaries.
A worldwide resurgence of the disease has taken place since the
1960s, and the number of cases in the United States has apparently
increased since the early 1970s. However, good epidemiologic
data are not available because scabies is not a reportable disease.
The disease appears to be cyclical in nature with peaks at
irregular intervals. Unfortunately, this means that a generation
of physicians may be, for a time, unfamiliar with the disease.
The reasons for the resurgence of scabies are really unknown, but
the following have been submitted: poverty, poor hygiene, crowding, sexual promiscuity, migration, and loss of herd immunity.
Scabies generally is transmitted by close contact with an
infected person. This occurs in bedfellows, family members,
patients in chronic care institutions, and health workers. An
infected child may be initially identified, and then lesions are discovered on the mother, father, siblings, and maid. Schoolroom
transmission probably is not important. However, transmission
can occur where children exchange clothing or spend the night at
one another's homes. Scabies has been introduced into families by
the adoption of a foreign-born child who may have resided for a
time in an orphanage prior to entry into the United States.

CLINICAL MANIFESTATIONS

<u>Scabies in the Adult</u>

Following infestation the patient may be asymptomatic for several days to a month. The incubation period is much shorter in

previously infested individuals. It is believed that symptoms are a result of sensitization to the mite or its products. The history is generally of severe itching present for weeks or months. Characteristically, the itching is more intense at night. The mites generally burrow into the skin between the fingers and on the volar aspects of the wrists. The burrows also are commonly found on the penis and scrotum, elbows, and buttocks. Less common locations are the axillary folds, the umbilicus, the beltline, and the areola and nipple. In men, the combination of pruritic lesions on the genitalia and hands suggests the diagnosis of scabies. In adults, the face, scalp, neck, upper back, palms of the hands, and soles of the feet are rarely involved.

The diagnostic lesion is the burrow. Burrows are several millimeters to a few centimeters in length, and a small vesicle may be present at the terminal end above the mite. The burrow is slightly elevated, threadlike, and grayish white in color. It may be present prior to symptoms. A magnifying glass aids in identifying burrows. On the male genitalia, burrows may be raised, slightly elongated, nodular lesions. Scabies rarely is seen on the female genitalia.

Scratching frequently obscures the original character of the lesions. Other lesions, including papules, pustules, vesicles, and excoriations, are not diagnostic, although their distribution is suggestive. Urticaria has been described in some patients with scabies. Furuncular lesions may be present on the elbows. Secondary infection with bacteria is common in the excoriated lesions. In light infestations or in the "clean" patient, the burrows are difficult to find. Scabies may be extremely difficult to diagnose in patients who have received topical steroids. Histopathologic lesions may not be specific. The burrow is within the stratum corneum, except at the distal end, which may lie over the stratum malpighii. The latter layer may be edematous just below the mite and show lymphocytic infiltration. Asymptomatic chronic carriage undoubtedly occurs, but there is little information on this subject.

Scabies in Children

In children, the distribution of the scabies lesions is not the same as in the adult. Burrows are difficult to identify. The head, neck, palms, and soles may be involved as well as the rest of the body. Also, in children, eczematous eruptions are found in untreated scabies. Blister formation or bulla, although unusual in adults, may be present in infant infestations.

Norwegian Scabies

This form of scabies has been described in immuno-compromised or institutionalized individuals. It occurs classically in two groups, the mentally retarded (especially male Down's syndrome patients) and patients with lepromatous leprosy. Itching is not necessarily a prominent feature of the disease. The disease consists of hyperkeratotic lesions of the hands, feet, ears, and scalp. The crusting lesions are teeming with mites, which may easily be shed on the exfoliating scales into the surrounding environment. Whereas the usual number of female mites is 12 per patient, patients with Norwegian scabies may have hundreds to thousands of mites. As in any patient with scabies, isolation precautions should be observed. Eosinophilia may be present.

Nodular Scabies

Nodular scabies occurs in about 7% of all patients with scabies. Nodules are more frequently present in patients with severe scabies. The lesions are reddish brown and pruritic and vary in size from a grain of wheat to a kernel of corn. Nodules are present on the parts of the skin where the stratum corneum is thin. They are infrequently observed on the hands and forearms but are seen in the axillary region and on the scrotum, genitalia, groin, and other covered parts of the body. The lesions may persist for months to more than a year despite appropriate therapy. In one series nodules were present for 1-3 months in 44% of the cases. Mites infrequently are identified in the older lesions.

The nodules may be a response to cell-mediated defense mechanisms to retained or absorbed mite antigens. The histologic characteristics of the lesions are those of a small-cell infiltrate in all parts of the dermis consisting mostly of lymphocytes and some eosinophiles. In the middle and deep dermis, the infiltrate have a perivascular arrangement. Itching may be less intense in this form of scabies, but patients do complain of paroxysms of nocturnal itching.

Scabies Transmitted by Animals

This form of scabies is caused by animal mites that are indistinguishable morphologically from the mites infesting humans. Dogs (usually puppies) are the most common vector. The infestation in man is self-limited unless reexposure occurs. In dogs

(mange), the ear is the common infection site. The lesions appear
on the hand in man. In canine-acquired scabies, the incubation
period is short and burrows are uncommon.

The differential diagnosis in scabies is depressingly large.
The nondermatologist must keep this disease in mind when con-
fronted with rashes in sexually active patients. As with all sexually transmitted disease, the discovery of one case will lead to the
diagnosis in others. With scabies, members of the family, as
well as sexual partners, are at risk. Scabies can mimic a number
of dermatologic conditions including dermatitis herpetiformis,
lichen planus, secondary syphilis, etc. Lesions treated with topical steroids may be especially difficult to recognize. Patients who
are treated with immunosuppressive or antineoplastic chemotherapy also may have atypical lesions that are diagnostic problems.

DIAGNOSIS

The diagnosis is made by the identification of the mite, its
smaller developmental forms, its egg, or inspissated excrement
(scybala) from a typical skin lesion. Mite scybala are oval in
shape, about 20 μm in size, and brown-black in color. All of the
above may be found in punch biopsies or skin shavings (see Figs.
13.1-13.2). However, other methods are less traumatic. Material must be obtained from an early papule or burrow. The ideal
lesion is slightly raised and oval or linear without surface discoloration. The latter, in the form of a crust or tiny dot, indicates
that the mite has departed from the burrow. The patient usually
can select an appropriate lesion based on symptoms.

A hand lens is useful in delineating the anatomy of the lesions.
Use a sterile surgical blade with a drop of mineral oil on it. Apply
the scalpel to the surface of the lesion so that the mineral oil goes
onto the surface of the lesion. The purpose of the oil is to prevent
the loss of diagnostic material in flying skin scales. Also, the
mites, eggs, scybala, etc. are well preserved and visualized,
presumably due to the refractive index of mineral oil. The scalpel
is scraped vigorously about six to seven times to remove the top
of the lesion. Stop when tiny flecks of blood appear in the oil. The
skin scales in the mineral oil are removed with the blade and placed
on a glass slide.

The procedure is repeated on four or five lesions, and the
scrapings are collected on the same slide. A cover slip is carefully placed over the oil, and then the scrapings are examined

initially under low power to look for movement of the mites. Due to the relatively large size (0.3-0.4 mm) of the mites, microscopic magnifications of 40× are adequate. The lesions with a decreasing magnitude of yield are burrows, eczematous lesions, papules and, finally, vesicles. Scrapings should be positive in 80% of patients thought to have scabies. Potassium hydroxide is not suitable as an examination vehicle as it kills the adult and larval organisms and dissolves the scybala.

Orkin and Maibach suggest identifying the burrows by filling them with ink. The scabitic papule is covered with ink from the underside of the nib of a fountain pen. The ink is wiped off immediately with an alcohol pad. If the test is positive, the ink will enter the burrow and form a zigzag line leading away from the papule. Although this test may be falsely negative, a positive test can be followed by shaving the epidermis with a scalpel blade held parallel to the skin surface.

Suggestive features of scabies are the distribution of the lesions, the presence of the burrows, the nocturnal itching, the presence of contact cases, the response to specific therapy, or the pathologic picture of a skin biopsy.

TREATMENT

Patients may be successfully treated with a number of topical compounds. Because of the epidemiology of scabies, members of the patient's immediate household, as well as the patient's sexual contacts, should be treated. The incubation period in uninfected individuals may be 1 month. Thus asymptomatic carriers are a potential source of the mites. Casual contacts need not be treated. Systemic antibodies are indicated if the scabies lesions are secondarily infected with bacteria and there is evidence of pyoderma, cellulitis, or furunculosis. These lesions may harbor nephritogenic group A streptococci. Although antibiotic therapy of the streptococcal pyoderma will not prevent glomerulonephritis, it will prevent the spread of these organisms to siblings or other family members.

Fortunately, mites survive for only a few days when removed from their hosts. Intimate articles of clothing, pajamas, and bedding are the only items that have to receive special attention in relation to a patient's therapy. These articles may be rid of mites by processing in an automatic washer and drier (hot cycle in each), boiling, or laundering and ironing. Reinfection is more likely to occur from a venereal source. Resistance to scabicides has not been conclusively demonstrated. The following are some effective topical treatments for scabies.

Gamma Benzene Hexachloride (GBH)

This drug should be used only for older children and adults. In high doses GBH is potentially dangerous, particularly in small children. GBH, a chlorinated hydrocarbon, is an insecticide (lindane). Deaths in young animals dipped in this insecticide have been reported in the veterinary literature. Also, convulsions and death have been reported in weanling rabbits. One experimental study using human subjects showed that when GBH was applied to the skin for 24 hr without washing, 9.3% was ultimately recovered in the urine. However, in that study the GBH was dissolved in acetone. Thus the risk in humans is not well documented. Other therapies are appropriate for infants and small children. Because of possible overuse, avoid giving too much. GBH is available in a 1% lotion or 1% ointment in a washable base. Approximately 30 g (1 oz) of the topical preparation is adequate to cover the trunk and extremities of an average adult.

Prior to therapy the patient should have a warm soapy bath and scrub with a soft brush. The lotion should be applied evenly in a thin coat from the neck downward over the trunk and extremities with attention to the hands, feet, and intertriginous areas. It is an error to limit the application to obvious lesions only. The lotion should be kept away from the eyes and mucous membranes. The GBH is left on the skin for 12-24 hr, and then a second bath is taken. Freshly laundered sheets, pajamas, pillowcases, and underclothing should be used following the initial and final baths.

A second application of GBH is recommended 1 week after the first. It has not been shown that any of the agents capable of killing the juvenile or mature mites also are capable of killing the eggs. Thus the second application will destroy any recently hatched nymphs and larvae from eggs present at the initial therapy. Allergic reactions to GBH can occur, as can local skin irritation from too frequent applications.

Crotamiton

This scabicide, N-ethyl-o-crotonotoluide, is available in a 10% cream and is also an effective antipruritic agent. Crotamiton in the form of .a vanishing cream is massaged into the skin. All topical agents are applied to the body from the neck down. A second

application is made 24 hr later. The following morning, the
clothing and bed linen are changed. A soap and water bath is taken
24–48 hr after the last application. Skin sensitization has been
reported with prolonged use and in patients with eczema.

Sulfur

Precipitated sulfur 6% in petrolatum is the drug of choice
for infants and small children. In its favor is its relative safety;
however, the preparation is smelly, messy, and stains clothing.
It should be applied nightly for three nights following a bath. The
child should be bathed 24 hr after the final application. Handling
of personal items of clothing and bedding is the same as previously
described.

Benzyl Benzoate

Benzyl benzoate is not commercially available in the United
States, although it is an effective scabicide. Benzyl benzoate is
available in the form of a lotion or emulsion and may be compounded
by a pharmacist. The U.S.P. Lotion (25%) is composed of the following ingredients: benzyl benzoate 25 ml, triethanolamine 0.5 g,
oleic acid 2.0 g, and water 75 ml. The lesions are first scrubbed
with soap and water, and then the lotion is immediately applied on
the body from the neck down. After the first application is dry, a
second application is applied to the active lesion. Children require
60–90 ml of the lotion, while adults require 120–180 ml for a single
treatment. The bedding and clothes are handled as described for
the other therapies. Twenty-four hours following the application,
the patient should bathe and dress in clean clothes. Two or three
treatments may be required. Side effects include a slight transi-
tory burning sensation in some patients with sensitive skin.
Following effective therapy for scabies, some patients may
continue to have symptoms and signs, although often to a lesser
degree. This is thought to be a hypersensitivity reaction to the
dead mites or mite antigens. Oral antipyretics, antihistamines,
or salicylates may provide some relief. One may see erythematous
papules or nodules as described in an earlier section. In severe,
persistent cases, corticosteroid injection into the lesion or surgical
incision may be the only methods to provide relief. Norwegian
scabies is treated in the conventional manner. In resistant cases,
sequential scabicides may be used following keratolytic agents.

BIBLIOGRAPHY

Ackerman AB, Stewart R, Stillman M. Scabies masquerading as dermatitis herpetiformis. J Amer Med Assoc, 33:53-54, 1975.

Anolik MA, Rudolph RI. Scabies stimulating Darier disease in an immunosuppressed host. Arch Dermatol, 112:73-74, 1976.

Bean SF. Bullous scabies. J Amer Med Assoc, 230:878, 1974.

Brown HW. Basic Clinical Parasitology, 4th ed., Appleton-Century-Crofts, New York, 1975.

Burkhart CG. Scabies: An epidemiologic reassessment. Ann Int Med, 98:498-503, 1983.

Chapel TA, Krugel L, Chapel J, Segal A. Scabies presenting as urticaria. J Amer Med Assoc, 246:1440-1441, 1981.

Espy PD, Jolly HW. Norwegian scabies, occurrence in a patient undergoing immunosuppression. Arch Dermatol, 112:193-196, 1976.

Feldmann RJ, Maibach HI. Percutaneous penetration of some pesticides and herbicides in man. Toxicol Appl Pharmacol, 28:126-132, 1974.

Food and Drug Administration: Gamma benzene hexachloride (Kwell and other products) alert, FDA Drug Bulletin, 6:28, 1976.

Ginsburg CM, Lowry W, Reisch JS. Absorption of lindane (gamma benzene hexachloride) in infants and children. J Ped, 91:998-1000, 1977.

Greaves WL, Juraneck DD, Washington AE. Treatment of scabies and pediculosis pubis. Rev Infect Dis, 4(Suppl.):S857-S863, 1982.

Hubler WF, Clabaugh W. Epidemic Norwegian scabies. Arch Dermatol, 112:179-181, 1976.

Hurwitz S. Scabies in babies. Amer J Dis Child, 126:226-228, 1973.

Konstantinov D, Stanoeva L. Persistent scabious nodules. Dermatologica, 147:321-327, 1973.

Lipitz R, Tur E, Brenner S, Krakowski A. Norwegian scabies following topical corticosteroid therapy. Israel J Med Sci, 17: 1165-1168, 1981.

Melton LJ, Brazin SA, Damm SR. Scabies in the United States Navy. Amer J Public Health, 68:776-778, 1978.

Muller G, Jacobs PH, Moore NE. Scraping for human scabies. A better method for positive preparations. Arch Dermatol, 107:70, 1973.

Orkin M. Today's scabies. J Amer Med Assoc, 233:882-885, 1975.

Orkin M. Resurgence of scabies. J Amer Med Assoc, 217:593-597, 1971.

Orkin M, Epstein E, Maibach HI. Treatment of today's scabies and pediculosis. J Amer Med Assoc, 236:1136-1139, 1976.

Orkin M, Maibach HI. Scabies. In McCormack WM (ed). Diagnosis and Treatment of Sexually Transmitted Diseases. John Wright, PSG Inc., Boston, 1983, Chapter 11.

Orkin M, Maibach HI. Current conception parasitology. This scabies pandemic. New Eng J Med, 298:496-498, 1978.

Parlette HL. Scabietic infestations in man. Cutis, 16:47-52, 1975.

Pratt HD. Mites of Public Health Importance and Their Control, Public Health Service Publication No. 772, Insect Control Series: Part IX, U.S. Government Printing Office, Washington, DC, 1963.

Rasmussen JE. The problem of lindane. J Amer Acad Dermatol, 5:507-516, 1981.

Shacter B. Treatment of scabies and pediculosis with lindane: An evaluation. J Amer Acad Dermatol, 5:517-527, 1981.

Shaw PR, Juranek DD. Recent trends in scabies in the United States. J Infect Dis, 134:414-416, 1976.

Shelly WB. Larval papule as a sign of scabies. J Amer Med Assoc, 236:1144-1145, 1976.

Solomon LM, Fahrner L, West DP. Gamma benzene hexachloride toxicity: A review. Arch Dermatol, 113:353-357, 1977.

Svartman M, Potter EV, Finklea JF, et al. Epidemic scabies and acute glomerulonephritis in Trinidad. Lancet, 1:249-251, 1972.

Wilson JW. Scabies (letter). Arch Dermatol, 104:223, 1971.

Chapter 14

PELVIC INFLAMMATORY DISEASE

ETIOLOGY

Pelvic inflammatory disease is a term that loosely embraces
a number of infectious diseases of the female genital tract. The
portions of the genital tract involved are the endometrium, the sal-
pinx, the ovaries, and the peritoneal cavity. Abscess formation
is a complication. <u>Neisseria gonorrhoeae</u> and <u>Chlamydia tracho-
matis</u> are the most frequent causes in patients with initial attacks
of pelvic inflammatory disease. <u>Mycobacterium tuberculosis</u> also
is an etiologic agent for pelvic inflammatory disease, however,
more frequently outside of North America and Europe. The role
of <u>Ureaplasma urealyticum</u> and <u>Mycoplasma hominis</u> as a pathogen
in this disease remains controversial. In many cases the disease
is polymicrobial in etiology, with anaerobes playing an important
role.

An overwhelming list of micro-organisms has been isolated
from patients in published reports. The major problem with
establishing a clear-cut microbiologic etiology in these patients is
the inaccessibility of the infected area. Blood cultures, culture of
the cul-de-sac by means of needle aspiration through the vagina,
and culture of the peritoneal cavity by means of laparoscopic examination have demonstrated multiple bacterial pathogens. Although
infection by <u>N. gonorrhoeae</u> may play an important role in the initiation of pelvic inflammatory disease, both aerobic and anaerobic
bacteria also have been implicated. A partial list of other micro-
organisms isolated from patients with pelvic inflammatory disease
includes anaerobic peptococci, peptostreptococci, <u>Bacteroides</u>
species, <u>Veillonella</u>, <u>Fusobacterium</u> species, <u>Clostridium</u> species,
gram-positive nonsporulating rods, streptococci, enterococci,
staphylococci, and Enterobacteriaceae including <u>E. coli.</u>

Frequently, the cultures reveal mixed infections rather than a single micro-organism. Most patients with pelvic inflammatory disease in the United States have infections with N. gonorrhoeae or anaerobic bacteria. However, in Sweden, Finland, and England, C. trachomatis has been identified as an etiologic agent in approximately one-third of patients with pelvic inflammatory disease. To date Chlamydia has not been commonly isolated from patients in the United States with pelvic inflammatory disease. The reason for this discrepancy is not known. It is believed, however, that some of the differences may be explained because the Swedish investigators are studying patients with milder disease. Pelvic inflammatory disease caused by C. trachomatis produces milder symptoms than that caused by N. gonorrhoeae.

CLINICAL MANIFESTATIONS

Pelvic inflammatory disease is a poorly defined entity, and this chapter is directed at infectious diseases produced by micro-organisms ascending from the endocervix through the endometrium to the fallopian tubes in otherwise normal women. Thus the chapter does not include infections that occur following childbirth, surgical procedures, or secondary infections resulting from direct spread from a nearby pelvic organ such as the appendix. The spread of micro-organisms into the fallopian tubes may be facilitated by menstruation. As a result of infection, the epithelium of a fallopian tube may be severely damaged, and the fimbriated ostia may be occluded, resulting in a hydrosalpinx. Rupture of a fallopian tube abscess or extrusion of inflammatory exudate via the os into the peritoneal cavity may result in peritonitis. Eschenbach points out that pelvic inflammatory disease is the most common serious infection among sexually active women.

One adverse consequence of pelvic inflammation is damage to the reproductive organ with the possibility of sterility. Long-term problems such as chronic pelvic pain and ectopic pregnancy also may be a result of scarring, adhesions, and tubal occlusion. With each repeat infection, the likelihood of damage to the salpinges increases. In the United States the increase in the incidence of gonorrhea in the 1960s was associated with increases in the 1970s in nonsurgical sterility and the occurrence of ectopic pregnancy in women. Although the yearly costs of pelvic inflammatory disease in the United States are estimated to be in the millions of dollars, the real tragedy lies not in the number of dollars but in

Table 14.1   Salpingitis: Clinical Criteria for Diagnosis[a]

Abdominal direct tenderness, with or without rebound tenderness	⎫	
Tenderness with motion of cervix and uterus	⎬ All three necessary for diagnosis	
Adnexal tenderness	⎭	

plus

Gram stain of endocervix: positive for gram-negative intracellular diplococci	⎫	
Temperature (greater than 38°C)		
Leukocytosis (greater than 10,000)	⎬ One or more necessary for diagnosis	
Purulent material (WBC[b] present) from peritoneal cavity by culdocentesis or laparoscopy		
Pelvic abscess or inflammatory complex on bimanual examination or by sonography	⎭	

[a] Reprinted with permission of The American College of Obstetricians and Gynecologists. Obstet Gynecol, 61(1):113-114, 1983.
[b] WBC = white blood cell count.

Table 14.2   Severity of Disease by Laparoscopic Examination[a]

Mild	Erythema, edema, no spontaneous purulent exudate;[b] tubes freely movable
Moderate	Gross purulent material evident; erythema and edema more marked. Tubes may not be freely movable, and fimbria stoma may not be patent.
Severe	1. Pyosalpinx or inflammatory complex 2. Abscess[c]

[a] Reprinted with permission from The American College of Obstetricians and Gynecologists. Obstet Gynecol, 61(1):113-114, 1983.
[b] The tubes may require manipulation to produce purulent exudate.
[c] The size of any pelvic abscess should be measured.

Table 14.3   Grading of Salpingitis by Clinical Examination[a]

1. Uncomplicated: limited to tubes and/or ovaries, without pelvic peritonitis or with pelvic peritonitis.

2. Complicated: inflammatory mass or abscess involving tubes and/or ovaries, without pelvic peritonitis or with pelvic peritonitis.

3. Spread to structures beyond pelvis, i.e., ruptured tubo-ovarian abscess.

[a] Reprinted with permission from The American College of Obstetricians and Gynecologists. Obstet Gynecol, 61(1):113–114, 1983.

the number of young women who desire children but are unable to have them as a result of pelvic inflammatory disease. The risk of involuntary infertility is nearly 20% in women who have had one or more episodes of pelvic inflammatory disease compared with women who have had no episodes.

Recently Hager et al. have offered criteria for diagnosis and grading of salpingitis. These are shown in Tables 14.1, 14.2, and 14.3.

Recurrent pelvic inflammatory disease is common, and the two most frequent predisposing factors are previous pelvic infection and the presence of an intrauterine device. For some unexplained reason, the use of barrier methods of contraception and oral contraceptives is associated with a decreased risk of pelvic inflammatory disease. Pelvic inflammatory disease is unusual in women who are not sexually active. Women with multiple sex partners are at increased risk for acquiring pelvic inflammatory disease. The incidence of pelvic inflammatory disease is four times higher in nonwhite than in white women. About 5–10% of women with gonorrhea will develop pelvic inflammatory disease. Women who have had pelvic inflammatory disease have an increased incidence of abdominal pain, longer and more painful menstruation, and more frequent pain during sexual intercourse in comparison to disease-free women.

DIAGNOSIS

Pelvic inflammatory disease usually is diagnosed by the presence of certain clinical signs and symptoms, and the clinical criteria for diagnosis may be found in Table 14.1. These include the presence of acute pelvic pain, often a few days duration; lower abdominal direct tenderness or rebound tenderness; tenderness with displacement of the uterine cervix; a fever of 38-39°C; a tender adnexal swelling or mass; and an elevation of the erythrocyte sedimentation rate and polymorphonuclear leukocyte count. Given these clinical criteria, the diagnosis will be correct about two-thirds of the time.

In clinically suspected cases that are negative by laparoscopic examination, other diagnoses include acute appendicitis, endometriosis, corpus luteum bleeding, ectopic pregnancy, ovarian tumor, chronic salpingitis, acute cholecystitis, hemorrhagic or torsion of an ovarian cyst, acute pyelonephritis, mesenteric lymphadenitis, and pelvic vein thrombophlebitis. Generally women with gonococcal pelvic inflammatory disease are sicker when they are first seen but respond more favorably to antibiotic therapy and appear to have fewer long-term complications than women with nongonococcal pelvic inflammatory disease.

It is difficult to arrive at a precise microbiologic diagnosis because of the inaccessibility of the involved structures. Several sites may be cultured with varying results. The following are some of the cultures that may help in a microbiologic diagnosis:

1. Blood cultures: Blood cultures are positive in only a small percentage of the patients.
2. Endocervical cultures: There is frequent disagreement between endocervical cultures and cultures taken from the cul-de-sac or from the peritoneal cavity via a laparoscope. Perhaps the only isolates from the endocervix that have any meaning therapeutically are N. gonorrhoeae and C. trachomatis. Even the presence of these micro-organisms in the endocervix does not rule out the presence of other microbes in deeper structures.
3. Cul-de-sac cultures: Culdocentesis may be performed in the following manner. The posterior vaginal wall below the cervix is washed with a 2% povidone iodine solution and then dried with several large cotton-tipped applicator sticks. Aspiration of fluid is accomplished under direct visualization with an 18-gauge needle and syringe. Usually 1-4 ml of specimen may be withdrawn. The syringe is corked, and the fluid is immediately

taken to the diagnostic microbiology laboratory. It is very important that the specimen be protected from contact with air and that the anaerobic culturing is performed quickly since anaerobic organisms are susceptible to atmospheric oxygen. The microbiologic media and technology in this area are undergoing constant change and improvement, and clinicians are urged to elicit the close cooperation and advice of the microbiology laboratory before attempting to collect anaerobic specimens. Aspiration of the cul-de-sac also may be performed by means of a small catheter that is inserted into the abdominal cavity through a 14-gauge needle which is placed through the posterior inferior fornix. Despite careful technique, cultures from the cul-de-sac may be contaminated by vaginal flora and thus may not accurately reflect the microbial flora in the fallopian tubes.

4. Laparoscopy cultures: Laparoscopy involves less risk from contamination when obtaining material for cultures. Exudates from the fallopian tubes may be obtained via laparoscopy. Specimens also may be taken from the lumina of the tubes. If the abdominal ostia of the fallopian tube is closed, then it is possible to puncture the os and aspirate the material. Physicians in the United States have been cautious about using the laparoscope as a routine method in the diagnosis of pelvic infections. In contrast, Swedish and other European physicians have used this instrument routinely in patients with suspected pelvic inflammatory disease.

Other diagnostic methods not generally available to venereal disease clinics include ultrasound, radio nuclides, and computerized tomography. These techniques may be helpful in identifying pelvic abscesses, a complication of pelvic inflammatory disease.

Perihepatitis or the Fitz-Hugh-Curtis syndrome is a complication of salpingitis caused both by <u>Neisseria gonorrhoeae</u> and <u>Chlamydia trachomatis</u>. In Scandinavian countries, perihepatitis is thought to be present in 5-10% of patients with acute pelvic inflammatory disease. The patients are women (with rare case reports in men) in their teens to mid-30s who may or may not have pelvic inflammatory disease. They typically have abrupt right or middle upper quadrant pain and signs of peritoneal irritations. Pain may be referred to the right shoulder. There is frequently hepatic tenderness or enlargement.

The liver function tests are elevated. Nausea, vomiting, low-grade fever, and a perihepatic friction rub also may be present.

As the disease progresses, "violin-string" adhesions appear between the anterior surface of the liver capsule and the anterior abdominal wall. This syndrome has to be distinguished from cholecystitis. The diagnosis is established in part by the presence of a positive gonococcal or chlamydial culture from a genital site, the clinical picture, and the response to therapy. Where available, laparoscopy is definitive. The liver surface may show fibrinous plaques, small hemorrhagic spots, and ultimately the "violin-string" adhesion.

TREATMENT

The treatment of pelvic inflammatory disease ideally should be directed to a specific microbial etiology. Unfortunately, the microbial causes of pelvic inflammatory disease do not produce distinct clinical syndromes in individual patients. Because of the diversity of etiologic agents and the paucity of definitive clinical studies, there are no universally agreed upon antibiotic regimens for the treatment of patients with pelvic inflammatory disease. In addition to antibiotic therapy, patients with pelvic inflammatory disease may require hospitalization. The indications for hospitalizing women with presumed acute salpingitis are outlined in Table 14.4.

The antibiotic therapies described below are taken from the Centers for Disease Control 1982 guidelines. There are undoubtedly regional differences in the etiology of pelvic inflammatory disease, and some centers have successfully treated their patients with one of the penicillin, ampicillin, or amoxicillin regimens. However, physicians are recognizing that Chlamydia trachomatis and anaerobes as well as gonococci are significant pathogens. Precision in therapy awaits precision in diagnosis in the collection of illnesses called pelvic inflammatory disease.

ANTIBIOTIC THERAPY FOR OUTPATIENTS

When the patient is not hospitalized, one of the following combination regimens is recommended:

Cefoxitin, 2.0 g, IM; or amoxicillin, 3.0 g, by mouth; or ampicillin, 3.5 g, by mouth; or aqueous procaine penicillin G,

Table 14.4   Indications for Hospitalization of Women with
Acute Salpingitis

---

1. Rebound tenderness indicating a possible surgical emergency
   (appendicitis)

2. Suspicion of a pelvic abscess or ectopic pregnancy

3. The patient is pregnant

4. The patient is too ill or otherwise unable to follow out-patient
   antibiotic therapy

5. The patient is not responsive to outpatient antibiotic therapy in
   48 hr

6. Clinical follow-up cannot be arranged after 48–72 hr of oral
   antibiotic therapy

7. The diagnosis is uncertain (e.g., mesenteric lymphadenitis,
   cholecystitis, pyelonephritis, or endometriosis)

4.8 million units, IM, at two sites; each along with probenecid
1.0 g, by mouth.

FOLLOWED BY

Doxycycline: 100 mg, by mouth, twice a day for 10–14 days

Tetracycline HCl 500 mg, by mouth, four times a day also
can be used but is less active against certain anaerobes and requires more frequent dosing; both represent drawbacks in the
treatment of PID.

Comment: Cefoxitin or an equivalently effective cephalosporin plus doxycycline (or tetracycline) provides activity against
N. gonorrhoeae, including PPNG, and C. trachomatis. PPNG-
associated PID, is not adequately treated with the combination of
either amoxicillin, ampicillin, or aqueous procaine penicillin plus
doxycycline.

ANTIBIOTIC THERAPY FOR
HOSPITALIZED PATIENTS

1. Doxycycline: 100 mg, IV, twice a day
                   PLUS
    Cefoxitin: 2.0 g, IV, four times a day

Continue drugs IV for at least four days and at least 48 hr after the patient defervesces. Continue doxycycline 100 mg, by mouth, twice a day after discharge from the hospital to complete 10-14 days of therapy.

Comment: This regimen provides optimal coverage for N. gonorrhoeae including PPNG, and C. trachomatis. It may not provide optimal treatment for anaerobes, pelvic mass, or PID associated with an intrauterine device (IUD).

2. Clindamycin: 600 mg, IV, four times a day
                   PLUS
    Gentamicin or tobramycin: 2.0 mg/kg, IV, followed by 1.5 mg/kg, IV, three times a day in patients with normal renal function.

Continue drugs IV for at least four days and at least 48 hr after the patient defervesces. Continue clindamycin 450 mg, by mouth, four times a day after discharge from the hospital to complete 10-14 days of therapy.

Comment: This regimen provides optimal activity against anaerobes and facultative gram-negative rods but may not provide optimal activity against C. trachomatis and N. gonorrhoeae.

3. Doxycycline: 100 mg, IV, twice a day
                   PLUS
    Metronidazole: 1.0 g, IV, twice a day

Continue drugs IV for at least four days and at least 48 hr after the patient defervesces. Then continue both drugs at same dosage orally to complete 10-14 days of therapy.

Comment: This provides excellent coverage for anaerobes and C. trachomatis. Both drugs can be continued for oral therapy. Activity against some strains of N. gonorrhoeae, including PPNG, and some facultative gram-negative rods is not optimal.

4. If the patient has pelvic inflammatory disease caused by penicillinase-producing <u>N. gonorrhoeae</u>, the patient ideally should be treated in the hospital. Based on limited information, the following therapies appear successful. For outpatients, give spectinomycin, 2 g IM daily for 7-10 days. For hospitalized patients, give cefoxitin, 2 g IM or IV every 8 hr for 7-10 days.

ANTIBIOTIC THERAPY FOR
PREGNANT PATIENTS

Because pelvic inflammatory disease in pregnancy is unusual, the best mode of therapy is unknown. Goodrich suggests that the penicillin regimens are safe and probably effective in the dosages recommended but that the tetracyclines (including doxycycline) are contraindicated. For penicillin-allergic patients he recommends a single IM dose of spectinomycin followed by IV erythromycin and then oral therapy until the patient is well. Estolate preparations of erythromycin should not be used in pregnant women.

MANAGEMENT OF SEXUAL PARTNERS

All persons who are sexual partners of patients with PID should be examined for STD and treated promptly with a regimen effective against uncomplicated gonococcal and chlamydial infection.

FOLLOW-UP

All patients treated as outpatients should be clinically reevaluated in 48-72 hr. Those not responding favorably should be hospitalized. For test of cure, a culture should be done as appropriate for pathogens initially isolated.

INTRAUTERINE DEVICE

The IUD is a risk factor for the development of PID. Although the exact effect of removing an IUD on the response of acute salpingitis to antimicrobial therapy and on the risk of recurrent salpingitis is unknown, removal of the IUD is recommended soon after antimicrobial therapy has been initiated. When an IUD is removed, contraceptive counseling is necessary.

Finally, patients should be counseled as to the recurrent nature and the adverse consequences of pelvic inflammatory disease.

BIBLIOGRAPHY

Adler MW, Belsey EH, O'Connor BH. Morbidity associated with pelvic inflammatory disease. Br J Vener Dis, 58:151-157, 1982.

Bowie WR, Jones H. Acute pelvic inflammatory disease in outpatients: Association with Chlamydia trachomatis and Neisseria gonorrhoeae. Ann Int Med, 95:685-688, 1981.

Burkman RT. Association between intrauterine device and pelvic inflammatory disease. Obstet Gynecol, 57:269-276, 1981.

Chow AW, Malkasian KL, Marshall JR, Guze LB. The bacteriology of acute pelvic inflammatory disease. Value of cul-de-sac cultures and relative importance of gonococci and other aerobic or anaerobic bacteria. Amer J Obstet Gynecol, 122:876-879, 1975.

Cunningham FG, Hauth JC, Gilstrap LC, Herbert WNP, Kappus SS. The bacterial pathogenesis of acute pelvic inflammatory disease. Obstet Gynecol, 52:161-164, 1978.

Cunningham FG, Hauth JC, Strong JD, Herbert WNP, Gilstrap LC, Wilson RH, Cappus SS. Evaluation of tetracycline or penicillin and ampicillin for treatment of acute pelvic inflammatory disease. N Eng J Med, 296:1380-1383, 1977.

Curran JW. Management of gonococcal pelvic inflammatory disease. Sex Transm Dis (Suppl.), 6:174-180, 1979.

Dalaker K, Gjønnaess H, Kville G, Urnes A, Anestad G, Bergan T. Chlamydia trachomatis as a cause of acute perihepatitis associated with pelvic inflammatory disease. Br J Vener Dis, 57: 41-43, 1981.

Darougar S, Forsey T, Wood JJ, Bolton JP, Allan A. Chlamydia and the Curtis-Fitz-Hugh syndrome. Br J Vener Dis, 58:391-394, 1981.

Eschenbach DA. New concepts of obstetric and gynecologic infection. Arch Int Med, 142:2039-2044, 1982.

Eschenbach DA, Buchanan TM, Pollack HM, Forsyth PS, Alexander ER, Lin JS, Wang SP, Wentworth BB, McCormack WM, Holmes KK. Polymicrobial etiology of acute pelvic inflammatory disease. N Eng J Med, 293:166-171, 1975.

Eschenbach DA, Harnisch JP, Holmes KK. Pathogenesis of acute pelvic inflammatory disease: Role of contraception and other risk factors. Amer J Obstet Gynecol, 128:838-850, 1977.

Gilstrap LC, Herbert WNP, Cunningham FG, Hauth JC, van Patton HG. Gonorrhea screening in male consorts of women with pelvic infection. J Amer Med Assoc, 238:965-966, 1977.

Goodrich JT. Pelvic inflammatory disease: Considerations related to therapy. Rev Infect Dis, 4(Suppl.):S778-S787, 1982.

Gump DW, Gibson M, Ashikaga T. Evidence of prior pelvic inflammatory disease and its relationship to Chlamydia trachomatis antibody and intrauterine contraceptive device use in infertile women. Amer J Obstet Gynecol, 146:153-159, 1983.

Hager WD, Eschenbach DA, Spence MR, Sweet RL. Criteria for diagnosing and grading salpingitis. Obstet Gynecol, 61:113-114, 1983.

Harding GKM, Buckwold FJ, Ronald AR, et al. Prospective randomized comparative study of clindamycin, chloramphenicol, and ticarcillin, each in combination with gentamicin, in therapy for intraabdominal and female genital tract sepsis. J Infect Dis, 142: 384-393, 1980.

Kaufman DW, Shapiro S, Rosenberg L, Monson RR, Miettinen OS, Stolley PD, Slone D. Intrauterine contraceptive device use in pelvic inflammatory disease. Amer J Obstet Gynecol, 136:159-162, 1980.

Kaufman DW, Watson J, Rosenberg L, et al. The effect of different types of intrauterine devices on the risk of pelvic inflammatory disease. J Amer Med Assoc, 250:759-762, 1983.

230 / Pelvic Inflammatory Disease

Kelaghan J, Rubin GL, Ory HW, Layde PM. Barrier-method contraceptives and pelvic inflammatory disease. J Amer Med Assoc, 248:184-187, 1982.

Koehler PR, Moss AA. Diagnosis of intra-abdominal and pelvic abscesses by computerized tomography. J Amer Med Assoc, 244: 49-52, 1980.

Lee NC, Rubin GL, Ory HW, Burkman RT. Type of intrauterine device and the risk of pelvic inflammatory disease. Obstet Gynecol, 62:1-6, 1983.

Litt IF, Cohen MI. Perihepatitis associated with salpingitis in adolescents. J Amer Med Assoc, 240:1253-1254, 1978.

Mårdh PA, Møller BR, Ingerselv HJ, Nüssler E, Weström L, Wølner-Hanssen P. Endometritis caused by Chlamydia trachomatis. Br J Vener Dis, 57:191-195, 1981.

Mårdh PA, Møller BR, Paavonen J. Chlamydial infection of the female genital tract with emphasis on pelvic inflammatory disease. A review of Scandinavian studies. Sex Transm Dis, 8(Suppl.):140-155, 1981.

McCormack WM, Nowroozi K, Alpert S, Sackel SG, Lee YH, Lowe BW, Rankin JS. Acute pelvic inflammatory disease. Characteristics of patients with gonococcal and nongonococcal infection and evaluation of their response to treatment with aqueous procaine penicillin G and spectinomycin hydrochloride. Sex Transm Dis, 4:125-131, 1977.

Møller BR, Mårdh P-A, Ahrons S, Nüssler E. Infection with Chlamydia trachomatis, Mycoplasma hominis and Neisseria gonorrhoeae in patients with acute pelvic inflammatory disease. Sex Transm Dis, 8:198-202, 1981.

Monif GRG. Significance of polymicrobial bacterial superinfection in the therapy of gonococcal endometritis-salpingitis-peritonitis. Obstet Gynecol, 55:154S-161S, 1980.

Monif GRG, Welkos SL, Baer H, Thompson RJ. Cul-de-sac isolates from patients with endometritis-salpingitis-peritonitis and gonococcal endocervicitis. Amer J Obstet Gynecol, 126:158-161, 1976.

Ossler S, Liedholm P, Gullberg B, Sjoberg HO. Risk of pelvic inflammatory disease among intrauterine-device users irrespective of previous pregnancy. Lancet, 2:386-388, 1980.

Ossler S, Persson K. Epidemiologic and serodiagnostic aspects of chlamydial salpingitis. Obstet Gynecol, 59:206-209, 1982.

Paavonen J, Saikku P, Vesterinen E, Aho K. Chlamydia trachomatis in acute salpingitis. Br J Vener Dis, 55:203-206, 1979.

Paavonen J, Saikku P, von Knorring J, Aho K, Wang SP. Association of infection with Chlamydia trachomatis with Fitz-Hugh-Curtis syndrome. J Infect Dis, 144:176, 1981.

Rendtorff RC, Curran JW, Chandler RW, Wiser WL, Robinson H. Economic consequences of gonorrhea in women: Experience from an urban hospital. J Amer Vener Dis Assoc, 1:40-47, 1974.

Rubin GL, Ory HW, Layde PM. Oral contraceptives and pelvic inflammatory disease. Amer J Obstet Gynecol, 144:630-635, 1982.

St. John RK (ed.). International symposium on pelvic inflammatory disease. Amer J Obstet Gynecol, 138(7):845-1112 (Part 2), 1980.

St. John RK, Blount J, Jones O. Pelvic inflammatory disease in the United States: Incidence and trends in private practice. Sex Transm Dis, 8:56-61, 1981.

St. John RK, Jones OG, Blount JH, Zaidi AA. Pelvic inflammatory disease in the United States: Epidemiology and trends among hospitalized women. Sex Transm Dis, 8:62-66, 1981.

Schafer MAB, Irwin CE, Sweet RL. Medical progress. Acute salpingitis in the adolescent female. J Ped, 100:339-350, 1982.

Sparks RA, Purrier BGA, Watt PJ, Elstein M. Bacteriological colonization of uterine cavity: Role of tailed intrauterine contraceptive device. Br Med J, 282:1189-1191, 1981.

Spence MR, Genadry R, Raffel L. Randomized prospective comparison of ampicillin and doxycycline in the treatment of acute pelvic inflammatory disease in hospitalized patients. Sex Transm Dis, 8:164-166, 1981.

Svensson L, Weström L, Mårdh P-A. Acute salpingitis with
Chlamydia trachomatis isolated from the Fallopian tubes: Clinical,
cultural and serologic findings. Sex Transm Dis, 8:51–55, 1981.

Sweet RL. Pelvic inflammatory disease; etiology, diagnosis, and
treatment. Sex Transm Dis, 8:308–315, 1981.

Sweet RL, Mills J, Hadley KW, Blumenstock E, Schacter J, Robbie MO, Draper DL. The use of laparoscopy to determine the
microbiologic etiology of acute salpingitis. Amer J Obstet Gynecol, 134:68–74, 1979.

Sweet RL, Schachter J, Robbie MO. Failure of beta-lactam antibiotics to eradicate Chlamydia trachomatis in the endometrium
despite apparent clinical cure of acute salpingitis. J Amer Med
Assoc, 250:2641–2645, 1983.

Thompson WE, Hager WD. Acute pelvic inflammatory disease.
Sex Transm Dis, 4:105–113, 1977.

Thompson SE, Hager WD, Wong KH, Lopez B, Ramsey C, Allen
SD, Stargel MD, Thornsberry C, Benigo BB, Thompson JD, Shul-
man JA. The microbiology and therapy of acute pelvic inflammatory disease in hospitalized patients. Amer J Obstet Gynecol, 136:
179–186, 1980.

Treharne JD, Ripa KT, Mårdh P-A, Svensson L, Weström L,
Darougar S. Antibodies to Chlamydia trachomatis in acute salpingitis. Br J Vener Dis, 55:26–29, 1979.

Vine HS, Birnholz JC. Ultrasound evaluation of pelvic pain.
J Amer Med Assoc, 244:2540–2542, 1980.

Weström L, Iosif S, Svensson L, Mårdh P-A. Infertility after
acute salpinigitis: Results of treatment with different antibiotics.
Curr Ther Res, 26:752–759, 1979.

Wølner-Hanssen P, Mårdh P-A, Svensson L, Weström L.
Laparoscopy in women with chlamydial infection and pelvic pain:
A comparison of patients with and without salpingitis. Obstet
Gynecol, 61:299–303, 1983.

Wølner-Hanssen P, Weström L, Mårdh P-A. Perihepatitis and
chlamydial salpingitis. Lancet, 1:901–904, 1980.

Chapter 15

PELVIC ACTINOMYCOSIS

ETIOLOGIC AGENT

Pelvic actinomycosis usually is the result of infection by
Actinomyces israelii, a gram-positive, nonspore-forming, fila-
mentous bacterium that is best grown anaerobically. Other pathogenic actinomyces species include Actinomyces naeslundii, Actinomyces odontolyticus, and Arachnia propionica (formally designated
as an Actinomyces). Actinomyces infections are believed to be
endogenous infections since these bacilli inhabit the oral cavity,
gastrointestinal tract, genitourinary tract, and skin. Cervico-
facial infections generally follow dental infections. Thoracic infection follows aspiration of infected oral material. Abdominal actinomycosis generally results from some disruption of the intestine or
abdominal surgery. Actinomyces israelii is not known to be sexually transmitted; however, pelvic infections with this organism
occur in women who are using intrauterine contraceptive devices.

CLINICAL MANIFESTATIONS

Colonization of the cervix by Actinomyces-like organisms is
more common in women who wear plastic in comparison to copper-
containing intrauterine contraceptive devices. The reason for this
is unknown. The longer the time that the intrauterine device is in
place, the higher the incidence of colonization with Actinomyces
species. The incidence of Actinomyces-like organisms in cervical
smears of women wearing intrauterine devices is approximately
10-30%. Recent reports show that 20-27% of women without intrauterine devices also may be colonized by Actinomyces species.

Patients who are colonized have no symptoms. Disease by <u>Actino-myces</u> species is uncommon but may occur in women wearing both the plastic and the metal devices. Pelvic actinomycosis causes chronic suppurative granulomatous lesions in soft tissue with the development of sinus tracts. There are few signs that are diagnostic of pelvic actinomycosis. Presentations may include pain associated with a lower abdominal mass, postmenopausal bleeding, pelvic inflammatory disease, or abdominal abscess. The findings of pelvic examination may be indistinguishable from those seen in chronic pelvic inflammatory disease. Because of the indolent nature of the disease, pelvic actinomycosis may progress to the point of irreversible damage by the time of diagnosis.

DIAGNOSIS

A presumptive diagnosis may be made by pap smear of vaginal or cervical secretions or histologic section. The gross lesions found by surgical exploration usually are single or multiple abscesses or indurated masses with firm fibrous walls and soft central locations containing white or yellow pus. Microscopically, a typical abscess has an outer zone of granulation surrounding central purulent loculations containing one to six granules. In most cases large macrophages with foamy cytoplasm accumulate around the purulent centers. The "sulfur granules" are visible manifestations of aggregated micro-organisms. Macroscopically, they are yellow to dull white in color and are hard in consistency. They average approximately 2 mm in diameter. Microscopically, those seen in actinomycosis infections are round or oval in shape and have a radiating fringe of eosinophilic club-like structures on the surface. Unfortunately, not all actinomycosis infections result in granule formation. In many cases the granules are few and hard to find, particularly in vaginal infections. Sulfur granules also are not specific for actinomycosis but may be found with certain fungi, <u>Nocardia</u>, <u>Streptomyces</u>, and other organisms including <u>Staphylococcus aureus</u>. The pathologic diagnosis of pelvic actinomycosis may not be made until multiple sections of material are carefully examined under the microscope.

The definitive diagnosis is made by means of a positive culture. Material taken for culture requires meticulous handling in that the organisms require anaerobic conditions. However, <u>A. israelii</u> sometimes will grow under microaerophilic conditions. Commonly abscesses may contain a number of other anaerobic

organisms in addition to the <u>Actinomyces</u> species. Material taken
from abscesses also may be gram-stained, and the diagnosis may
be suspected if branching gram-positive filaments are identified.
Where available, direct immunofluorescent isothiocyanate-labeled
antisera against <u>A. israelii</u> is both sensitive and specific and may
be a method of choice for positive identification of material taken
from a cervical swab.

There are no serologic tests nor is there a skin test for actinomycosis. The presence of an abdominal abscess may be localized
by means of radionuclides or computerized tomography.

THERAPY

If there is evidence of <u>Actinomyces</u> colonization in a vaginal
smear of a woman who is using an intrauterine device, the device
should be removed and some other means of contraception substituted. The risk of colonization in these women is unknown.
Vaginal cytology should be repeated in 1 month to 6 weeks after
removal of the device to ascertain if the colonization still persists.
Removal of the device in a colonized patient may be the safest
course given the indolent and progressive nature of the disease.
Antibiotic therapy probably is not indicated in such asymptomatic
women. The standard therapy for patients with local or systemic
disease includes excision of the necrotic, infected tissue and intensive and prolonged antibiotic therapy. In patients who have intrauterine devices in place, these should be removed and some other
form of contraception advised.

Although many forms of actinomycosis do not require surgery,
pelvic actinomycosis generally requires surgical drainage of
abscesses and removal of sinuses if they are present. Penicillin
is a drug of choice. Penicillin G, 10-20 million units per day, is
given intravenously for 1 month to 6 weeks followed by oral phenoxy-
methyl penicillin, 2-4 g per day for another 6 months or a year.
Some patients may not be able to tolerate this much oral penicillin,
and the dosage may have to be reduced. In patients who fail on
penicillin therapy or who are allergic to penicillin, other drugs
may be attempted. These include erythromycin, chloramphenicol,
and tetracycline.

BIBLIOGRAPHY

Brenner R, Gehring SW. Pelvic actinomycosis in the presence of an endocervical contraceptive device. Obstet Gynecol, 29:71-73, 1967.

Brown JR. Human actinomycosis. A study of 181 subjects. Hum Pathol, 4:319-330, 1973.

Brown R, Bancewicz J. Ureteric obstruction due to pelvic actino-mycosis. Br J Surg, 69:156, 1982.

Curtis EM, Pine L. Actinomyces in the vaginas of women with and without intrauterine contraceptive devices. Amer J Obstet Gynecol, 140:880-883, 1981.

Duguid HLD, Parratt D, Traynor R. Actinomyces-like organisms in cervical smears from women using intrauterine contraceptive devices. Br Med J, 281:534-537, 1980.

Grice GC, Hafiz S. Actinomyces in the female genital tract. A preliminary report. Br J Vener Dis, 59:317-319, 1983.

Gupta PB, Woodruff JD. Actinomyces in vaginal smears. J Amer Med Assoc, 247:1175-1176, 1982.

Gupta PK, Hollander DH, Frost JK. Actinomycetes in cervico-vaginal smears: An association with IUD usage. Acta Cytol, 20:295-297, 1976.

Keebler C, Chatwani A, Schwartz R. Actinomycosis infection associated with intrauterine contraceptive devices. Amer J Obstet Gynecol, 145:596-599, 1983.

Kelly J, Aaron J. Pelvic actinomycosis and usage of intrauterine contraceptive devices. Yale J Biol Med, 55:453-461, 1982.

Luff RD, Gupta PK, Spence MR, Frost JK. Pelvic actinomycosis and the intrauterine contraceptive device. A cyto-histomorphologic study. Amer J Clin Pathol, 69:581-586, 1978.

de la Monte SM, Gupta PK, White EL. Systemic actinomyces infection. A potential complication of intrauterine contraceptive devices. J Amer Med Assoc, 248:1876-1877, 1982.

Pine L, Malcolm GB, Curtis EM, Brown JM. Demonstration of
Actinomyces and Arachnia species in cervicovaginal smears by
direct staining with species-specific fluorescent-antibody conjugate.
J Clin Microbiol, 13:15-21, 1981.

Schiffer MA, Elguezabal A, Sultana M, Allen AC. Actinomycosis
infections associated with intrauterine contraceptive devices.
Obstet Gynecol, 45:67-72, 1975.

Sonnenwirth AC, Dowell VR, Jr. Gram-positive nonsporeforming
anaerobic bacilli. In Lennette EH, Balows A, Hausler WJ, Truant
JP (eds.), Manual of Clinical Microbiology, 3rd ed., American
Society for Microbiology, Washington, DC, 1980, pp. 440-445.

Valicenti JF, Pappas AA, Graber CD, Williamson HO, Willis NF.
Detection and prevalence of IUD-associated Actinomyces colonization and related morbidity. A prospective study of 69,925 cervical
smears. J Amer Med Assoc, 247:1149-1152, 1982.

Chapter 16

CYTOMEGALOVIRUS INFECTIONS

ETIOLOGIC AGENT

The cytomegalovirus is a member of the herpesvirus family.
It is DNA virus that was discovered in 1956 in children with cyto-
megalic inclusion disease. The virus exhibits a marked degree of
host specificity. For example, viruses found in Old World mon-
keys do not infect humans. The cytomegaloviruses of humans,
however, are not all alike. Unfortunately, there is no useful taxonomic subdivision which has clinical utility, such as that of the
type 1 and type 2 herpesviruses.

EPIDEMIOLOGY

Cytomegalovirus is widely distributed in human populations
in all areas of the world. The majority of adult individuals have
serologic evidence of cytomegalovirus infection. The age at which
an individual acquires the virus is not always the same, and individuals living in crowded conditions are more likely to have cytomegalovirus infection early in life. Once infection takes place,
viral excretion may continue for many weeks, months, or years.
Cytomegalovirus has been identified in urine, cervical secretions,
semen, saliva, breast milk, blood, and feces. As far as long-
term excretion is concerned, urine and perhaps cervical secretions
and semen may be the most important epidemiologically. Urine
may contain as many as 1 million infectious units of cytomegalovirus per milliliter. In large population studies, the virus has
been found in approximately 5% of children, 1-2% of young adults,
10% of pregnant women, and more than half of renal transplant

recipients or other immunocompromised patients. Cytomegalovirus infection is common in homosexual men.

There is some evidence indicating that the condition of pregnancy may change the host-parasite relationship. In the first trimester of normal pregnancy, the cervix is positive on culture in 0-2%. By the third trimester, the cervix is positive in approximately 12-28%. The latter figures are more consistent with excretion in individuals in the nonpregnant state. Investigators have argued that cytomegalovirus, rather than becoming active from a latent state during pregnancy, is in fact suppressed early in pregnancy.

Cytomegalovirus may be transmitted by sexual intercourse. The importance of this mode of transmission with respect to the widespread nature of this virus is unknown. The evidence for sexual transmission rests on case reports identifying cytomegalovirus in the urine, semen, and cervical secretions of the affected individuals and the development of a clearly identifiable syndrome associated with the virus cytomegalovirus mononucleosis. Case reports have indicated that cytomegalovirus may be present in the semen for more than 1 year. About 5-10% of women attending venereal disease clinics excrete cytomegalovirus. The percentage of black women excreters is higher than in comparable white women attending venereal disease clinics. Other evidence that cytomegalovirus may be transmitted sexually comes from studies of nuns. Nuns do not show the expected abrupt rise in antibody prevalence during young adulthood, and the prevalence of antibody to cytomegalovirus in this group is significantly lower than in other groups at all but the lowest comparable age range. Serologic evidence for cytomegalovirus infection is more frequent in homosexual than in heterosexual men.

CLINICAL MANIFESTATIONS

Cytomegalovirus infection was first identified in infants. Surveys in the United States and England indicate that approximately 1% of infants have active infection demonstrated by the presence of viruria. Approximately one in ten of these infants will have clinical manifestations, and these are not always apparent at birth. The full-blown syndrome of cytomegalovirus infection in infants includes splenomegaly, hepatomegaly, microcephaly, mental retardation, motor disability, petechiae, jaundice, chorioretinitis, and cerebral calcification. As the child grows older, hearing loss and minor neurologic or developmental abnormalities may be noticed that ultimately cause learning difficulties. Congenitally acquired infections may occur in consecutive pregnancies. Acquired cytomegalovirus infection in children between 3 and 6 months of age may manifest intself with pneumonitis, hepatosplenomegaly, or adenopathy.

Cytomegalovirus in adults may be transmitted by oral secretions, sexual contact, or blood transfusion. Cytomegalovirus in young adults may cause a syndrome that may be confused with infectious mononucleosis. The illness is characterized by malaise, fatigue, myalgia, mild sore throat, and fever, often as high as 39.4°C (103°F). The liver is regularly affected, but jaundice or hepatomegaly is uncommon. The illness may last from 2 to 6 weeks. In a small percentage of patients there may be splenomegaly. The commonest signs are pharyngeal erythema, lymphadenopathy and, occasionally, rash. A morbilliform rash frequently occurs in individuals with cytomegalovirus infection who receive ampicillin. The mechanism for this is not known.

Most individuals with cytomegalovirus mononucleosis are able to return to their regular activities within 8 weeks of the onset of the illness. The major laboratory finding in these patients is the presence of lymphocytosis with abundant atypical lymphocytes. The white blood cell count ranges from 6000 to 38,000 with a mean of 13,000. The percentage of lymphocytes ranges from 55 to 86% with a mean of 71%. The percentage of atypical lymphocytes ranges from 12 to 55% with a mean of 22%. Relative and absolute lymphocytosis without the appearance of atypical lymphocytes may persist for many months. Also, abnormal liver function tests occur in the majority of individuals, and these return to normal in about 4-6 weeks without residual damage.

Certain patients with cytomegalovirus mononucleosis develop abnormal serologic reactions including antinuclear antibodies, rheumatoid factor, cold agglutinins, and cryoglobulins. Lung involvement is uncommon in normal hosts. Myocarditis and pericarditis also are infrequent. Urinary retention has been described as a complication of acute cytomegalovirus infection. Cytomegalovirus infections are quite common in renal and bone marrow transplant recipients. The most common manifestation in these compromised individuals is pneumonitis. In such individuals it is quite common to have infections with a number of pathogens, and the contribution of individual agents often is hard to define.

DIAGNOSIS

Cytomegalovirus mononucleosis may be suspected because of
the clinical manifestations as well as the laboratory findings of
lymphocytosis, atypical lymphocytes, and abnormal liver function
tests. However, confirmation of the diagnosis rests on virus isolation or the results of virus serologic testing. The isolation of
cytomegalovirus presents some difficulties, because this virus is
heat-labile (56°C for 30 min), unstable at pH < 5, and susceptible
to freezing and thawing in the absence of stabilizers. The virus
can be stored at -90°C in the presence of 35% sorbitol. Because of
this instability, it is preferable to culture fresh specimens. The
specimens should be delivered to the virus diagnostic laboratory
as quickly as possible after collection. Until processed, the specimens may be kept at 4°C in a refrigerator. Samples of semen,
urine, saliva, or cervical fluid on swabs are likely to yield the
highest return.

Viruria has been detected for 22-51 weeks in some patients
following cytomegalovirus mononucleosis. Cytomegalovirus can
be recovered from blood early in the course of the illness. The
best results are when both lymphocytes and neutrophils are cultured by means of a density gradient system. This virus can be
isolated and propagated only in human fibroblast cells derived from
embryonic tissues. These cells are grown in medium containing
antibiotics to prevent bacterial contamination. Another problem
associated with cytomegalovirus isolation is that the virus may
require many days for detection of the characteristic cytopathic
effect on the tissue culture cells. The cytopathic effect may take
from 3 to 30 days or longer to be seen. The development of cytopathic effect is related to the amount of virus in the inoculum.
Once the cytopathic effect is seen, many laboratories will confirm
its identity as a cytomegalovirus by means of serologic tests.

The serologic diagnosis of cytomegalovirus is most commonly performed by complement fixation or neutralization tests.
Fluorescent antibody tests for the detection of IgG or IgM antibody
also are available. In both the complement fixation test and the
neutralization test, a titer of 1:8 or greater is considered positive
for cytomegalovirus antibody. Because this antibody is so widespread in the population, a single serologic titer is of little diagnostic value in establishing infection by cytomegalovirus. Approximately 80% of adults over the age of 35 are seropositive. Evidence
for diagnosis is the appearance of a fourfold or greater rise in

complement fixation antibody titer. In patients with cytomegalovirus mononucleosis, the maximum antibody titer rise may take 6
weeks. The presence in the fluorescent antibody test of IgM antibody to cytomegalovirus is suggestive of a recent infection if the
titer is 1:16 or greater. Because of the ubiquity of this virus, one
should be cautious in ascribing disease unless the serologic diagnosis is confirmed by virus isolation.

Cytologic methods may be used to identify cells containing
intranuclear inclusions in urinary sediment or tissue sections.
However, this method is neither very sensitive nor very specific
for the diagnosis of cytomegalovirus infection. The electron
microscope may be used to identify the virus in urine samples.
Although this method may be performed very rapidly, it is not as
sensitive or as specific as culture of the virus.

THERAPY

At the moment there is no effective therapy for cytomegalovirus infection. Prevention by vaccination has been proposed, and
an experimental live virus vaccine has been developed for renal
transplant candidates. It is too early to say if this approach will
have general applicability.

BIBLIOGRAPHY

Chretien JH, McGinniss CG, Muller A. Venereal causes of cytomegalovirus mononucleosis. J Amer Med Assoc, 238:1644-1645,
1977.

Clarke J, Craig RM, Saffro R, Murphy P, Yokoo H. Cytomegalovirus granulomatous hepatitis. Amer J Med, 66:264-269, 1979.

Davis LE, Stewart JA, Garvin S. Cytomegalovirus infection: A
seroepidemiologic comparison of nuns and women from a venereal
disease clinic. Amer J Epidemiol, 102:327-330, 1975.

Drew WL, Mintz L, Miner RC, Sands M, Ketterer B. Prevalence
of cytomegalovirus infection in homosexual men. J Infect Dis, 143:
188-192, 1981.

Glazer JP, Friedman HM, Grossman RA, Starr SE, Barker CF, Perloff LJ, Huang ES, Plotkin SA. Live cytomegalovirus vaccination of renal transplant candidates. A preliminary trial. Ann Int Med, 91:676-683, 1979.

Jordan MC, Rousseau WE, Noble GR, Stewart JA, Chin TDY. Association of cervical cytomegalovirus with venereal disease. N Eng J Med, 288:932-934, 1973.

Jordan MC, Rousseau WE, Steward JA, Noble GR, Chin TDY. Spontaneous cytomegalovirus mononucleosis. Clinical and laboratory observations in nine cases. Ann Int Med, 79:153-160, 1973.

Klemola E, Von Essen R, Wager O, Haltia K, Koivuniemi A, Salmi I. Cytomegalovirus mononucleosis in previously healthy individuals. Five new cases and follow-up of 13 previously published cases. Ann Int Med, 71:11-20, 1969.

Lang, DL. Cytomegalovirus immunization: Status, prospects, and problems. Rev Infect Dis, 2:449-458, 1980.

Lang DJ, Kummer JF. Cytomegalovirus in semen: Observations in selected populations. J Infect Dis, 132:472-473, 1975.

Lee FK, Nahmias AJ, Stagno S. Rapid diagnosis of cytomegalovirus infection in infants by electron microscopy. N Eng J Med, 299:1266-1270, 1978.

Levin MJ, Rinaldo CR, Leary PL, Zaia JA, Hirsch MS. Immune response to herpes virus antigens in adults with acute cytomegaloviral mononucleosis. J Infect Dis, 140:851-857, 1979.

Luby JP, Shasby DM. A sex difference in the prevalence of antibodies to cytomegalovirus. J Amer Med Assoc, 222:1290-1291, 1972.

Michaelson RA, Benson GS, Friedman HM. Urinary retention as the presenting symptom of acquired cytomegalovirus infection. Amer J Med, 74:526-528, 1983.

Mintz L, Drew WL, Miner RC, Braff EH. Cytomegalovirus infections in homosexual men. An epidemiological study. Ann Int Med, 99:326-329, 1983.

Osborn JE. Cytomegalovirus: Pathogenicity, immunology, and vaccine initiatives. J Infect Dis, 143:618-630, 1981.

Smith TF. Cytomegalovirus infections: Current diagnostic methods. Mayo Clin Proc, 56:767, 1981.

Stagno A, Reynolds DW, Huang ES, Thames SD, Smith RJ, Alford CA, Jr. Congenital cytomegalovirus. Occurrence in an immune population. N Eng J Med, 296:1254-1258, 1977.

Stagno S, Reynolds D, Tsiantos A, Fuccillo DA, Smith R, Tiller M, Alford CA. Cervical cytomegalovirus excretion in pregnant and nonpregnant women: Suppression in early gestation. J Infect Dis, 131:522-527, 1975.

Waner JL, Hopkins DR, Weller TH, Alfred EN. Cervical excretion of cytomegalovirus: Correlation with secretory and humoral antibody. J Infect Dis, 136:805-809, 1977.

Willmott FE. Cytomegalovirus in female patients attending a VD clinic. Br J Vener Dis, 51:278-280, 1975.

Chapter 17

CHANCROID

ETIOLOGIC AGENT

Chancroid is the result of an infection with the microorganism
Haemophilus ducreyi. H. ducreyi is a small, pleomorphic, nonmotile, nonsporulating gram-negative rod. Until recently it has
been difficult to cultivate, and not much is known about its metabolism and pathophysiology. Recent improvements in laboratory
media have made diagnosis easier.

EPIDEMIOLOGY

Chancroid may be found in Southeast Asia, Africa, and the
West Indies but is uncommon in the United States. The Centers for
Disease Control reported 850 cases in the year 1981. However,
240 patients with culture-confirmed chancroid were identified in
1982 in Orange County, California. The majority of the men were
Hispanic, recent immigrants from Mexico, and most had recent
sexual contact with a prostitute.

In past years in the United States, the disease was seen more
commonly in blacks than in whites. The male-to-female ratio is
approximately 10:1. Why this is so is not clear. Possibly women
may have unrecognized asymptomatic cervical or vaginal lesions,
or some women may constitute a reservoir of the bacillus while
remaining free of the disease. A more recent study by Lykke-
Olesen et al. showed a male to female ratio of 1.6:1, and they did
not believe that symptom-free female carriers were an important
reservoir of infection. In Nairobi, Kenya, prostitutes are the
most important reservoir of the disease.

Plasmids with various molecular weights have been used to "fingerprint" H. ducreyi isolates. By use of this molecular epidemiology, Hansfield et al. showed person-to-person transmission of this micro-organism.

Infection is more common in uncircumcised men. Previous chancroid infection does not result in immunity to reinfections. Chancroid probably is not transmitted by fomites or other nonsexual contact. Postcoital washing does not prevent chancroid.

CLINICAL MANIFESTATIONS

H. ducreyi is inoculated into the skin at sites of sexual contact. The incubation period from inoculation to the appearance of

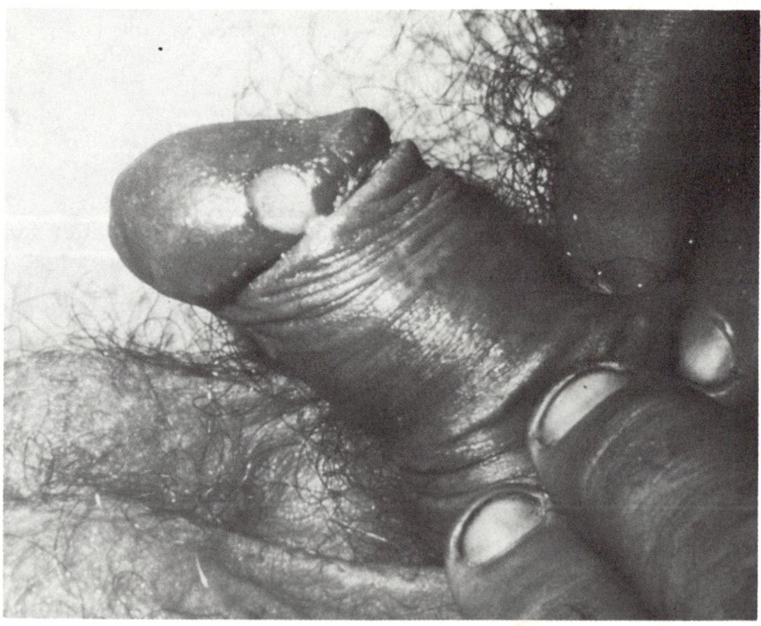

Figure 17.1 Ulcer of chancroid on the penis. Chancroid is caused by Haemophilus ducreyi and is uncommon in the United States. The ulcer of chancroid is usually a sharply circumscribed ulcer with an irregular edge. The base may be covered with a purulent exudate. Photograph courtesy of the Venereal Disease Control Program, CDC, USPHS.

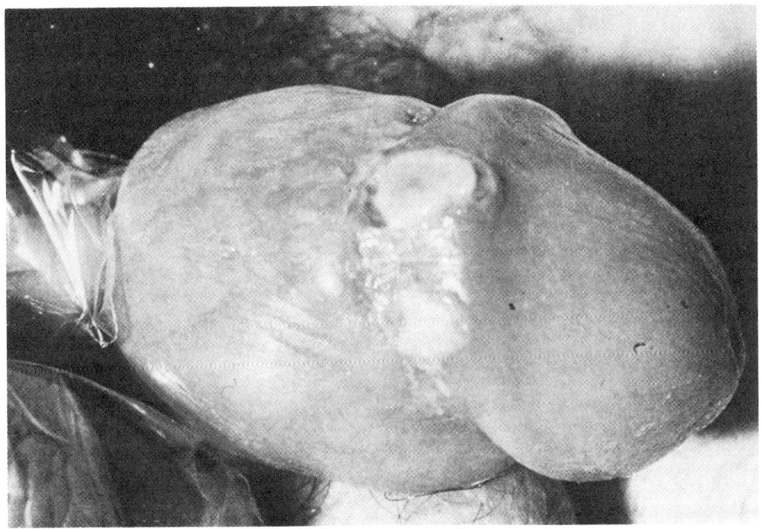

Figure 17.2   Ulcer of chancroid in the coronal sulcus of the penis.
The edge of the ulcer is soft and not indurated. Multiple lesions
are present in at least one-third of patients. Photograph courtesy
of E. Stolz and J. van der Stek.*

a lesion is four to five days, but may take up to 2 weeks. There is
a rapid progression from an initial vesicle-like pustule covered by
a fragile membrane to a sharply circumscribed ulcer with an irregular edge. The base of the ulcer may be covered with a gray
purulent exudate. The ulcer edge is soft and not indurated. There
is some surrounding inflammation. Multiple lesions are present
in at least one-third of the patients, and apposing lesions from
autoinoculation are common. In men the ulcers commonly are
located on the frenulum and sulcus, the internal surface of the prepuce, the preputial margin, the glans penis, the corona, and the
shaft of the penis (see Figs. 17.1 and 17.2). In women the ulcers
are present most frequently on the labia, clitoris, fourchette,
vestibule, the perianal area and the medial aspect of the thighs.
The oropharynx may be a reservoir of both symptomatic and asymptomatic H. ducreyi infection.

The ulcers average 0.5 cm in diameter but may vary in size
from 1 mm to 2 cm. A pathologic description of an ulcer of 2-3
weeks duration is as follows. The ulcer is shallow and only 2 or
3 mm in depth. There is a surface zone of necrotic tissue

containing largely polymorphonuclear leukocytes and debris. Beneath the surface zone there is an area of edematous tissue and proliferating blood vessels with occasional thrombosis. Below this is a deep layer of cellular infiltration with large numbers of plasma cells and, in older lesions, lymphocytes.

Pain caused by a genital ulceration may be the patient's presenting complaint. Men may have edema of the prepuce, phimosis, and paraphimosis. Unilateral inguinal adenopathy is present in one-quarter to one-half of patients with chancroid. Enlarged lymph nodes appear approximately 1 week after the ulcer and may form bubos which may suppurate. In patients with bubos, one-fifth are bilateral. Enlarged nodes are not necessarily tender to palpation, but bubos are. Ulcerating lesions may ring the coronal sulcus.

The complications of chancroid are destructive and disfiguring. Scars may narrow the preputial opening, requiring circumcision. Secondary infection may result in destructive ulceration. The prepuce may have triangular defects resulting from destructive ulceration. Destructive ulceration also may cause a urethral fistula in the glans penis. Matted inguinal nodes may rupture to form a large ulcerating skin lesions.

DIAGNOSIS

With the advent of newer media, the chance of a diagnosis of chancroid has improved. The genital ulcers are invariably superinfected with a myriad of other bacteria, predominantly gram-negative rods. At present there is no universally accepted diagnostic culture medium to enhance the growth of H. ducreyi and suppress the other competing micro-organisms. Despite the contamination with gram-negative rods, Gram stains of the exudate from ulcers are of some value. The "school-of-fish" configuration of gram-negative rods in the exudate of the ulcer is found in less than half of cases of chancroid. Pus aspirated from a bubo should be attempted as a source of material for culture.

Before a sample is taken, the ulcer base must be thoroughly cleaned with a gauze pad moistened with normal saline. The sample is taken from the cleaned ulcer base with a cotton swab moistened with saline, which is then immediately streaked on the surface of a plate containing chocolate ager, 1% iso VitaleX, and vancomycin, 3 μg/ml. Other investigators advise the use of culture media containing defibrinated rabbit blood, human blood, haemoglobin or haemin. H. ducreyi is identified in Gram-stained smears following growth in the laboratory medium. Microscopically, it is a small coccoid-bacillary rod, 1-2 μm in length and 0.5 μm wide. When observed from an in vivo source, H. ducreyi is present in pairs and short chains, often paralleling shreds of mucus. In liquid cultures the organisms appear in chains and in long parallel rows ("school of fish" pattern). Consultation with a microbiologist prior to collecting the specimen is imperative since H. ducreyi is so difficult to isolate.

Biopsy as a method of diagnosis should be reserved for resistant cases or when a malignancy is suspected. Currently there is no available serologic test or skin test antigen. Autoinoculation as a method of diagnosis has fallen into disrepute. A dark-field examination and serologic test for syphilis should be performed on all patients with genital ulcers. It is possible that a fluorescent antibody test for H. ducreyi may be available in the future.

TREATMENT

Patients should be treated with local cleansing and soaks of the ulcer and with measures to reduce edema of the prepuce if this is a problem. Retraction of a foreskin is contraindicated in the presence of preputial edema. If circumcision is required it should be delayed until after antibiotic therapy because of the possibility of autoinoculation into the suture line.

Sulfonamides, because of the development of resistance, are no longer the drug of choice. Erythromycin is effective: 500 mg by mouth four times a day. Trimethoprim/sulfamethoxazole, double strength tablet (160/800 mg), is also effective when given by mouth twice a day. For both erythromycin and trimethoprim/ sulfamethoxazole the therapy should be continued for a minimum of ten days and until ulcers and/or lymph nodes have healed. If the patient does not respond to the antibiotic therapy, then susceptibility testing should be performed on the H. ducreyi isolate. Plummer et al. showed that a single dose of trimethoprim-sulfametrole (640/3200 mg) taken orally is inexpensive and effective.

Undoubtedly there may be regional variation in susceptibility of H. ducreyi to various antibiotic regimens. Other antimicrobial agents to which most H. ducreyi are susceptible include clindamycin, rifampin, the aminoglycosides (gentamicin, tobramycin, and amikacin), cefotaxime, and cefoxitin. Appropriate regimens for these antibiotics have not been clearly defined.

Ampicillin and penicillin are ineffective in <u>H. ducreyi</u> infection because many isolates contain beta-lactamase-producing plasmids. However, amoxicillin given with clavulanic acid, a potent beta-lactamase inhibitor, is useful in the therapy of beta-lactamase producing <u>H. ducreyi</u>. The drugs are present in a capsule containing a fixed combination: amoxicillin 250 mg and clavulanic acid 125 mg. The patient takes two capsules orally three times a day for seven days.

Bubos have been observed to develop during treatment, and treatment may not prevent suppuration of the bubo. For this reason bubos should be frequently aspirated with a large-bore needle during therapy. Aspiration may prevent spontaneous drainage.

Sexual partners of patients with chancroid should be examined for a sexually transmitted disease. Those without chancroid should be epidemiologically treated with erythromycin or trimethoprim-sulfamethoxazole for ten days as described above.

BIBLIOGRAPHY

Bilgeri YR, Ballard RC, Duncan MO, Mauff AC, Koornhof HJ. Antimicrobial susceptibility of 103 strains of <u>Haemophilus ducreyi</u> isolated in Johannesburg. Antimicrob Agents Chemother, 22:686-688, 1982.

Brunton JL, MacLean I, Ronald AR, Albritton WL. Plasmid-mediated ampicillin resistance in <u>Haemophilus ducreyi</u>. Antimicrob Agent Chemother, 15:294-299, 1979.

Carpenter JL, Back A, Gehle D, Oberhoffer T. Treatment of chancroid with erythromycin. Sex Transm Dis, 8:192-197, 1981.

Centers for Disease Control. Chancroid-California. Morbid Mortal Weekly Rep, 31:173-175, 1982.

Centers for Disease Control. Sexually transmitted diseases treatment guidelines-1982. Morbid Mortal Weekly Rep, 31:35S-60S, 1982.

Duncan MO, Bilgeri YR, Fehler HG, Ballard RC. Treatment of chancroid with erythromycin. Br J Vener Dis, 59:265-268, 1983.

Fast MV, Nsanze H, D'Costa LJ, et al. Antimicrobial therapy of chancroid: An evaluation of five treatment regimens correlated with in vitro sensitivity. Sex Transm Dis, 10:1-6, 1983.

Fast MV, Nsanze H, D'Costa LJ, et al. Treatment of chancroid by clavulanic acid with amoixicillin in patients with B-lactamse-positive Haemophilus ducreyi infection. Lancet, 2:509-511, 1982.

Fast MV, Nsanze H, Plummer FA, D'Costa LJ, MacLean IW, Ronald AR. Treatment of chancroid. A comparison of sulphameth-oxazole and trimethoprim-sulpha-methoxazole. Br J Vener Dis, 59:320-324, 1983.

Fitzpatrick JE, Tyler H, Gramstand D. Treatment of chancroid. Comparison of sulfamethoxazole-trimethoprim with recommended therapies. J Amer Med Assoc, 246:1804-1805, 1981.

Hafiz S, Kinghorn GR, McEntegart MG. Chancroid in Sheffield. A report of 22 cases diagnosed by isolating Haemophilus ducreyi in a modified medium. Br J Vener Dis, 57:382-386, 1981.

Hammond GW, Lian CJ, Wilt JC, Albritton WL, Ronald AR. Determination of the hemin requirement of Haemophilus ducreyi: Evaluation of the porphyrin test and media used in the satellite growth test. J Clin Microbiol, 7:243-246, 1978.

Hammond GW, Lian CJ, Wilt JC, Ronald AR. Antimicrobial sus-ceptibility of Haemophilus ducreyi. Antimicrob Agent Chemother, 13:608-612, 1978.

Hammond GW, Lian CJ, Wilt JC, Ronald AR. Comparison of specimen collection and laboratory techniques for isolation of Haemophilus ducreyi. J Clin Microbiol, 7:39-43, 1978.

Hammond GW, Slutchuk M, Scatliff J, Sherman F, Wilt SC, Ron-ald AR. Epidemiologic, clinical, laboratory, and therapeutic fea-tures of an urban outbreak of chancroid in North America. Rev Infect Dis, 2:867-879, 1980.

Hannah P, Greenwood JR. Isolation and rapid identification of Haemophilus ducreyi. J Clin Microbiol, 16:861-864, 1982.

Hansfield HH, Totten PA, Fennel CL, Falkow S, Holmes KK. Molecular epidemiology of Haemophilus ducreyi infections. Ann Int Med, 95:315-318, 1981.

Hart G. Chancroid, donovanosis and lymphogranuloma venereum. Department of Health, Education and Welfare, Publication No. CDC, 75:8302, Centers for Disease Control, Atlanta, 1975.

Kilian M. Haemophilus. Chapter 25 in EH Lennette, A Balows, WJ Hausler, JP Truant (eds.). Manual of Clinical Microbiology, 3rd ed. American Society for Microbiology, Washington, DC, 1980.

Kinghorn GR, Hafiz S. McEntegart MG. Oropharyngeal Haemophilus ducreyi infection. Br Med J, 287:650, 1983.

Kinghorn GR, Hafiz S, McEntegart MG. Pathogenic microbial flora of genital ulcers in Sheffield with particular reference to herpes simplex virus and Haemophilus ducreyi. Br J Vener Dis, 58: 377-380, 1982.

Kraus SJ, Kaufman HW, Albritton WL, Thomsberry C, Biddle JW. Chancroid therapy: A review of cases confirmed by culture. Rev Infect Dis, 4(Suppl.):S848-S856, 1982.

Kraus SJ, Werman BS, Biddle JW, Sottnek FO, Ewing EP. Pseudogranuloma inguinale caused by Haemophilus ducreyi. Arch Dermatol, 118:494-497, 1982.

Latif AS. Thiamphenicol in the treatment of chancroid in men. Br J Vener Dis, 58:54-55, 1982.

Luders G, Braun J, Pietzcker F, Schule D. Neue therapeutische Gesichtspunkte beim Ulcus molle. Hautartz, 26:35-40, 1975.

Lykke-Olesen L, Larsen L, Pedersen TG, Gaarslev K. Epidemic of chancroid in Greenland 1977-78. Lancet, 1:654-655, 1979.

Meheus A, van Dyck E, Ursi JP, Ballard RC, Piot P. Etiology of genital ulcerations in Swaziland. Sex Transm Dis, 10:33-35, 1983.

Messing M, Sottnek FO, Biddle JW, Schlater LK, Kramer MA, Kraus SJ. Isolation of Haemophilus species from the genital tract. Sex Transm Dis, 10:56-61, 1983.

Nayyar KC, Stolz E, Michel MF. Rising incidence of chancroid in Rotterdam. Epidemiological, clinical, diagnostic and therapeutic aspects. Br J Vener Dis, 55:439-441, 1979.

Nobre GN. Identification of Haemophilus ducreyi in the clinical laboratory. J Med Microbiol, 15:243-245, 1982.

Oberhofer TR, Back AE. Isolation and cultivation of Haemophilus ducreyi. J Clin Microbiol, 15:625-629, 1982.

Plummer FA, D'Costa LJ, Nsanze H, et al. Antimicrobial therapy of chancroid: Effectiveness of erythromycin. J Infect Dis, 148:726-731, 1983.

Plummer FA, Nsanze H, D'Costa LJ, et al. Single-dose therapy of chancroid with trimethoprim-sulfametrole. N Eng J Med, 309: 67-71, 1983.

Sanson-LePors MJ, Casin I, Ortenberg M, Perol Y. In vitro susceptibility of thirty strains of Haemophilus ducreyi to several antibiotics including six cephalosporins. J Antimicrob Chemother, 11: 271-280, 1983.

Sng EH, Lim AL, Rajan VS, Goh AJ. Characteristics of Haemophilus ducreyi. A study. Br J Vener Dis, 58:239-242, 1982.

Sottnek FO, Biddle JW, Kraus SJ, Wever RE, Stewart JA. Isolation and identification of Haemophilus ducreyi in a clinical study. J Clin Microbiol, 12:170-174, 1980.

Chapter 18

LYMPHOGRANULOMA VENEREUM

ETIOLOGY

Lymphogranuloma venereum is a result of infection by sero-
groups L1, L2, and L3 of <u>Chlamydia trachomatis</u>. These particular LGV strains of <u>C. trachomatis</u> are more virulent than other
<u>Chlamydia</u> strains, and they infect macrophages and have a predi-
lection for lymph nodes. They do not infect the squamocolumnar
cells in contrast to the other <u>C. trachomatis</u> strains.

EPIDEMIOLOGY

Lymphogranuloma venereum is uncommon and appears to be
decreasing in the United States. In 1981 the U.S. Centers for Disease Control reported only 263 civilian cases. Much of the transmission appears to be among homosexual men. Many cases occur
in military personnel or travelers returning from endemic areas
such as Southeast Asia, Africa, South America, and the West Indies.
In the past the disease was endemic in blacks of lower socioeconomic status in the southeastern United States. Lymphogranuloma
venereum is acquired by sexual contact and is more common in
men than women by a ratio of at least 2:1. The frequency of
asymptomatic carriage and duration of infection of the lymphogranuloma <u>Chlamydia</u> in women is not known. Men are thought to
be noninfectious following healing of the primary lesion.

CLINICAL MANIFESTATIONS

Following exposure to an infected patient, the incubation
period ranges from 1 to 3 weeks. The first manifestation of disease

may be the appearance of a primary lesion on the genitalia. A primary lesion, however, can be identified in only 10-40% of patients. The primary lesion is most commonly herpetiform in nature, resulting in a shallow ulcer 5-6 mm in diameter. In men the ulcer commonly appears on the coronal sulcus, is painless, and heals in a few days without scar formation. In women a common site is the posterior aspect of the vulva. Uncommon presentations of a primary lesion include small papules or nodules or the appearance of urethritis with a small nodule in the urethra that may be identified by palpating the penis.

The second stage of the disease, inguinal adenopathy, also may be the patient's presenting complaint. The presentation of enlarged inguinal lymph nodes is much more frequent in men (>10:1) than in women. This is believed to be the result of the difference in lymph node drainage of the penis versus the labia or vagina where the initial lesions are likely to appear. The lymph node drainage of the penis is to the inguinal area, and the lymph node drainage of the labia and vagina is to the retroperitoneal area. If inoculation occurs at the perineum, anus, or rectum below the pectinate line, inguinal adenopathy also may take place.

Inguinal adenopathy generally appears 1-3 weeks following the disappearance of the primary lesion. The medial nodes are first involved and, as the disease progresses, enlarged lymph nodes on either side of Poupart's ligament may give rise to the "groove sign" (see Fig. 18.1). In one-third of the patients the lymphadenopathy is bilateral. During the course of the disease, the enlarged lymph nodes may regress in size or spontaneously suppurate. The skin over the matted nodes may have a violaceous hue. Although the inguinal nodes are the ones most commonly involved, this is not always the case. Where oral-genital contact with infected individuals has occurred, enlarged lymph nodes may be present in the cervical lymphatics. Such a presentation may lead to an initial diagnosis of lymphoma or Hodgkin's disease. Lymphogranuloma is a systemic disease, and constitutional symptoms may accompany the lymphadenopathy. These include fever, chills, sweats, headache, malaise, arthralgia, myalgia, and anorexia.

Rectal infections may occur in women and homosexual men. Infection may occur both with LGV and non-LGV serotypes C. trachomatis. Although infection may be present in asymptomatic patients, generally infection with the LGV serotypes produces more severe disease. Acute proctitis due to lymphogranuloma venereum serotypes of C. trachomatis may result in a bloody,

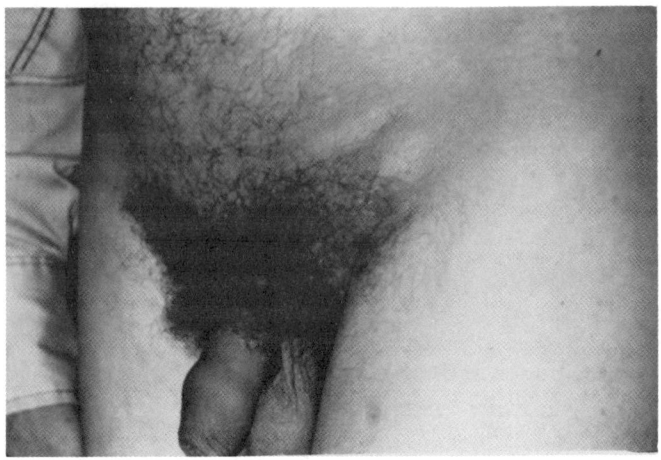

Figure 18.1   Lymphogranuloma venereum. This sexually transmitted disease is infrequently diagnosed in the United States. Infection with a <u>Chlamydia trachomatis</u> species, the etiologic agent,
results in a transient shallow ulcer followed by inguinal adenopathy.
Enlarged inguinal lymph nodes on either side of Poupart's ligament
result in the groove sign, as depicted here in a 20-year-old man.
To our embarrassment, aspiration of an enlarged node in this patient following unsuccessful therapy with oral tetracycline revealed
tetracycline-resistant <u>Staphylococcus aureus</u> in pure culture. This
patient emphasized to us the importance of establishing the correct
diagnosis. His CF serology to the psittacosis lymphogranuloma
group was 1:16; his wife's was 1:32.

mucopurulent discharge from the rectum. Anoscopy is essential
in the examination of these patients. There may be a wide variety
of findings, including mild mucosal inflammation or granular or
follicular or ulcerative changes on the rectal mucosa. The clinical
findings are not definitive and cultures are required for the diagnosis. Other infectious causes of proctitis include <u>Shigella</u>, <u>Campylo-
bacter</u>, <u>E. histolytica</u>, herpes simplex virus, <u>N. gonorrhoeae</u>, and
syphilis. The <u>Chlamydia</u> causing LGV, if untreated, may persist
in the patient for a considerable period of time. Dan reported a
patient with lymphogranuloma venereum of 20 years duration. Not
all buboes are the result of lymphogranuloma. Figure 18.1 shows
our misadventure with a bubo caused by <u>S. aureus</u>. Plague, herpesvirus infection, chancroid, granuloma <u>inguinal</u>, and lymphoma

are some of the other causes of buboes. Table 18.1 lists seven
lessons of Murphy and Fred for distinguishing infectious lymphadenitis and lymphoma.

The late manifestations of lymphogranuloma venereum may
be both debilitating as well as disfiguring. Two late manifestations
are the development of rectal strictures and lesions resulting from
impeded lymphatic flow. Men uncommonly develop urethral fis-
tulae and genital edema with resulting skin ulcerations. Women

Table 18.1   Seven Lessons of Murphy and Fred When Deciding
Whether It Is Infectious Lymphadenitis or Lymphoma[a]

---

1. Painful lymph nodes do not always mean infection.
    "Painful nodes are the presenting complaint in 4-13% of pa-
    tients with lymphoma."

2. Inguinal lymph nodes do not always mean infection.
    "Inguinal adenopathy is the earliest expression of illness in 8-
    12% of patients with lymphoma."

3. Fever does not always mean infection.
    "Fever is a cardinal feature of lymphoma and may precede all
    other manifestations."

4. Nondiagnostic lymph node biopsies do not rule out lymphoma.
    "Multiple lymph node biopsies may be necessary to establish
    the diagnosis of lymphoma."

5. Complications of a lymph node biopsy do not always mean
    infection.
    "Incisional therapy can spread not only infection but also
    lymphoma."

6. "Cutaneous lymphoma can mimic cutaneous infection."

7. The groove sign does not always mean lymphogranuloma
    venereum.
    "Signs sometimes point in the wrong direction."

---

[a] Adapted from J. F. Murphy and H. L. Fred, Infectious lymphadenitis or lymphoma? Seven lessons. J Amer Med Assoc, 235:
742-743, 1976.

may develop an ulcerative lesion of the vulva surrounded by fibrous induration and edema. This lesion is called esthiomene, named for the Greek word for "eaten" or "eroded." With lymphatic drainage of the lower rectum impaired, lymphorrhoids may appear. These appear as anal tags that may be confused with hemorrhoids, but the tags are actually dilated lymphatic channels. Rectal strictures as a result of lymphogranuloma venereum infection are more common in women than in men. The strictures may take the form of an annular band above the rectal orifice or a tubular constriction several centimeters into the lower bowel with marked thickening and fibrosis of the bowel wall.

DIAGNOSIS

The diagnosis of lymphogranuloma venereum may be made on the basis of a typical clinical picture, a positive culture for C. trachomatis of an LGV serotype, and serologic conversion to a serologic test for C. trachomatis. As shown below, this ideal world is not always achieved because of inherent technical difficulties in culturing Chlamydia and problems with the Chlamydia serology. Not the least of these is the general lack of Chlamydia culture facilities and the unavailability in general of the more specific serologic tests. The intradermal skin test (Frei test) is not specific for infection with Chlamydia of the LGV serotype. It is not recommended.

Chlamydia are grown in less than 50% of patients that are cultured. Material from culture should be aspirated from involved lymph nodes and taken from biopsies and swabs of involved rectal sites. Isolation of the LGV Chlamydia is best performed in a special tissue culture system such as that using cyclohexamide-treated McCoy cells.

The standard serologic test for the diagnosis of lymphogranuloma venereum is a complement fixation (CF) test that utilizes a group-specific chlamydial antigen. Thus the test measures antibodies to infection with both C. trachomatis and C. psittaci. Because chlamydial infections are common in some patient populations, a positive serologic test may assist in the diagnosis, but it does not establish the diagnosis of lymphogranuloma venereum. A serologic indication of infection would be a fourfold rise in titer in the acute and convalescent paired sera. However, many patients have been ill for several weeks prior to their initial visit, and because of this a rise in serologic titer may not be demonstrated.

Although a single titer of 1:8 or 1:16 may be significant, a titer of 1:64 or greater is a much stronger indication of disease. The <u>Chlamydia</u>-causing nongonococcal urethritis may result in a serologic response in the CF test, but the response is generally lower than that in patients with lymphogranuloma venereum. Thus in men with chlamydial urethritis, a CF titer of above 1:16 is rare. A falling convalescent titer does not necessarily support the diagnosis, and the serologic response does not always correlate with a response to antibiotic therapy.

Another diagnostic test is the microimmunofluorescent test. This test measures specific antibodies to different <u>Chlamydia</u> antigens, and it is more sensitive than the CF test. However, the microimmunofluorescent test is not routinely available in diagnostic laboratories.

The histologic picture of an involved lymph node is not diagnostic. There is capsular thickening, edema, disorganized architecture, and cellular infiltration with lymphocytes, eosinophiles, plasma cells, histiocytes, and epithelioid cells. Micro-abscesses or stellate abscesses containing thick yellow pus occur in a number of cases. A culture and gram stain of the bubo aspirate should be examined to rule out staphylococcal or other bacterial causes of lymphadenitis.

THERAPY

There are few studies that compare antibiotic therapies for lymphogranuloma venereum. Therapy should be given in suspected cases prior to the return of the culture or serologic results. Patients may be treated with tetracycline, 500 mg orally, 1 every 6 hr for 3 weeks, or sulfisoxazole, 4 g initially, followed by 1 g every 6 hr for 3 weeks. Fluctuant lymph nodes should be aspirated frequently to diminish the possibility of spontaneous drainage. In advanced or late disease, surgery may be required to correct deformities. Surgery, on occasion, has resulted in worsening of the lymphedema.

BIBLIOGRAPHY

Abrams AJ. Lymphogranuloma venereum. J Amer Med Assoc, 205:199-202, 1968.

Andrada MT, Dhar JK, and Wilde H. Oral lymphogranuloma venereum and cervical lymphadenopathy. Milit Med, 139:99-101, 1974.

Becker LE. Lymphogranuloma venereum. Int J Dermatol, 15:26-33, 1976.

Bolan RK, Sands M, Schachter J, Miner RC, and Drew WL. Lymphogranuloma venereum and acute ulcerative proctitis. Amer J Med, 72:703-706, 1982.

Dan M, Rotmensch HH, Eylan E, et al. A case of lymphogranuloma venereum of 20 years duration. Br J Vener Dis, 56:344-346, 1980.

Goldmeier D, Darougar S. Isolation of <u>Chlamydia trachomatis</u> from throat and rectum of homosexual men. Br J Vener Dis, 53: 184-185, 1977.

Grayson JT, Wang S. New knowledge of chlamydiae and the diseases they cause. J Infect Dis, 132:87-105, 1975.

Hart G. Chancroid, donovanosis, lymphogranuloma venereum. Department of Health, Education, and Welfare Publication No. CDC 75-8302, Centers for Disease Control, Atlanta, 1975.

Hirschberg SM, Horton CE. Radical perineal resection for far-advanced lymphogranuloma venereum. Plast Reconstr Surg, 51: 217-219, 1973.

Holder WR, Duncan WC. Lymphogranuloma venereum. Clin Obstet Gynecol, 15:1004-1009, 1972.

Hopsu-Havu VK, Sonek CE. Infiltrative, ulcerative, and fistular lesions of the penis due to lymphogranuloma venereum. Br J Vener Dis, 49:193-202, 1973.

Kampmeier RH. The genito-anal-rectal syndrome: Late manifestation of lymphogranuloma inguinal (Historical article). Sex Transm Dis, 10:47-50, 1983.

Klotz SA, Drutz DJ, Tam MR, and Reed KH. Hemorrhagic proctitis due to lymphogranuloma venereum serogroup L2. N Eng J Med, 308:1563-1565, 1983.

Koteen H. Lymphogranuloma venereum. Medicine, 24:1-69, 1945.

Lassus A, Mustakallio KK, and Wagner O. Autoimmune serum factors and IgA elevation in lymphogranuloma venereum. Ann Clin Res, 2:51-56, 1970.

Mathewson C. Inflammatory strictures of the rectum associated with venereal lymphogranuloma. J Amer Med Assoc, 110:709-714, 1938.

McLelland BA, Anderson PC. Lymphogranuloma venereum. Outbreak in a university community. J Amer Med Assoc, 235:56-57, 1976.

Murphy JF, Fred HL. Infectious lymphadenitis or lymphoma? Seven lessons. J Amer Med Assoc, 235:742-743, 1976.

Osoba AO, Beetlestone CA. Lymphographic studies in acute lymphogranuloma venereum infection. Br J Vener Dis, 52:399-403, 1976.

Philip RN, Casper EA, Gordan FB, and Quan AL. Fluorescent antibody responses to chlamydial infection in patients with lymphogranuloma venereum and urethritis. J Immunol, 112:2126-2134, 1974.

Ripa KT, Mårdh P-A. Cultivation of *Chlamydia trachomatis* in cyclohexamide-treated McCoy cells. J Clin Microbiol, 6:328-331, 1977.

Schachter J. Confirmatory serodiagnosis of lymphogranuloma venereum proctitis may yield false-positive results due to other chlamydial infections of the rectum. Sex Transm Dis, 8:26-28, 1981.

Schachter J, Causse G, and Tarizzo ML. Chlamydiae as agents of sexually transmitted diseases. Bull World Health Org, 54:245-254, 1976.

Schachter J, Osoba AO. Lymphogranuloma venereum. Br Med Bull, 39:151-154, 1983.

Schachter J, Smith DE, Dawson CR, Anderson WR, Deller JJ, Hoke AW, Smith WH, and Meyer KF. Lymphogranuloma venereum I. Comparison of the Frei Test, complement fixation test, and isolation of the agent. J Infect Dis, 120:372-375, 1969.

Sigel MM (ed.). Lymphogranuloma venereum. University of Miami Press, Coral Gables, 1962.

Sowmini CN, Gopalan KN, and Rao GC. Minocycline in the treatment of lymphogranuloma venereum. J Amer Vener Dis Assoc, 2:19-22, 1976.

Thompson SE, Washington AE. Epidemiology of sexually transmitted Chlamydia trachomatis infections. Epidem Rev, 5:91-123, 1983.

Thorsteinsson SB, Musher DM, Min KW, and Gyorkey F. Lymphogranuloma venereum. A cause for cervical lymphadenopathy. J Amer Med Assoc, 235:1882, 1976.

Walzer PD, Armstrong D. Lymphogranuloma venereum presenting as supraclavicular and inguinal adenopathy. Sex Transm Dis, 4:12-14, 1977.

Wang SP, Grayson JT, Alexander ER, and Holmes KK. A simplified microimmunofluorescence test with trachoma-lymphogranuloma venereum (Chlamydia trachomatis) antigens for use as a screening test for antibody. J Clin Microbiol, 1:250-255, 1975.

Chapter 19

GRANULOMA INGUINALE (DONOVANOSIS)

ETIOLOGIC AGENT

Granuloma inguinale frequently is confused with lymphogranuloma venereum, another sexually transmitted disease. Many clinicians and investigators argue that the term granuloma inguinale should not be used and that the disease should be called donovanosis, which recognizes Donovan as the discoverer and designates the etiologic agent. Unfortunately for Donovan, the etiologic agent has been renamed. What clinicians knew as Donovania granulomatis is now called Calymmatobacterium granulomatis.

C. granulomatis was discovered by Donovan in 1905 and is a gram-negative bacterium measuring approximately 1.5×0.7 μm. It is a coccobacillus, nonmotile, encapsulated, and does not form spores. Although the organism has been placed in the family Brucellaceae, little is known about it. It is antigenetically related to some Klebsiella species including K. pneumoniae. Unfortunately, C. granulomatis is difficult to grow in isolates taken from clinical material.

EPIDEMIOLOGY

Donovanosis is uncommon in the United States today. In the past it was more common in the southern states east of the Mississippi and in the area around the Gulf of Mexico. The disease is endemic in India, Southeast Asia, North Australia, New Guinea, Central Africa, and Central and South America. Donovanosis probably is spread by sexual intercourse. However, it appears to be a disease of low infectivity. Sexual partners do not invariably contract it, despite unprotected contact for long periods of time. Even in endemic areas, the incidence is low when compared with that of syphilis and gonorrhea.

The incidence of donovanosis is different with respect to race and sex. Donovanosis is twice as common in men as in women, and it is more common in blacks than whites. The racial differences in the incidence of donovanosis may reflect standards of personal hygiene and social habits associated with a lower socioeconomic status. As with other sexually transmitted diseases, the greatest incidence falls within the age period of maximum sexual activity. Despite numerous attempts, there is no animal model for the disease.

CLINICAL MANIFESTATIONS

The incubation period is not precisely known, but probably ranging from several days to 4 or 5 months. In over 90% of the cases, the primary lesion is located on the genitalia. In men the most common sites are the prepuce, the frenulum, or the glans penis. In women, lesions are generally present on the labia minora, the mons veneris, or the fourchette.

Early lesions are small papules, subcutaneous nodules, or ulcers approximately 0.5 cm in size. All lesions soon become ulcers of varying size. The ulcers are generally painless, and when fully developed are of different types. The hypertrophic verrucous type is found in both men and women and may involve extensive areas on both the genitalia and adjacent areas. Granulation tissue on the base of the ulcer may protrude above the surrounding skin. The skin at the edge of the ulcer is thickened and grayish white. There is little or no exudate, and Donovan bodies are easily located in the granulation tissue.

Sclerotic or cicatrical donovanosis is more common in women and results from extensive formation of fibrous tissue. Donovan bodies are infrequently seen, and the fibrous tissue may deform the genitalia.

Donovanosis also may be present as a fleshy, exuberant type. These lesions are painful, and the projecting granulation tissue produces a serosanguineous foul-smelling liquid. The early forms of Donovan bodies predominate, and they may be seen both inside and outside macrophages. When lesions are superinfected with fusospirochetal organisms, destructive necrotic lesions may occur.

These lesions are characterized by a gray exudate, and there may
be rapid destruction of tissue.

Extragenital lesions generally are located on the head, neck,
and oral cavity. There is evidence of hematogenous spread with
involvement of bone and liver, but this is unusual. Spread to the
lymphatics may result in the formation of psuedobubos. Aspiration
of these may reveal typical cells of the disease. Spread via the
lymphatics is disputed by some workers who believe that enlarged
lymph nodes in patients with this disease suggest superinfection,
lymphogranuloma venereum, syphilis, or malignant metastasis.
There is an association between donovanosis and carcinoma that is
not well documented. Both lesions may resemble one another.
Anal lesions are seen in women and homosexual men.

Donovanosis is indolent, and the lesions spread slowly over
a period of months. Patients commonly may have lesions for 2 or
more months prior to seeking medical aid. This may be due to the
socioeconomic setting in which the disease occurs. There is no
evidence that lesions spontaneously regress without therapy.
Complications of the disease are related to the anatomic sites
involved. Pseudoelephantiasis of the genitalis may be present in
15-20% of patients with donovanosis and is more common in women.
Also common are various deformities resulting from the scars
and adhesions. These include stenosis of the urethral, vaginal,
and anal orifices. Hypopigmentation of the skin is present at the
sites of healed ulcers.

DIAGNOSIS

The differential diagnosis should include genital carcinoma,
lymphogranuloma venereum, chancroid, syphilis, and anogenital
cutaneous amebiasis. The diagnosis of donovanosis rests on the
demonstration of the micro-organisms in macrophages in tissue
smears or in biopsies taken from the patient (see Fig. 19.1). It
is essential to get a fragment of granulation tissue in order to make
a proper examination. Material collected on cotton swabs or scalpel scrapings is inadequate. Prior to collecting the specimen, the
lesion should be wiped clear of exudate with numerous saline-
soaked gauzes and then dried. A small amount of granulation tissue is then collected by means of punch biopsy, forceps, or other
instrument, such as nasal punch biopsy forceps. The small bit of
tissue is then crushed between two glass slides and spread by
means of a circular motion.

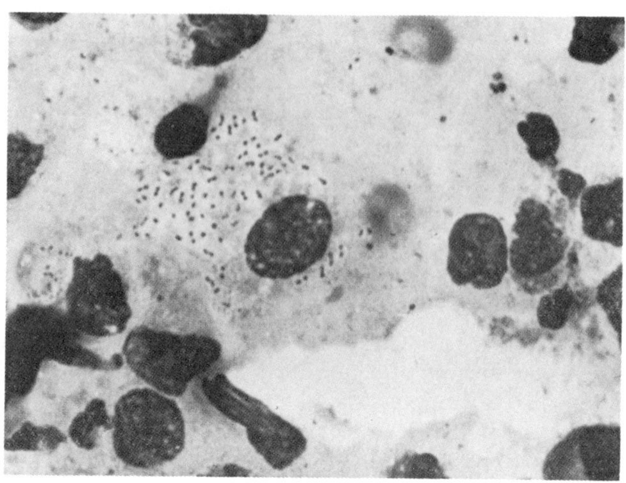

Figure 19.1   Granuloma inguinale (donovanosis). Donovanosis is also rare in the United States. Since the organism is difficult to grow, the diagnosis is established pathologically. Here Donovan bodies are seen in a smear of a small piece of granulation tissue from a lesion with Wright stain. Photograph from I. Maddocks et al., Br J Vener Dis, 52:190, 1976.

Staining of the tissue is performed with Wright or Giemsa stain. The stain is applied for 1-2 min, then diluted with distilled water, and the dilute stain is continued for 5 min. Another stain that can be used is 1% pinacyanole. This stain is applied for 2 min, followed by another 2 min with the same stain diluted 1:1 with water. Formalin-fixed tissue and hematoxylin eosin stain both give inadequate results.

The pathognomonic component of donovanosis is the demonstration of Donovan bodies within phagocytic cells. These are large mononuclear cells with round, oval, or bean-shaped nuclei. The phagocytosed organisms may be encapsulated or nonencapsulated. Encapsulated bacilli are ovoid or bean-shaped bodies 1-1.5 μm in length and 0.5-0.7 μm in width. In Wright-stained material the encapsulated organisms are dark blue and surrounded by a well-defined dense pinkish substance. Dark blue or blue-black chromatin inclusions may be present. The minute inclusions in the body of the organisms are more frequently seen in the younger forms. Nonencapsulated forms, 0.6-1.0 μm in size, may have varying morphology and may resemble a closed safety pin in appearance. They also may be surrounded by a halo of unstained material. Generally the encapsulated forms are associated with older lesions. A single vacuole in a mononuclear cell may contain 20-30 organisms. A mononuclear cell may contain many such vacuoles. The size of the mononuclear cell varies from 25 to 90 μm in diameter.

The histopathology of donovanosis includes the following features: The ulcerated area consists of luxuriant granulation tissue, with infiltrates consisting of predominantly polymorphonuclear leukocytes. The marginal epithelium has acanthosis and irregular elongation of the rete pegs. The elongated pegs form an interlacing network enclosing islands of exudates containing plasma cells, a smaller number of polymorphonuclear leukocytes, eosinophiles, monocytes, and occasional lymphocytes. Pseudoepithelial hyperplasia may be a predominant feature. In older lesions fibroblasts may predominate. Certain lesions may be suggestive of malignancy.

Although <u>Calymmatobacterium granulomatis</u> has been cultivated in the yolk sac of chicken eggs, the organism does not grow on ordinary laboratory media. Thus routine culturing is of no benefit and the diagnosis must be established by the examination of tissue smears or biopsies. Skin test antigens and serologic tests are not available. A biopsy always should be performed when there is a strong suspicion of malignancy. The differential diagnosis may be influenced by geographic location but could include syphilis, chancroid, lymphogranuloma venereum, epithelioma, filariasis, cutaneous tuberculosis, or cutaneous amoebiasis.

TREATMENT

The lesions of donovanosis should be cleaned at least twice daily with soap and water. A number of antibiotic regimens have been effective in curing donovanosis, and antibiotic therapy should be continued for at least 3 weeks. If the drug therapy is effective, peripheral epithelialization should be evident in about 1 week. The following antibiotic regimens are effective: tetracycline 500 mg orally every 6 hr for 3 weeks; chloramphenicol 500 mg orally three times per day for 3 weeks; gentamicin 40 mg intramuscularly twice daily for 3 weeks; ampicillin 500 mg orally every 6 hr for 3 weeks; and cotrimoxazole, two tablets (each tablet containing trimethoprim 80 mg and sulfamethoxazole 400 mg) orally twice daily for 10-15 days. Only a small number of patients have been treated with lincomycin. There are a number of patients in whom ampicillin was ineffective in eradicating the lesions. Streptomycin, 2 g daily, also is effective but should not be used because of a high incidence of toxicity. In some patients a 2-week course of antibiotics may be sufficient. Fortunately, there appears to be no relationship to the size of the lesion and the antibiotic response.

BIBLIOGRAPHY

Anderson K, DeMonbreun WA, Goodpasture EW. An etiologic consideration of _Donovania granulomatis_ cultivated from granuloma inguinale (three cases) in embryonic yolk. J Exp Med, 81:25-40, 1945.

Anderson K, Goodpasture EW, DeMonbreun WA. Immunologic relationship of _Donovania granulomatis_ to granuloma inguinale. J Exp Med, 81:41-50, 1945.

Ashdown LR, Kilvert GT. Granuloma inguinale in Northern Queensland. Med J Aust, 1:146-148, 1979.

Breschi LC, Goldman G, Shapiro SR. Granuloma inguinale in Vietnam: Successful therapy with ampicillin and lincomycin. J Amer Vener Dis Assoc, 1:118-120, 1975.

Davis CM. Granuloma inguinale, a clinical, histological and ultrastructural study. J Amer Med Assoc, 211:632-636, 1970.

Davis CM, Collins C. Granuloma inguinale: An ultrastructural study of _Calymmatobacterium granulomatis_. J Invest Dermatol, 53:315-321, 1969.

Dienst RB, Reinstein CR, Kupperman HS, Greenblatt RB. Studies on the causal agent of granuloma inguinale. Amer J Syph Gonor Vener Dis, 31:614-617, 1947.

Dodson RF, Fritz G, Hubler WR, Rudolph AH, Knox JM, Chu LW. Donovanosis: A morphologic study. J Invest Dermatol, 62:611-614, 1974.

Endicott JN, Kirkconnell WS, Bean D. Granuloma inguinal of the orbit with bony involvement. Arch Otolaryngol, 96:457-459, 1972.

Fritz GS, Hubler WH, Dodson RF, Rudolph A. Mutilating granuloma inguinale. Arch Dermatol, 111:1464-1465, 1975.

Garg RB, Lal S, Bedi BMS, Ratnam DV, Naik DN. Donovanosis (granuloma inguinale) of the oral cavity. Br J Vener Dis, 51:136-137, 1975.

Hart G. Chancroid, donovanosis and lymphogranuloma venereum. Department of Health, Education, and Welfare, Publication No. CDC 75-8302, Centers for Disease Control, Atlanta, 1975.

Kuberski T. Review. Granuloma inguinale (Donovanosis). Sex Transm Dis, 7:29-36, 1980.

Kuberski T, Papademitriou JM, Phillips P. Ultrastructure of Calymmatobacterium granulomatis in lesions of granuloma inguinale. J Infect Dis, 142:744-749, 1980.

Lal S. Continued efficacy of streptomycin in the treatment of granuloma inguinale. Br J Vener Dis, 47:454-455, 1971.

Lal S, Garg BR. Further evidence of the efficacy of cotrimoxazole in granuloma venereum. Br J Vener Dis, 56:412-413, 1980.

Lal S, Nicholas C. Epidemiological and clinical features in 165 cases of granuloma inguinale. Br J Vener Dis, 46:461-463, 1970.

Maddocks I, Anders EM, Dennis E. Donovanosis in Papua, New Guinea. Br J Vener Dis, 52:190-196, 1976.

Murugan S, Venkatram K, Renganathan PS. Vaginal bleeding in granuloma inguinale. Br J Vener Dis, 58:200-201, 1982.

Rajam RV, Rangiah PN. Donovanosis. World Health Organization, Geneva, 1954.

Subramanian S. Sclerosing granuloma inguinale. Br J Vener Dis, 57:210-212, 1981.

Thew MA, Swift JT, Heaton CL. Ampicillin in the treatment of granuloma inguinale. J Amer Med Assoc, 210:866-867, 1969.

Chapter 20

REITER'S SYNDROME

ETIOLOGIC AGENT

There is no established etiologic agent for this illness. In
1916 Hans Reiter, a German physician, described a young soldier
with nongonococcal urethritis, conjunctivitis, and arthritis, all of
which appeared eight days following an episode of bloody diarrhea.
The young man denied sexual exposure. Mycoplasma and _Chlamydia_
species are suspected as etiologic agents.

CLINICAL MANIFESTATIONS

Reiter's syndrome occurs most commonly in young men and
is uncommon in women of any age. Neuwelt disputes this and believes the incidence in the civilian population is similar in men and
women. Patients with Reiter's syndrome have an increased frequency of HLA-B27 histocompatibility antigen, as do patients with
ankylosing spondylitis. Reiter's syndrome may appear following
sexual exposure or bacterial gastroenteritis. Of men with nongonococcal urethritis, 1% or less may have Reiter's syndrome as a
complication. Reiter's syndrome has been described following
gastroenteritis with the following bacteria: _Salmonella_, _Shigella_,
Yersinia, and _Campylobacter_. The incidence of Reiter's syndrome
following bacterial gastroenteritis is also 1% or less. Women, who
otherwise rarely have the syndrome, constitute about 10% of the
patients with postgastroenteritis Reiter's syndrome.

Urethritis

Most patients with Reiter's syndrome experience urethritis
that begins 1-2 weeks following sexual intercourse. The urethral

discharge has no special characteristics. It may be purulent, mucopurulent, or thin and watery. Dysuria is not always present. The other elements of the syndrome usually appear 1-5 weeks after the onset of the urethritis.

Arthritis

Typically the arthritis is asymmetrical and begins about 2 weeks after the urethritis has appeared. The joints involved in order of frequency are knees, ankles, metatarsophalangeal joints, sacroiliac joints, and spine. Most patients who are positive for the HLA-B27 histocompatibility antigen and who develop Reiter's syndrome will have ankylosing spondylitis as a complication. About one-fourth of patients will have had pain as a result of the development of a spur on the calcaneus. Those patients seem to have a poor prognosis. Tendonitis may develop in the plantar fascia and the Achilles tendon. A physical finding present in some patients is swelling of the fingers and toes resulting in a sausage shape. The arthritis may persist as long as 6 months after the other elements of the syndrome have disappeared.

Mucocutaneous Skin Lesions

Mucocutaneous skin lesions are present in 80% of the patients with Reiter's syndrome. The lesions most characteristically develop over the soles and palms. They start as tiny vesicles which enlarge to pustules. As the material in the pustule dries and the inflammatory reaction at the base of the lesion continues, heaped up keratotic and painless scaling lesions called keratosis blennorrhagica are formed (Fig. 20.1). Similar scaling lesions may appear on the skin, scalp, scrotum, and penis. Erosive and exudative plaques may be present on the penis and scrotum.

About one-fourth of patients will have a mucosal lesion on the penis called balanitis circinata sicca (see Fig. 20.2). This is an erythematous, moist, and slightly elevated or eroded lesion present on the glans penis. Similar erythematous patches and erosions may develop in the oropharynx or buccal mucosa. Painless erosions may occur on the tongue. Shallow, circinate lesions may be present on the vulva in women with Reiter's syndrome. Reiter's syndrome also affects the nails. Pustules may develop under the nail. These are yellow in color and may enlarge and erode through the nail plate. The nail may be loosened and deformed by this process and ultimately may be shed.

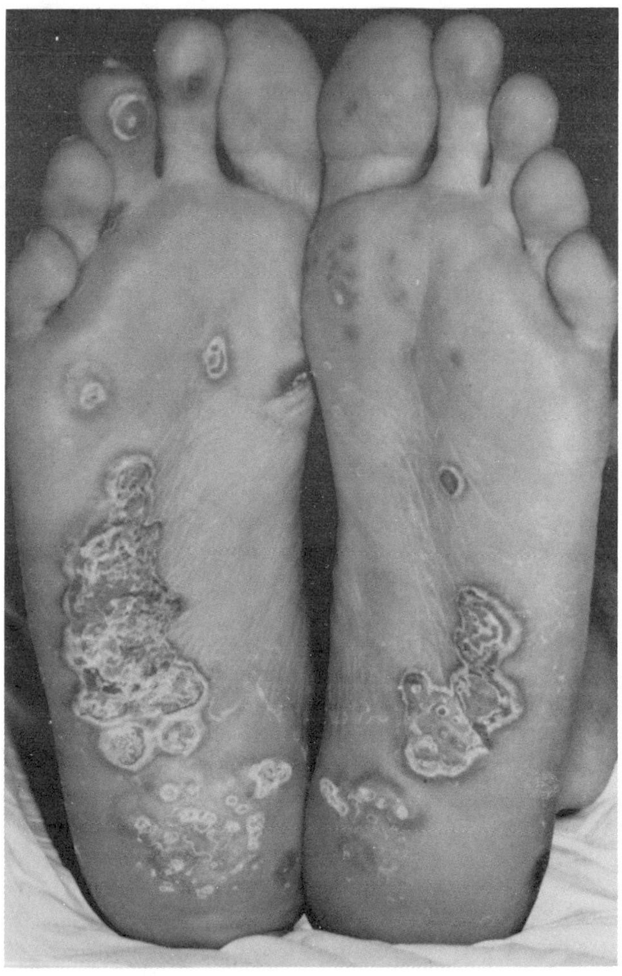

Figure 20.1　Soles of feet of patient with Reiter's syndrome. The hyperkeratotic and scaling lesions are called keratosis blennorrhagia.

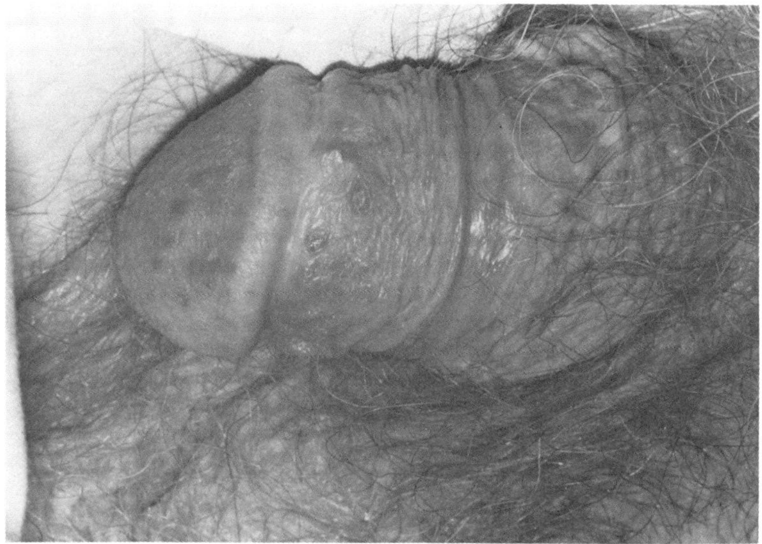

Figure 20.2   Penis of patient with Reiter's syndrome.   Of the
mucosal lesions, one of the more characteristic is balanitis circinata sicca.   The lesions are moist, slightly elevated papules that
may sometimes be eroded.

Eye Findings

The eye findings occur least frequently in comparison to the
other manifestations of Reiter's syndrome.   They also may be
present for only a few days.   The patients may have a bilateral
purulent conjunctivitis.   In patients with more severe disease, inflammation of the iris and cornea may occur, and this ultimately
may result in blindness.

Reiter's syndrome may develop over a few days with arthritis
as the most prominent manifestation, and the first attack may last
for several months.   The skin manifestations heal without scarring.
Approximately 80% of the patients will have some continuous symptoms with arthritis as the most disabling manifestation.   Of the
individuals with recurrent disease, half will have permanent joint
damage.   Patients who are HLA-B27 positive have an increased
prevalence of sacroiliitis and chronic uveitis.

Some of the more unusual manifestations of Reiter's syndrome
are pericarditis, myocarditis with atrioventricular heart block,

aortitis which may lead to aortic insufficiency, acute meningoencephalitis, seizures, and polyneuritis. First-degree heart block
is the most commonly reported EKG abnormality.

DIAGNOSIS

The diagnosis of Reiter's syndrome is dependent upon the
recognition of the constellation of its clinical features. The principal features are urethritis, arthritis, conjunctivitis, circinate
balanitis, shallow ulcerations of the buccal mucosa, and kerato-
derma blennorrhagicum. A combination of at least three of these
findings should have taken place in order to make the diagnosis.
The findings may not be present all at the same time. There is no
diagnostic laboratory test or diagnostic pathologic picture. About
80% of whites and 50% of blacks with Reiter's syndrome are HLA-
B27 positive. The absence of the HLA-B27 histocompatibility antigen does not exclude the diagnosis. A negative test in a black patient has much less clinical value than does a negative result in a
white patient. This test is of little practical value in the diagnosis
of Reiter's syndrome. The erythrocyte sedimentation rate is generally elevated. The examination of the joint fluid reveals an inflammatory response, yellow to opalescent in color with a low
viscosity. The leukocyte counts range from 2000 to 100,000. Fifty
percent or more of the cells are polymorphonuclear leukocytes.
The mucin clot is friable, and the joint fluid glucose is generally
greater than 25 mg/100 ml but lower than that of the blood.
Roentgenograms may show severe demineralization of the
bone next to involved joints and less commonly destructive changes
in the joints themselves. Sacroiliac involvement may be present
roetgenographically, and periosteal formation may be seen at
the insertion of the Achilles tendon. Also, calcification of the
paraspinus ligaments may take place. The spondylitis (arthritis of the spine) associated with Reiter's disease is similar to the
spondylitis associated with psoriasis, and this may be a confusing
diagnostic point since both diseases have joint as well as skin manifestations. Other diseases to be included in a differential diagnosis
are gonococcal arthritis, ankylosing spondylitis, or spondylitis
associated with regional enteritis or ulcerative colitis.

TREATMENT

There is no specific therapy for Reiter's syndrome. Antiinflammatory agents are not always effective. Aspirin, if used, should be administered so that blood levels of 20 mg/100 ml are achieved. Prednisone may be administered in an initial dosage of 60 mg daily followed by tapering to a maintenance level. Indomethacin also may be administered in dosages ranging from 75 to 150 mg/day. Some physicians treat patients with a course of tetracycline, 500 mg orally every 6 hr for 10 days. There is no evidence that this is effective in shortening the course of the disease. Nonsteroidal anti-inflammatory agents also are worthy of trial.

BIBLIOGRAPHY

Butler MJ, Russell AS, Percy JS, Lentle BC. A follow-up study of 48 patients with Reiter's syndrome. Amer J Med, 67:808-810, 1979.

Calin A. HLA-B27 in 1982: Reappraisal of a clinical test. Ann Int Med, 96:114-115, 1982.

Calin A. HLA-B27: To type or not to type? Ann Int Med, 92: 208-211, 1980.

Calin A, Fries JF. An "experimental" epidemic of Reiter's syndrome revisited: Follow-up evidence on genetic and environmental factors. Ann Int Med, 84:564-566, 1976.

Daunt SO'N, Kotowski KE, O'Reilly AP, Richardson AT. Ulcerative vulvitis in Reiter's syndrome. A case report. Br J Vener Dis, 58:405-407, 1982.

Fox R, Calin A, Gerber RC, Gibson D. The chronicity of symptoms and disability in Reiter's syndrome: An analysis of 131 consecutive patients. Ann Int Med, 91:190-193, 1979.

Good AE. Reiter's disease: A review with special attention to cardiovascular and neurologic sequellae. Sem Arthr Rheum, 3: 253-286, 1974.

Grumet FC, Fendly BM, Engleman EG. Monoclonal anti-HLA-B27 antibody (B27M'): Production and lack of detectable typing difference between patients with ankylosing spondylitis, Reiter's syndrome, and normal controls. Lancet, 2:174-176, 1981.

Hochberg MC, Bias WB, Arnett FC. Family studies in HLA-B27 associated arthritis. Medicine, 57:463-475, 1978.

Kanerva L, Kousa M, Niemi K-M, et al. Ultrahistopathology of balanitis circinata. Br J Vener Dis, 58:188-195, 1982.

Keat A. Reiter's syndrome and reactive arthritis in perspective. N Eng J Med, 309:1606-1615, 1983.

Khan MA. Clinical application of the HLA-B27 test in rheumatic diseases. A current perspective. Arch Int Med, 140:177-180, 1980.

Khan MA, Askari AD, Braun WE, Aponte CJ. Low associations of HLA-B27 with Reiter's syndrome in blacks. Ann Int Med, 90: 202-203, 1979.

Khan MA, Khan MK. Diagnostic value of HLA-B27 testing in ankylosing spondylitis and Reiter's syndrome. Ann Int Med, 96: 70-76, 1982.

Kousa M, Saikku P, Richmond S, Lassus A. Frequent association of chlamydial infection with Reiter's syndrome. Sex Transm Dis, 5:57-61, 1978.

McEwen C, DiTata D, Lingg C, Porini A, Good A, Rankin T. Ankylosing spondylitis and spondylitis accompanying ulcerative colitis, regional enteritis, psoriasis and Reiter's disease. Arch Rheum, 14:291-318, 1971.

Moll JMH, Haslock I, Macrae IF, Wright V. Associations between ankylosing spondylitis, psoriatic arthritis, Reiter's disease, the intestinal arthropathies, and Behcet's syndrome. Medicine, 53: 343-364, 1974.

Morris R, Metzger AL, Bluestone R, Terasaki PI. HLA-B27-A clue to the diagnosis and pathogenesis of Reiter's syndrome. N Eng J Med, 290:554-556, 1974.

Neuwelt CM, Borenstein DG, Jacobs RP. Reiter's syndrome: A male and female disease. J Rheumatol, 9:268-272, 1982.

Noer HR. An "experimental" epidemic of Reiter's syndrome. J Amer Med Assoc, 198:693-698, 1966.

Paronen I. Reiter's disease: A study of 344 cases observed in Finland. Acta Med Scand (Suppl.), 212:1-114, 1948.

Paulus HE, Pearson CM, Pitts W. Aortic insufficiency in five patients with Reiter's syndrome. A detailed clinical and pathologic study. Amer J Med, 53:464-472, 1972.

Rodman GP, McEwcn C, Wallace SL. Primer on rheumatic diseases. J Amer Med Assoc (Suppl.), 5:224, 1973.

Ruppert GB, Lindsay J, Barth WF. Cardiac conduction abnormalities in Reiter's syndrome. Amer J Med, 73:335-340, 1982.

Smith DL, Bennet RM, Regan MG. Reiter's disease in women. Arth Rheum, 23:335-340, 1980.

Thambar IV, Dunlop R, Thin RN, Huskisson EC. Circinate vulvitis in Reiter's syndrome. Br J Vener Dis, 53:260-262, 1977.

Urman JD, Zurier RB, Rothfield NF. Reiter's syndrome associated with Campylobacter fetus infection. Ann Int Med, 86:444-445, 1977.

Weinberger HW, Ropes MW, Kulka JP, Bauer W. Reiter's syndrome, clinical and pathologic observations: A long-term study of 16 cases. Medicine (Baltimore), 41:35-91, 1962.

Wilkens RF, Arnett FC, Bilter T, et al. Reiter's syndrome. Evaluation of preliminary criteria for definite disease. Arth Rheum, 24:844-849, 1981.

Wright V. Arthritis associated with venereal disease: A comparative study of gonococcal arthritis and Reiter's syndrome. Ann Rheum Dis, 22:77-90, 1963.

Yunus M, Calabro JJ, Miller KA, Masi AT. Family studies with HLA typing in Reiter's syndrome. Amer J Med, 70:1210-1214, 1981.

Chapter 21

BEHÇET'S DISEASE

ETIOLOGIC AGENT

The cause of Behçet's disease is not known.

EPIDEMIOLOGY

Behçet's disease was named for a Turkish dermatologist who
in 1937 described patients with recurrent oral and genital ulcerations and relapsing iridocyclitis. Behçet's disease is twice as
common in men than in women, and the illness occurs most often
in individuals between 19 and 40 years old. Geographically,
Behçet's disease most often is found in the Middle East, Israel,
Turkey, Greece, Cyprus, and Japan. The disease is also encount-
ered in North European countries, especially England and France.
Although likely to go unrecognized, this disease is infrequently
reported in the United States. There may be a genetic predisposi-
tion to Behçet's disease, and some investigators believe that the
manifestations are secondary to vascular immune complex deposi-
tion. If this is so, the nature of the antigen is unknown.

CLINICAL MANIFESTATIONS

Behçet's disease, as with many of the rheumatic diseases,
exists as it is defined. One diagnostic schema suggests the following as major manifestations of the disease: aphthous stomatitis,
genital ulceration, and iridocyclitis. Minor manifestations include
cutaneous lesions, recurrent thrombophlebitis, thrombosis of the

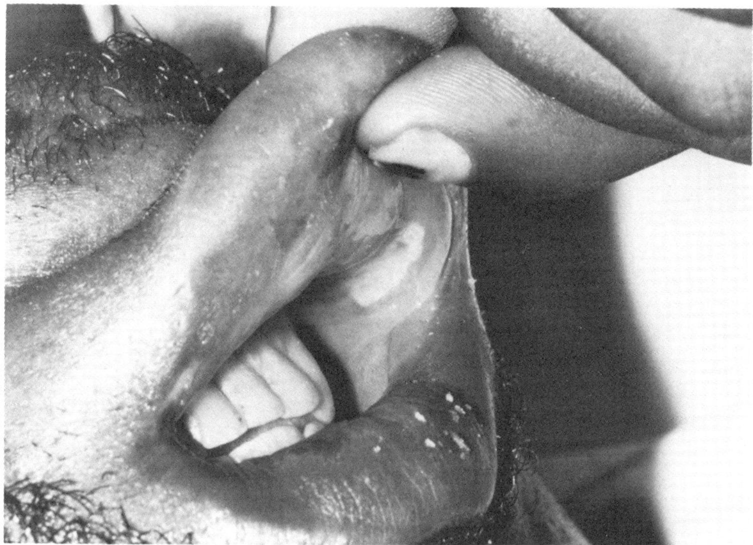

Figure 21.1   Aphthous stomatitis in a patient with Behçet's disease. Most patients have painful recurrent oral ulcers that persist for 1-2 weeks. This unfortunate patient also had neurologic involvement with his Behcet's disease manifesting as meningoencephalitis.

venae cavae, arteritis, and meningoencephalomyelitis. The diagnosis of Behçet's disease is established in this schema when two major and one minor manifestation are present. Another diagnostic schema includes the following suggested criteria: aphthous stomatitis, aphthous genital ulceration, uveitis, cutaneous vasculitis, synovitis, and meningoencephalitis. In this schema the diagnosis is established when three of the suggested criteria are present, one being recurrent aphthous ulceration. An incomplete form of Behcet's disease is diagnosed if there are two criteria present, one being recurrent aphthous ulceration. The major features of the disease often do not occur all at the same time, and their appearance may be transient in character (see Fig. 21.1).

Aphthous Stomatitis

Most patients have painful recurrent oral ulcers that persist for 1-2 weeks, heal spontaneously, and then reappear at irregular intervals between several weeks to several months. They may be present on the lips, buccal mucosa, tongue, gums, larynx, or tonsils. The ulcers may be present as a single lesion, or they may appear in clusters. The ulcers vary in diameter (2-10 mm) and depth. The deep ulcers may have a central necrotic base.

Genital Ulcers

The genital ulcers also are painful and have a similar appearance and course as the oral ulcers. The ulcers may be present on the vulva or vagina in women and on the penis and scrotum in men.

Other Skin Lesions

These include a nonspecific inflammatory response to injections and superficial scratches as well as a variety of other skin lesions. The latter include erythema-nodosum-like lesions, vesicles, papules, pustules, acne-like lesions, pyodermas, abscesses, and folliculitis. These nonspecific lesions also disappear in 1 or 2 weeks and recur irregularly.

Eye Findings

The patients may have anterior segment involvement (in order of frequency): relapsing iridocyclitis, conjunctivitis, and corneal ulceration. Posterior segment involvement includes choroiditis. Patients may complain of photophobia, blurred vision, and pain. They may have retinal vessel involvement (phlebitis and/or arteritis), optic papillitis, and inflammatory or hemorrhagic involvement of the vitreous humor. The retinal veins may be engorged and permeable to fluorescein dye. Unfortunately, some patients may be blinded by this disease, approximately one-third of those with uveitis. Other patients may have cataracts and glaucoma as a result of Behçet's disease.

Neurologic Involvement

Neurologic involvement is present in 10-25% of patients with Behçet's disease and usually occurs at the same time as the ulcerative lesions. Neurologic manifestations may not develop until several months after the appearance of the disease. Patients with neurologic involvement generally have fever, headache, and abnormal spinal fluid findings. The latter consist of mildly elevated

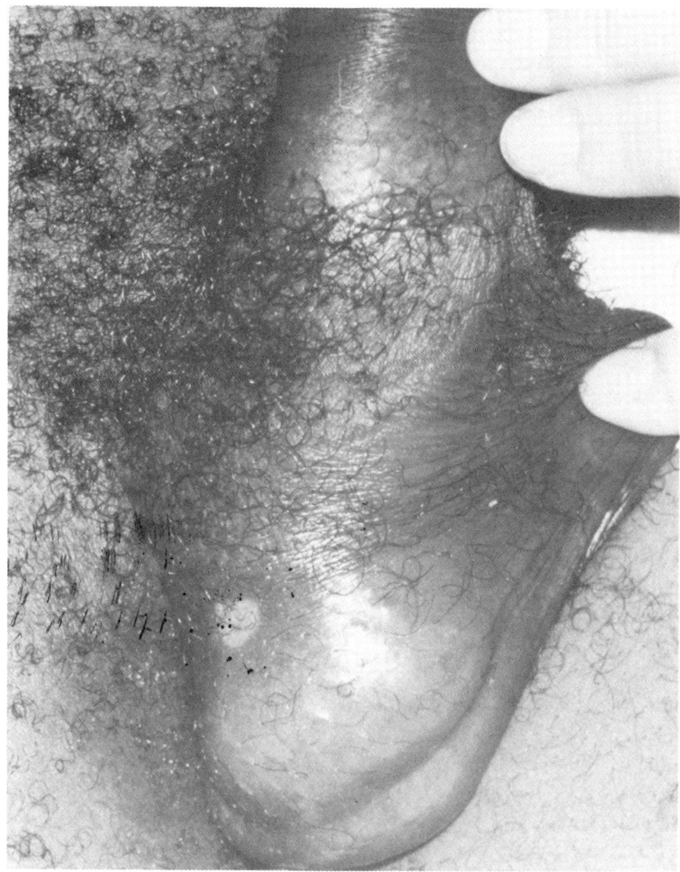

Figure 21.2   Ulcer on the scrotum of a patient with Behcet's disease. The genital ulcers also are painful and have a similar appearance to the oral ulcers. The ulcers may be present on the vulva or vagina in women and on the penis and scrotum in men.

protein concentrations and pleocytosis (5-500 cells/mm^3) with predominant lymphocytosis. The neurologic manifestations may be varied and include transient ocular palsies, corticospinal tract disease, pseudobulbar palsy, cerebellar ataxia, and meningoencephalitis. Papilledema may be present. The illness in some patients may resemble an organic confusional state. The mortality rate in patients with neurologic disease is approximately 40%.

Arthritis

Arthritis is one of the common features of Behçet's disease. Patients may have arthralgias initially that later develop into arthritis. The most frequently involved joints are the knees, followed by the ankles, fingers, wrists, elbows, and feet. The arthritis usually resolves without permanent damage to the joint, and only a minority of cases show radiologic evidence of cartilage destruction and bone erosion. The arthritis is generally accompanied by fever, mouth and genital ulcers, and other skin lesions including the erythema-nodosum-like lesions.

Other Manifestations

Other manifestations of this disease include thrombophlebitis, colon arterial thrombosis, colitis, aneurysm of the systemic and pulmonary circulations, orchitis, epididymitis, glomerulonephritis, recurrent pneumonitis, pericarditis, and amyloidosis.

Other Diseases That May Be Confused with Behçet's Disease

These include systemic lupus erythematosus, inflammatory bowel disease, Reiter's syndrome, herpetic infections, Mollaret's meningitis, sarcoidosis, Vogt-Kayanagi's syndrome, herpesvirus meningoencephalitis, confusional states, and small strokes.

DIAGNOSIS

The diagnosis of Behçet's disease depends on the recognition of the clinical manifestations of the disease previously described. These may not all appear at the same time. There are no diagnostic laboratory tests. Complete blood counts and blood chemical analysis are within normal limits. The plasma globulins may be slightly elevated, and the erythrocyte sedimentation rate also is generally elevated. The common histopathologic lesion of all of the clinical manifestations is a vasculitis characterized by perivascular infiltrates with mononuclear cells, resembling the lesion seen in a delayed hypersensitivity reaction to an intradermal antigen.

TREATMENT

Therapy of this disease is unsatisfactory and difficult to evaluate, in part because of the unpredictability of the natural course of Behcet's disease. Some investigators begin therapy with oral prednisone 50 mg daily. This drug is then tapered over several days to a maintenance dose between 5 and 20 mg. Other investigators add cytotoxic agents such as azathioprine to the prednisone. O'Duffy et al. recently reported favorable responses in patients with uveitis and meningoencephalitis whose Behcet's disease was treated with 0.1 mg/kg daily doses of chlorambucil for periods of 3 months to 4 years. However, no controlled studies are available that identify ideal medical therapy.

BIBLIOGRAPHY

Chajek T, Fainaru M. Behcet's disease: A report of forty-one cases and a review of the literature. Medicine, 54:179-196, 1975.

Comess KA, Zibelli LR, Gorden D, Frederickson SR. Acute, severe, aortic regurgitation in Behcet's syndrome. Ann Int Med, 99:639-640, 1983.

Durieux P, Bletry O, Huchon G, Wechsler B, Chretien J, Godeau P. Multiple pulmonary arterial aneurysms in Behcet's disease and Hughes-Stovin syndrome. Arch Surg, 115:736-738, 1980.

Eglin RP, Lehner T, Subak-Sharpe JH. Detection of RNA complementary to herpes-simplex virus in mononuclear cells from patients with Behcet's syndrome and recurrent oral ulcers. Lancet, 2:1356-1361, 1982.

France R, Buchanan RN, Wilson MW, Sheldon MB. Relapsing iritis with recurrent oral ulcers of the mouth and genitalia (Behcet's syndrome). Medicine, 30:335-355, 1951.

Gamble CN, Wiesner KB, Shapiro RF, Boyer WJ. The immune complex pathogenesis of glomerulonephritis and pulmonary vasculitis in Behçet's disease. Amer J Med, 66:1031-1039, 1979.

James DG. Behçet's syndrome. N Eng J Med, 301:431-432, 1979.

Kalbian VV, Challis MT. Behçet's disease. Report of twelve cases with three manifesting as papilledema. Amer J Med, 49: 823-829, 1970.

Kansu E, Deglin S, Cantor RI, Burke JF, Cho SY, Cathart RT. The expanding spectrum of Behçet syndrome. A case with renal involvement. J Amer Med Assoc, 237:1855-1856, 1977.

Ketch LL, Buerk CC, Liechty RD. Surgical implications of Behçet's disease. Arch Surg, 115:759-760, 1980.

Lehner R, Barnes CG (eds.). Behçet's Syndrome: Clinical and Immunological Features. Academic Press, London, 1979.

O'Duffy JD, Carney JA, Deodhar S. Behçet's disease. Report of ten cases, three with new manifestations. Ann Int Med, 75:561-570, 1971.

O'Duffy JD, Goldstein NP. Neurologic involvement in seven patients with Behçet's disease. Amer J Med, 61:170-178, 1976.

O'Duffy JD, Robertson DM, Goldstein NP. Chlorambucil in the treatment of uveitis and meningoencephalitis of Behçet's disease. Amer J Med, 76:75-84, 1984.

Petty TL, Scoggin CH, Good JT. Recurrent pneumonia in Behçet's syndrome. Roentgenographic documentation during 13 years. J Amer Med Assoc, 238:2529-2530, 1977.

Rogé J, Fabre M, Dursand B, et al. Les localisations intestinales du syndrome de Behçet. Étude anatomo-clinique de 2 cas avec lésions vasculaires. Gastroenterol Clin Biol, 6:872-878, 1982.

Rogé J, Durand B. Syndrome de Behçet et intestin. Gastroenterol Clin Biol, 6:886-891, 1982.

Rosenthal T, Bank H, Aladjem M, David R, Gafni J. Systemic amyloidosis in Behçet's disease. Ann Int Med, 83:220-223, 1975.

Scarlett JA, Kistner ML, Yang LC. Behçet's syndrome. Report of a case associated with pericardial effusion and cryoglobulinemia treated with indomethacin. Amer J Med, 66:146-148, 1979.

Smith GE, Kime LR, Pitcher JL. The colitis of Behçet's disease: A separate entity? Colonoscopic findings and literature review. Amer J Digest Dis, 18:987-1000, 1973.

Thach BT, Cummings NA. Behçet syndrome with "aphthous colitis." Arch Int Med, 136:705-709, 1976.

Wilkey D, Yocum DE, Oberley TD, Sundstrom WR, Karl L. Bud-Chiari syndrome and renal failure in Behçet disease. Report of a case and review of the literature. Amer J Med, 75:541-550, 1983.

Chapter 22

OTHER DISEASES AND CONDITIONS LIKELY TO BE
FOUND IN PATIENTS ATTENDING A CLINIC FOR
SEXUALLY TRANSMITTED DISEASES

ACUTE EPIDIDYMITIS

Acute epididymitis has a number of etiologic agents. Escherichia
coli, Klebsiella species, Proteus species, Pseudomonas aeruginosa.
Neisseria gonorrhoeae, and Chlamydia trachomatis are among the
identifiable causes of this illness. N. gonorrhoeae and C. trachomatis appear to be the more common etiologic agents in men under
35, and the gram-negative rod infections are found more commonly
in men over 35. The latter group also are more likely to have
some underlying genitourinary pathology.

The clinical diagnosis of acute epididymitis is based on the
finding of pain, swelling, and tenderness of the epididymis and
surrounding structures often accompanied by fever and scrotal
edema. Inguinal pain has been described in chlamydial epididymitis.
Patients with epididymitis may have a history of trauma. There is
usually an associated urethral discharge if the epididymitis is
caused by Chlamydia or gonococci. Dysuria may be absent.

Laboratory findings include the presence of ten or more leukocytes per 400× microscopic field in a first voided urine sediment.
Peripheral blood leukocytosis also may be present. The first
voided urine should be quantitatively cultured in addition to the
microscopic examination, and a urethral culture and Gram stain
of the discharge should be performed for gonococci. A Chlamydia
culture also should be performed where laboratory facilities permit
this. If patients are not responding to therapy or if the diagnosis
is uncertain, then an epididymal aspiration with a small needle and
syringe should be considered. In the differential diagnosis of

epididymitis, torsion, trauma, tumor, and tuberculosis should be included.

The treatment of acute epididymitis depends on the etiologic agent. As a general rule, tetracycline is the treatment of choice. In men over 35 who may have gram-negative bacilli more commonly as an etiologic agent, the therapy may have to be altered based on the results of the urine or epididymal aspirate culture and antibiotic susceptibility tests. The dose of tetracycline for acute epididymitis is 500 mg orally four times daily for ten days. Doxycycline, 100 mg orally twice daily, also is effective but is significantly more expensive. Epididymitis is a serious disease. Long-term fertility disturbances have been reported in approximately 20% of patients with a single attack.

TORSION OF THE TESTIS

Testicular torsion may be easily confused with epididymitis and if not quickly diagnosed and treated will result in loss of function of the testicle. Although torsion of the testis often is considered a disease of young boys, the peak incidence is at 14-28 years.

The onset of the illness is generally acute with radiation of pain into the groin or abdomen. Fever is uncommon as is urethritis as diagnosed by the presence of leukocytes in the microscopic examination of a first voided urine specimen. These findings do not reliably separate torsion from epididymitis. The involved testicle may be higher in the scrotum and lie horizontally as a result of shortening of the twisted cord. About one-third of patients will have histories of similar symptoms that resolved spontaneously.

Pain and swelling in the scrotum may make examination impossible and, if torsion is suspected, the patient should be quickly taken to a urologic surgeon for immediate surgical relief. Permanent damage can occur within 3 or 4 hours of ischemia.

Two newer diagnostic methods offer some help in identifying patients with testicular torsion: radionuclide scans and Doppler studies. Of the two, the radionuclide scan is the most accurate, while the Doppler study is undoubtedly the most convenient. Where there is confusion between epididymitis and torsion, remember that epididymitis patients generally have dysuria, pyuria, fever, epididymal swelling, and tenderness. If swelling obscures scrotal anatomy, then a radionuclide scan or Doppler study immediately should be considered. Testicular torsion is a surgical emergency, and any delay in diagnosis should be avoided.

MASSES IN THE SCROTUM

A number of intrascrotal swellings may present diagnostic problems to the examining clinician. Some of these are listed below with a short accompanying description.

Hydrocele

A hydrocele is a fluid-filled nontender sac that can be enclosed by the examining fingers. It is translucent when transilluminated with a small light.

Hernia

A hernia cannot be enclosed by the examining fingers and does not transilluminate.

Spermatocele and Cyst of the Epididymis

This is generally a mass found in the posterior testis. The cyst of the epididymis may be somewhat lobulated in shape and is generally firmer than the spermatocele. Both may be translucent by transillumination, although the spermatocele is less brilliant.

Varicose Veins of the Spermatic Cord

Varicose veins of the spermatic cord may form a varicocele. This feels to the palpating fingers like a "bag of worms." The soft mass is separate from the testes and epididymis. If the patient lies on his back and the scrotum is elevated, the mass will slowly decrease in size.

Neoplasm

Any painless nodule in the testes or epididymis should be considered a neoplasm until a more satisfactory explanation is forthcoming. If there is the slightest doubt, the patient should be referred to a surgeon for exploration and diagnosis. In malignant testicular tumors, the vas remains normal. The vas is generally thickened in inflammatory conditions.

Chronic Infectious Diseases

Syphilis may cause a smooth, painless enlargement of the body of the testis. A gumma, if present, may deform the testis into an irregular shape. Tuberculosis infection may result in irregularities in the shape of the epididymis and thickening of the vas. Pain is uncommon in tuberculous orchitis.

ACUTE PROSTATITIS

There are a variety of types of prostatitis caused by diverse etiologies. This discussion will concentrate on acute prostatitis. Acute prostatitis has a number of identifiable microbiologic causes. However, nonbacterial prostatitis, a more prevalent disease, is a condition of unknown cause. Bacterial causes of prostatitis include E. coli (the most common cause), Proteus, Klebsiella, Enterobacter, Pseudomonas, and Serratia species. Enterococci (Streptococcus faecalis), Trichomonas vaginalis, and the tubercle bacilli also are other uncommon causes. Gonococci may cause acute prostatitis, but the frequency at which this occurs is unknown. The role of C. trachomatis is uncertain. Brunner et al. believe that Ureaplasma urealyticum is of etiologic importance in patients with chronic prostatitis.

The patients with acute bacterial prostatitis generally complain of low back and perineal pain, chills, fever, malaise, urinary frequency and urgency, dysuria, and nocturia. Patients may complain of symptoms of bladder outlet obstruction. The prostate is enlarged, firm, and tender on rectal examination. Patients with acute nonbacterial prostatitis generally have less severe symptoms and do not have chills or fever.

Identifying the microbiologic etiology of acute prostatitis is not easy, given the inaccessibility of the gland. The most convenient method to date is the three-glass test, a comparison of quantitative cultures of samples of the urine from the urethra, bladder, and prostatic secretions. The patient should have a full bladder prior to this examination. Patients with presumed bacterial prostatitis (i.e., those with swollen, warm, and tender glands) probably should not have a prostatic massage, because the infecting bacteria are likely to be found in the urethral culture. Also, a bacteremia may result from a prostatic massage of an infected gland.

The first culture is taken from the first voided 10 ml of urine (VB1), the second is taken after about 200 ml of urine has been passed (VB2), the third is taken from the prostatic secretions (EPS) expressed by prostatic massage, and the fourth is taken from the first voided 10 ml immediately following the prostatic massage (VB3). The specimens are quantitatively cultured then. The cultures are interpreted in the following manner. If the bladder urine (VB2) sample is sterile, the pathogenic bacteria may be localized to the urethra (VB1) or prostate (EPS) by comparison of the bacterial counts. In urethritis, the bacterial colony counts in the urethral specimen (VB1) generally exceed the counts in the other specimens by a log or more.

In patients with bacterial prostatitis, the bacterial counts in the prostatic secretion (EPS) or the postmassage voided urine (VB3) should exceed by one log or more the quantitative bacterial count of the VB1 culture. If the urethral or postmassage urine cultures are similar in colony counts, the prostatic fluid culture should have a higher count if the infection is in the prostate. If the bladder urine (VB2) has an equally high count, the site of localization may not be accurately determined. In this case the examination may be repeated following a short course of ampicillin, penicillin G, or nitrofurantoin, which will sterilize the urine but not the prostatic secretions. Patients with nonbacterial prostatitis typically have a normal urinalysis. The prostatic exudate in patients with nonbacterial prostatitis has greater than 10 white blood cells per 400× microscopic field and also an abnormal number of lipid-laden macrophages.

Patients with acute bacterial prostatitis may require hospitalization and suprapublic tube bladder drainage if urinary obstruction is a significant problem. Antibiotic therapy with trimethoprim-sulfamethoxazole (TMP-SMX) should be initiated prior to the culture results unless cultures of previous episodes have demonstrated an organism resistant to TMP-SMX. The dose of TMP-SMX is two regular tablets (80 mg TMP and 400 mg SMX per tablet) or one double strength tablet (160 mg TMP and 800 mg SMX) twice daily until the results of the culture and sensitivity are known. If TMP-SMX is the appropriate drug, therapy should be continued for 30 days. In patients unable to take TMP-SMX, an alternative initial therapy is gentamicin or tobramycin 3-5 mg/kg/day divided into three intramuscular or intravenous doses, plus ampicillin, 2g, given intravenously every 6 hr. Patients with gonococcal prostatitis may be treated with minocycline 100 mg orally twice daily for 2 weeks followed by 100 mg daily for another 2 weeks.

The treatment of patients with nonbacterial prostatitis is less satisfactory. Because <u>C. trachomatis</u> and <u>U. urealyticum</u> may possibly cause nonbacterial prostatitis, a clinical trial of oral tetracycline or oral erythromycin is indicated. Unless a favorable response is achieved, further therapy is not indicated. Acute relapses may be managed with antiinflammatory agents and hot sitz baths. Sexual activity is not contraindicated.

INFECTION OF THE BARTHOLIN AND SKENE'S GLANDS

The Bartholin (greater vestibular) glands are small glands located on either side of the posterior vaginal orifice. Normally the glands are not palpable. If the glands are enlarged, they may be palpated between the thumb and index finger beneath the posterior portion of the labia majora. The ducts to these glands open into the inner surface of the labium minus. If they become blocked, an abscess may form. The diagnosis is generally obvious. Patients complain of pain, and the introitus is deformed by the swollen and tender gland.

Sarrel et al. described four patients who had unilateral introital pain on sexual arousal as a result of chronic occlusion of a Bartholin gland duct. In each case the gland was palpable and tender. The patients responded to surgical excision. Bartholinitis may be caused by a number of micro-organisms including <u>E. coli</u> and other aerobic gram-negative bacilli, <u>Bacteroides</u> species and and anaerobic streptococci, and gonococci. <u>Mycoplasma hominis</u> and <u>U. urealyticum</u> are only rarely found as causes of these abscesses, and data concerning <u>C. trachomatis</u> as a pathogen are limited. Davis et al. believe that <u>C. trachomatis</u> can infect the Bartholin duct alone and in conjunction with <u>N. gonorrhoeae</u>. Skene's glands are small glands located on either side of the female urethra. They may be infected with <u>Trichomonas</u> and other organisms that have been described as causing bartholinitis. Patients may complain of dysuria, and pus may be expressed from the ducts which empty into the distal urethra just inside the meatus (see Fig. 2.6).

Material expressed from the ducts of the Bartholin or Skene's glands should be Gram-stained and cultured for bacterial pathogens. An appropriate initial therapy is ampicillin or amoxicillin, 500 mg orally four times daily for 1 week. Repeated attacks of bartholinitis may occur, and surgery may be indicated if antibiotic therapy failure occurs.

NONVENEREAL DERMATOLOGIC CONDITIONS

Patients attending sexually transmitted disease clinics may have any number of puzzling dermatologic conditions on the skin of the genitalia and perineum. The purpose of this section is to list a selected number of skin lesions with a short description so that the clinician or nondermatologist might have a point of reference prior to consulting a dermatology text or deciding that the patient should be referred. Initially the examiner should ascertain whether the condition is confined to the genitalia. As a second generalization, when in doubt as to the nature of the lesion, a biopsy may provide an answer.

Trauma

Usually the results of trauma are obvious. The patient can supply the history, although sometimes a little encouragement is necessary because of the circumstances under which the trauma occurred. This may be especially true if the trauma has been the result of masturbation. On the other hand, patients may supply a history of trauma to explain an ulcer which is in reality a manifestation of syphilis or other sexually transmitted disease. Human bites are often quite serious and may require surgical management. Citron and Wade reported four patients with penile injuries as a result of using a vacuum cleaner for sexual excitement. They noted that the patients "were driven to new lengths by the novelty of the experience and came to grief."

Bacterial or Mycologic Skin Infections

Other than the sexually transmitted agents previously mentioned, patients may acquire a number of superficial fungal or bacterial skin infections. Staphylococcal folliculitis or furunculosis may be present. Group A streptococcal genital skin infections resulting in cellulitis or impetigo fortunately are not common but may result from fellatio from an infected partner. In some tropical countries, schistosomal infection of the genitalia may be confused with other sexually transmitted diseases. Cutaneous schistosomal lesions may present as painful nodules or warty growths on the vulva, clitoris, labia, and cervix. Edema and inflammation is commonly associated with the granulomatous growths. The diagnosis is made by identification of the ova in a biopsy specimen. Lesions seem to be more frequent with S. haematobium.

Candida albicans

These infections have been covered elsewhere. Superficial fungal (tinea cruris) infections generally itch, are scaly, and are commonly found in the groin. They may be diagnosed by means of a culture and a microscopic examination of a 10% potassium hydroxide preparation of skin scales.

Balanitis and Balanoposthitis

The former term describes inflammation of the glans penis or glans clitoridis; the latter, inflammation of the glans penis and the overlying prepuce. Balanitis and balanoposthitis in men are typically caused by Candida albicans. Kinghorn et al. reported that subpreputial carriage of Gardnerella vaginalis and Bacteroides species may be responsible for balanoposthitis in some men with phimosis or long redundant prepuces. With these infections comes a mild irritation of the prepuce and glans penis often associated with an excessive offensive-smelling preputial discharge.

Hidradenitis suppurativa

Hidradenitis suppurativa is a chronic disease resulting from obstruction of the apocrine ducts resulting in dilatation and secondary bacterial infection. The apocrine glands in the axillae and the anogenital areas are principally involved. The disease is most common in patients between puberty and middle age. Obesity, tight clothing, local trauma, or chemical irritation may be predisposing factors. Small inflammatory swellings unrelated to hair follicles appear in the apocrine areas. The axillae are more frequently involved in women, whereas in men it is the perineum (Fig. 22.1).

If patients do not receive therapy, the initial lesions become abscesses and drain purulent or seropurulent fluid. With the passage of time, new lesions and the healing process of old lesions cause sinus tracts and the appearance of bands of fibrous tissue. Fistulas may form in the perianal area. These tracts become infected with a number of bacteria including staphylococci, streptococci, and gram-negative rods including Escherichia coli, Proteus mirabilus, and Pseudomonas aeruginosa.

Hidradenitis should be differentiated from furuncles, carbuncles, infected dermal inclusion cysts, lymphadenitis, or perirectal abscess. Advanced disease can be confused with

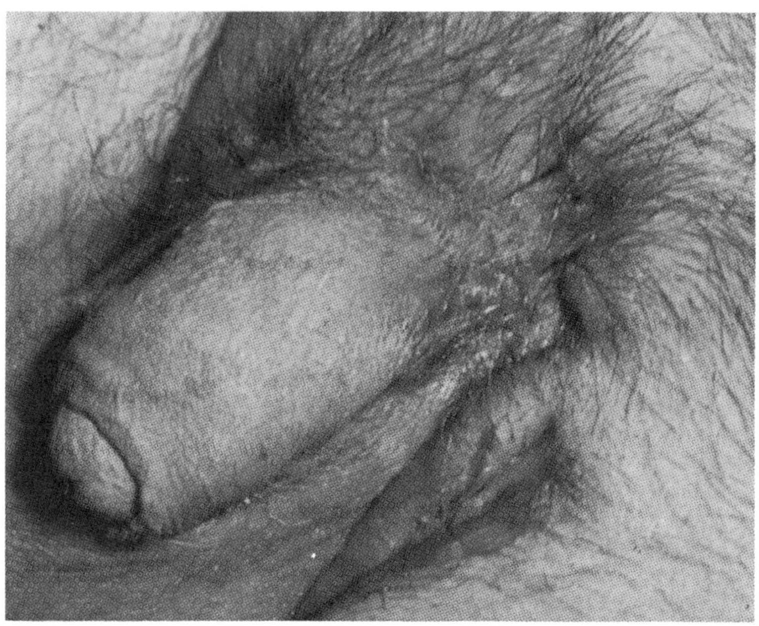

Figure 22.1   Hidradenitis suppuration may form draining sinus tracts and involve the perineum in men.   From T. B. Fitzpatrick, Atlas 9.   Disorders Primarily Affecting the Skin and Mucous Membranes; Ochronosis, p. 1827.   In T. B. Fitzpatrick, A. Z. Eisen, K. Wolff, I. M. Freedberg, and K. F. Austin.   Dermatology in General Medicine, 2nd ed., McGraw-Hill, New York, 1971.

lymphogranuloma venereum, granuloma inguinale, advanced tuberculosis, or actinomycosis.   The diagnosis is made by observation of the distribution of the lesions and their history.

Therapy should first be the removal of any inciting cause such as chemical irritants or skin-tight designer jeans.   Antibiotic therapy should be tailored to the offending organisms in the sinus tracts, and thrice daily hot tub soaks may be successful in treating early lesions.   In some cases intralesional steroids (triamcinolone, 10 mg/ml) may be administered.   Surgical drainage is required for advanced cases, and the open lesions may be treated with wet to dry saline dressings or a 1:40 dilution of Burow's solution three or four times daily.   Surgical therapy is required for medically unresponsive cases and is most successful if the involved tissue can be removed in a block. Untreated chronic lesions can result in fistula formation, fibrosis, and scarring, even to the point of inhibiting locomotion.

Seborrheic Dermatitis

Seborrheic dermatitis may involve the genital area, particularly in the crural and intergluteal folds. Maceration and erythema may be present in the intertriginous areas of fat people, and thus seborrheic dermatitis can be confused with <u>Candida</u> infection. However, the diagnosis usually is suggested by the presence of scalp lesions with scale and erythema. Often the lesions may be found in the fold behind the ear as well. Seborrheic dermatitis is treated with medicated shampoo.

Fournier's Gangrene

This rare infectious clinical entity is a fulminant disease of the scrotum and penis associated with prostration, systemic signs and symptoms of infection, swelling of the penis and scrotum, and local gangrene. Crepitation of the tissues of the perineum, genitalia, and sometimes the abdomen and thighs may be present. Fournier's gangrene is a surgical emergency. One unfortunate patient is shown in Fig. 22.2.

Lichen simplex chronicus

Lichen simplex chronicus or neurodermatitis is a poorly understood disorder causing itching and scratching, and resulting in skin thickening, hyperkeratosis, and deepening of skin folds. The labia major and minora and clitoral hood in women may become thickened and swollen. The scrotum in men may develop exaggerated rugosity, and the penile skin may become thickened. Itching of the anus is more common in men than in women and may result in lichenification of the skin. Contact dermatitis must be excluded.

Contact Dermatitis

Contact dermatitis is an acute or chronic eruption on the skin resulting from contact with a foreign substance. The eruption is a red, edematous rash with papules and vesicles. After chronic exposure the skin may be thickened and lichenified with hyper- or hypopigmentation. Erythema is generally the most prominent

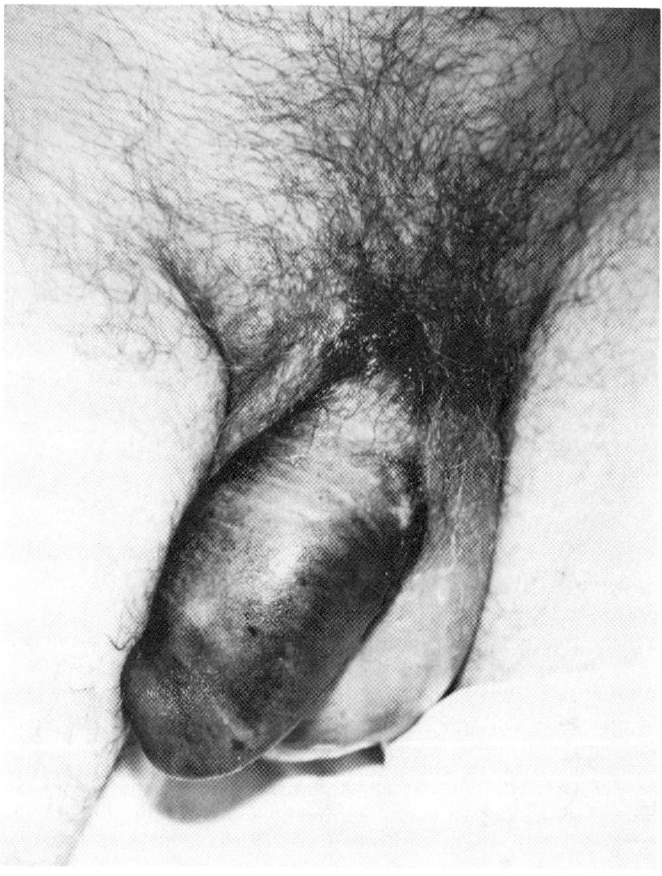

Figure 22.2   Fournier's gangrene of the penis is a surgical emergency.

feature on the penis and scrotum. Perspiration, friction, and pressure may influence both the appearance and the outcome of the rash.

Causes of contact dermatitis include a wide variety of agents including detergents, spermicidal jellies, diaphragms, condoms, colored or scented toilet paper, douches, vaginal deodorants, menstrual pads, or dye in clothes or undergarments.

Although the diagnosis is usually made on the clinical appearance of the rash, contact dermatitis can be confused with fungal infections or atopic and lichen simplex chronicus (neurodermatitis). A definitive diagnosis is made with a patch test of the suspected material along with suitable controls.

Treatment consists of identification and removal of the inciting agent and wearing loose-fitting clothing. Erythematous, painful rashes can be treated with thrice daily compresses of 1:40 dilute Burow's solution for several days.

Fixed Drug Eruptions

Certain drugs may result in a reaction on the genitals in some individuals. The drugs include tetracycline, penicillin, sulphonamides, phenolphthalein, antipyrine, quinine, quinidine, barbiturates, phenacetin, gold, phenylbutazone, chlordiazipoxide, and oxyphenbutazone.

The patient notices a burning sensation on the mucous membranes or skin followed by a well-demarcated circular or oval erythematous eruption that becomes dusky red in color. The lesions vary in diameter from a few millimeters to 3-4 cm in diameter, and bullae may occur (Fig. 22.3). With healing, the area becomes darkly pigmented and may remain so for several weeks to months. The lesions may be reproduced with readministration of the offending drug. Because vesicles are present, fixed drug eruption must be differentiated from genital herpes. In the fixed drug eruption, the vesicles are much larger than in herpes infection. Following withdrawal of the drug, the lesions resolve in a matter of days.

Psoriasis

Psoriasis is a chronic skin disease with epidermal hyperplasia and rapid rate epidermal turnover. White papules and plaques covered with silver scales are the characteristic lesions. The lesions have well-demarcated but irregular borders that start with an erythematous patch which elevates and develops scales. Maceration rather than scales may be present in lesions of the genitals. Psoriasis patches most frequently are found on the elbows, knees, intertriginous areas, scalp, and buttocks. Itching is more severe in erupting lesions, while older lesions may be asymptomatic. Half the patients will have abnormalities of their nails, and 10% will have arthritis.

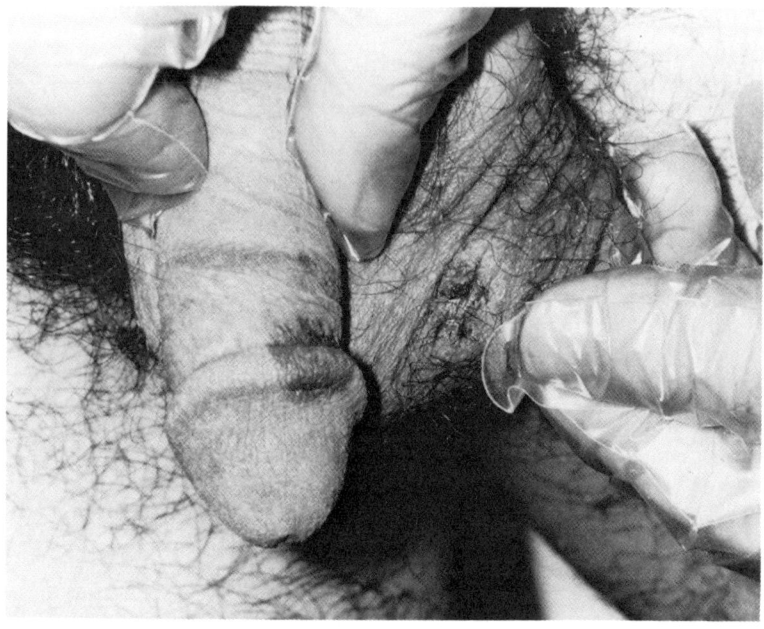

Figure 22.3   Fixed drug eruption.   A 26-year-old salesman noticed the sudden appearance of dark lesions on his scrotum and penis.   He believed that he might have AIDS.   Further history indicated that he had been taking tetracycline because of nongonococcal urethritis.   The lesions disappeared a few days after stopping the tetracycline.

Psoriasis can be confused with pityriasis rosea, lichen planus, superficial fungal infections, and seborrheic dermatitis.   If there is a question on the appearance of the lesions, a skin biopsy will resolve the diagnosis.   Therapy usually involves administration of topical steroids, keratolytic agents and, in severe cases, tar and possibly long-wave ultraviolet light.   The long-term effects of ultraviolet light treatments are unknown.

Pityriasis rosea

Pityriasis rosea is mentioned in this section because it is easily confused with the rash of secondary syphilis.   It occurs in all ages but most frequently between the ages of 10 and 35 years.

There is no known etiology, and the diagnosis is based on the clinical findings. A "herald patch" (2-6 cm) first appears anywhere on the body several days to weeks before the papulosquamous eruption that is generally distributed in the areas covered by clothing, sparing the face, hands, and feet in adults. The rash of secondary syphilis frequently involves the hands and feet. The lesions are oval, less than 2 cm, and light brown, tan, or pink in color with a central scale, "cigarette paper" in character. Lesions are distributed in skin folds and on the patient's back have a "fir tree" distribution. Most patients are symptomatic, but about 20% complain of itching. Itching may be worse after hot baths. The symptoms resolve in 2-14 weeks.

Lichen planus

No one knows what causes lichen planus, but it occurs in both sexes and all races. Most patients are 30-60 years old. Lichen planus may follow the use of certain drugs including antimalarials, thiazide diuretics, gold, phenolphthalein, and barbiturates. Lesions may disappear within 3 months or may last up to 3 years, although most resolve within 1 or 2 years.

The genitals may be involved, but usually the lesions are first seen on the upper extremities and the flexor surface of the wrist and forearm. Other involved areas include the sides of the neck, the back, the thighs, and shins. The face, palms, and soles are spared. The lesion of lichen planus is a small papule that is flat-topped with a central umbilication and covered with a thin scale. It also may be covered by a network of white lines called Wickham's striae. If the lesions are hypertrophic, they may be intensely pruritic. Scarring is uncommon, but hyperpigmentation can occur and remain for months. As in psoriasis, the isomorphic or Koebner phenomenon can be induced by trauma.

Genital lesions in men are usually papular in nature but may have an annular configuration (Fig. 22.4). Men with lichen planus have genital lesions in about one-fourth of cases with the glans most commonly involved. The anus may be involved as well. Lesions on the vulva and in the vaginal vault are similar to lesions found in the mouth.

Lichen planus may be confused with drug eruptions, psoriasis, leukoplakia, Candida infection, mucous patches of secondary syphilis, and seborrheic dermatitis. Itching penile lesions suggest scabies. Hypertrophic lesions must be differentiated from Kaposi's sarcoma, neurodermatitis, and cutaneous amyloid. If the lesions are not typical, a biopsy is in order to establish the diagnosis.

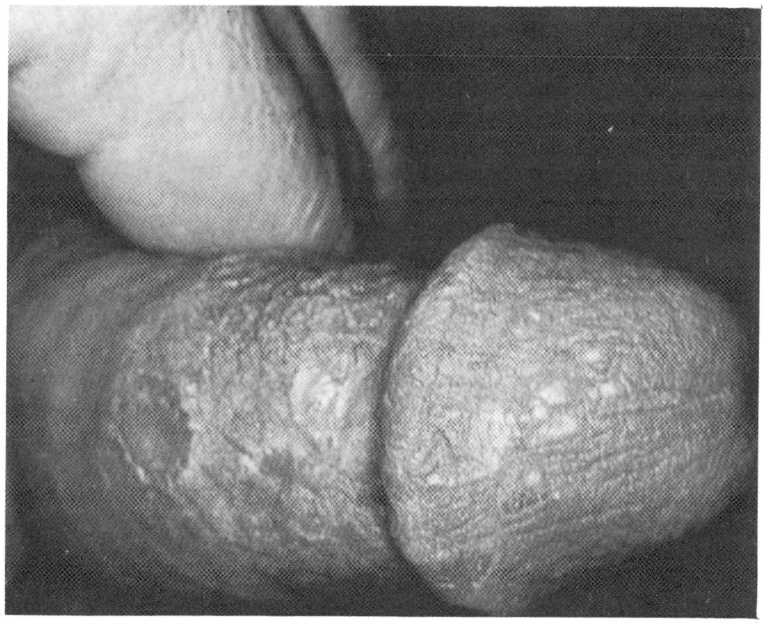

Figure 22.4 Lesions of lichen planus on the penis. Reprinted from S. M. Bluefarb. Dermatology. A Scope Publication. With permission from the Upjohn Company, Kalamazoo, Mich., 49001.

The passage of time is the best treatment, as the disease is benign and self-limited. Topical steroids under occlusive dressings may cause the lesions to regress. Offending drugs, if identified, should be discontinued.

Vitiligo

Vitiligo is a disease of unknown etiology resulting in the loss of melanin in the skin. The disease is more common in women than in men and affects all races equally. The patients are generally between the ages of 10 and 30 years old, and one-third have another family member with the disease.

The lesions are pale white macules a few millimeters to several centimeters in diameter with an oval or round shape that enlarge slowly over time. Small areas of pigment may surround hair follicles in the lesions. The genitalia may be involved, but the lesions have no particular predilection except possibly for the extensor bony surfaces such as the knees, elbows, and digits.

The diagnosis is rarely in question, and the therapy is generally trioxalen and timed exposure to ultraviolet irradiation or sunlight in an attempt to repigment the lesions.

Fox-Fordyce Disease

Fox-Fordyce disease is a disorder that results from plugging and/or rupture of the intraepidermal apocrine gland ducts, causing changes in the secretory tubule and dermis.

Patients complain of itching and skin-colored or pigmented follicular papules in the axilla, pubic area, and mammary areola. The disease is most common between the ages of 13 and 35, and women are affected nine times more frequently than men. The affected areas may have less hair as the result of excoriation, and the itching is aggravated by sweating. The diagnosis is made by biopsy, and there really is no effective therapy.

Angiokeratomas

Angiokeratomas are 2-3 mm multiple lesions found on the labia and scrotum. There are two types of angiokeratomas. The angiokeratomas of Fordyce have little keratin and are highly vascular. They are not associated with any internal vascular abnormality, although they may rupture and bleed superficially. The angiokeratoma corporis diffusum of Fabrey looks like the angiokeratoma of Fordyce but is related to a metabolic disorder of lipids. They may be distinguished histologically. The diagnosis is made by their characteristic appearance, and there is no therapy.

Pearly Penile Papules (Acral Angiofibromas)

Pearly penile papules are multiple lesions (1-4 mm in size) located in one to five rows around the coronal sulcus of the penis. The cause is unknown, and they have such a characteristic appearance that they are likely to be confused only with warts or lichen nitidis. The latter lesions appear on the penile shaft as well. Excision is the only therapy, and histologic examination provides the diagnosis.

Lichen nitidis

Lichen nitidis is a rare, chronic eruption that is characterized by asymptomatic, normally pigmented, small papules on the
genitals, anus, and abdomen. There is no predilection for any sex
or race. The papules are usually discrete, slightly raised, pin-
head, and polygonal or round, and their surface has a glistening
character. They are found most often on the glans and shaft of the
penis, the groin, the lower abdomen, the flexor surface of the
arms, the palmer surface of the wrists, and the breasts. Lichen
nitidis can be confused with flat warts, lichen planus, or pearly
penile papules. Warts are brown in color, lichen planus is violaci-
ous, and lichen nitidis is flesh colored. Biopsy is definitive, and
there is no therapy.

Ectopic Sebaceous Glands

On occasion sebaceous glands may be found on mucocutaneous
junctions high in the cutus and unrelated to hair follicles. They do
not generally cause any problems.

Benign Transient Lymphangiectasis of the Penis (Sclerosing Lymphangitis)

Benign lymphangiectasis of the penis, an uncommon condition
of unknown etiology, results in thickening of the connective tissue
in the wall of lymphatic vessels with partial or total occlusion. It
is most commonly seen in sexually active men between 20 and 40
years of age. It usually appears suddenly, after intercourse, as
painless, hard, nodular, translucent cord in the penis, sometimes
in the coronal sulcus. A number of the reported patients developed
their lesions after oral-genital sex. Stolz described similar lesions
in the labium majora and labium minora of two women. The condition may persist for 1-4 months but is self-limiting, and the patients
need only reassurance. A few days abstinence from intercourse
may help.

Penile Venereal Edema

This is a benign, uncommon, self-limited condition of sexually
active men presenting as a painless, boggy swelling of the prepuce
and penile shaft. Friction or trauma may play an etiologic role,
and the condition frequently is associated with urethritis or pyoderma.

Some patients believe that the condition results from intercourse with a partner who is poorly lubricated. Penile venereal edema is fairly characteristic, but lymphedema of the penis and scrotum can have a number of causes including filiariasis, severe congestive heart failure, hypoproteinemia, and radiation, surgical, or neoplastic obstruction of lymphatic flow. Lymphedema also may result from paraffin or silicone injections into the penis and trauma as a result of constrictive rubber bands or devices used to prolong erection. Penile venereal edema usually resolves spontaneously with abstinence from intercourse or after treatment of an underlying urethritis or skin infection.

Premalignant and Malignant Genital Lesions

The lesions described below are best treated by dermatologists, and the diagnosis is generally made by biopsy.

Note: Dermatologic terms have often been a problem for the nondermatologist, and the terms to diagnose vulvar disease are no exception. Friedrich and the Committee on Terminology of the International Society for the Study of Vulvar Disease have suggested that a number of terms used in this book be dropped including leukoplakia, lichen sclerosis et atrophicus, neurodermatitis, Bowen's disease, and erythroplasia of Queyrat. Since this advice is relatively new (1976) and some of the readers may be old, I have placed the new terms in parentheses as a transitional compromise.

Leukoplakia (Vulvar Dystrophy)

Leukoplakia is variously defined but originally described any white plaque that persisted on a mucous or mucocutaneous surface. Lesions appear in the mouth as a response to irritation. Leukoplakia in women occurs on the inner aspects of the labia majora, the anterior fourchette, the introitus, the labia minora, and the clitoris. Leukoplakia may be easily confused with lichen simplex, and it may be present along with lichen sclerosus.

Lichen sclerosus et atrophicus (Lichen sclerosus)

This is an uncommon disease most often found in whites and women. The lesions are small, white, and atrophic and most often are present on the genitalia, but they also may be found on the trunk. Lichen sclerosis et atrophicus may be confused with leuko-plakia and lichen planus. The lesions of the latter have a more violaceous color. When the vulva and perianal areas are involved together, they form an inverted keyhold distribution. LSA also may be present on the trunk and limbs and, if present before puber-ty, the lesions may resolve. Although LSA may be asymptomatic, women commonly complain of soreness, dyspareuria, and dysuria. Lesions on the outer aspects of the labia majora may become lichenified and, in anogenital LSA, lesions may become macerated and hyperkeratotic. LSA may result in atrophy of the labia minora and, in severe cases, there may be contracture of the introitus. In long-standing lesions, there may be transient ulceration and secondary infection. Small adjacent areas of leukoplakia may com-plicate LSA, and the patient may suffer with itching.

In men LSA is generally confined to the glans and prepuce. In circumcised men the lesions appear anywhere on the glans, in-cluding the urinary meatus (Fig. 22.5). This may result in restric-tion of the urinary flow.

Contractures of the foreskin may occur in uncircumcised men, resulting in phinosis and in a need for circumcision. One term given to this is balanitis xerotica obliterans (Fig. 22.6). Leuko-plakia and resulting carcinoma may be present in the preputial sac.

LSA in men and women may be easily confused with a number of other conditions. In men this includes any form of balanitis, erythroplasias, and leukoplakia. Involvement in premphigoid may cause severe atrophy and adhesions of the prepuce to the glands. In women the diagnosis is equally difficult because of the presence of dermatitis, maceration, and the effects of excoriation. Leuko-plakia may be confused with LSA and be present in addition to LSA. Lichen planus also may be confused with LSA. However, lichen planus usually is present at other sites on the body. Macerated and inflamed areas may be confused with <u>Candida</u> infections. Biopsy is necessary for a definitive diagnosis. Before biopsy it may be necessary to clear up any superficial infection and inflam-mation that would make interpretation difficult.

Itching is one of the most disturbing symptoms in women. Control of this may require the application of topical steroids. Unfortunately atrophy is a side effect of this medication, and the weakest preparation that will control the symptoms is the one that should be used. Intralesional steroids or freezing with liquid nitrogen has been effective.

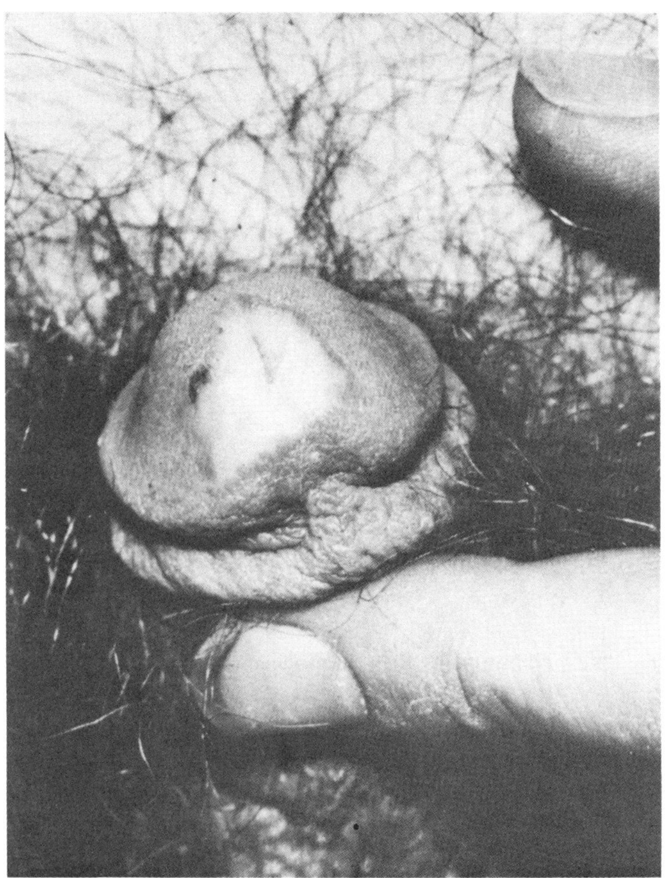

Figure 22.5   A linear white atrophic plaque of lichen sclerosis involving the urethral orifice.   From H. J. Wallace and A. B. Hyman, Disorders of the External Genitalia, Chapter 97, p. 919.   In T. B. Fitzpatrick, A. Z. Eisen, K. Wolff, I. M. Freedberg, and K. F. Austin, Dermatology in General Medicine, 2nd ed., McGraw-Hill, New York, 1971.

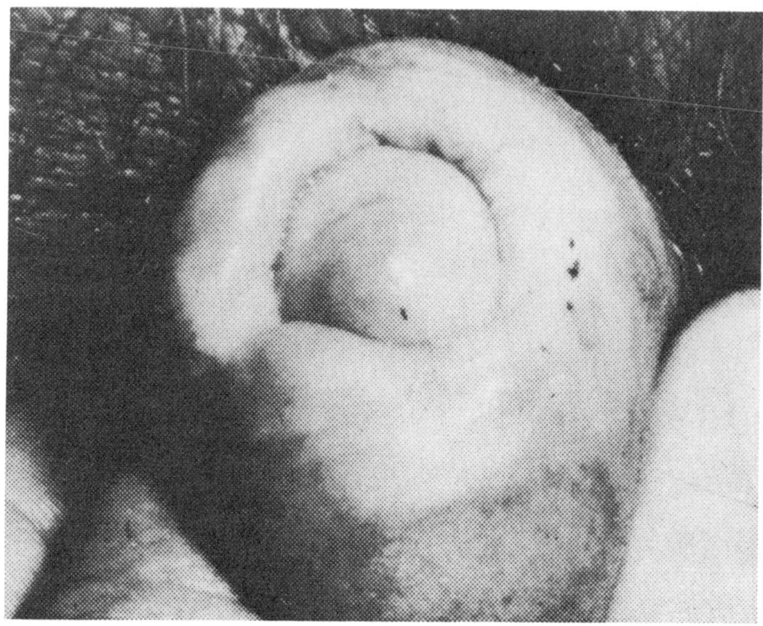

Figure 22.6 Balanitis xerotica obliterans. From H. J. Wallace
and A. B. Hyman, Disorders of the External Genitalia, Chapter
97, p. 919. In T. B. Fitzpatrick, A. Z. Eisen, K. Wolff, I. M.
Freedberg, and K. F. Austin. Dermatology in General Medicine,
2nd ed., McGraw-Hill, New York, 1971.

Zoon's Plasma Cell Balanitis

This is a condition more often found in middle-aged or elderly
men and is characterized by erythematous, shiny lesions. Benign
erythroplasia also may be present as an asymptomatic velvety,
red, moist, plaque-like lesion on the vulva in women (vulvar dys-
trophy) and in the buccal mucosa. It is not thought to be premalignant, but it must be distinguished from a rare premalignant lesion
described below.

Erythroplasia of Queyrat (Squamous
Cell Carcinoma in situ)

This is a well-defined, slightly raised, velvety, red plaque
found on the penis of men (Fig. 22.7) and the labia minora of women.

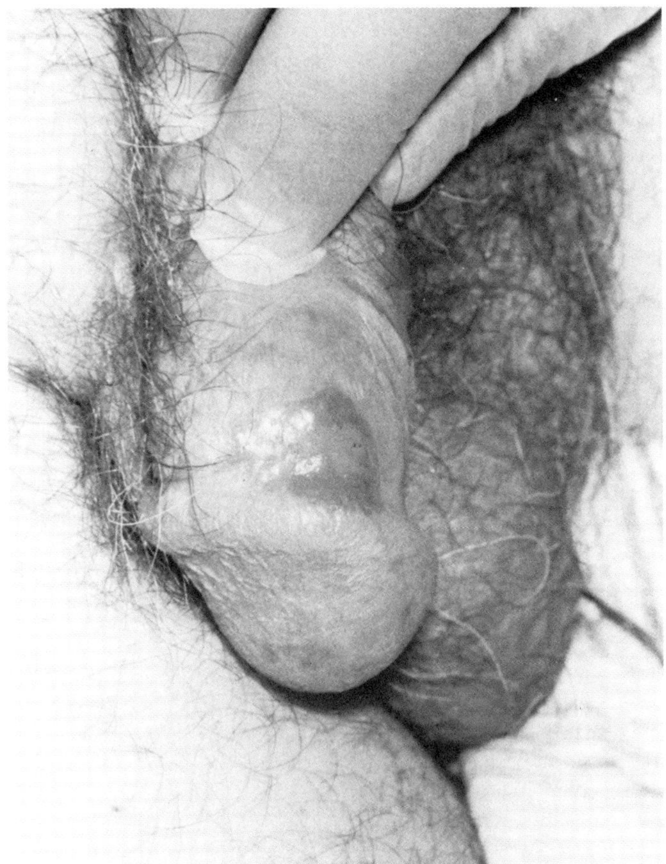

Figure 22.7 Erythroplasia of Queyrat versus Bowen's disease is what our urologists diagnosed when they saw this velvety, red, superficial marginated plaque on the penis of a 62-year-old white married man. A biopsy initially showed squamous cell carcinoma in situ, and the entire lesion subsequently was removed. The pathology report showed invasive squamous cell carcinoma in one lateral margin of the lesion. The patient was well, and the lesion was gone 1 year later.

In women lesions may itch or burn, causing dysuria and painful intercourse. Erythroplasia of Queyrat is more common later in life in men than in women, and it is unusual in men who have been circumcised as infants. Some authors believe that erythroplasia of Queyrat and Bowen's disease are histologically the same. However, not all erythroplastic lesions are the same, as some benign varieties do occur. Bowen's disease may be distinguished from erythroplasia of Queyrat if lesions are present on the other body areas.

Bowen's Disease (Squamous Cell Carcinoma in situ)

This is a term given to intraepidermal carcinoma. The lesions are sharply defined, thickened, and brown to brownish red plaques. There may be areas of hyperkeratosis resulting in skin scales. The lesions are not restricted to the genitalia. Excision is the treatment of choice.

Paget's Disease

Paget's disease generally is associated with the nipple and carcinoma of the breast. However, Paget's disease of the genitalia can occur, usually in older adults. It presents as a white, irregularly shaped, hyperkeratotic plaque with or without areas of erosion. In men the scrotum is the most commonly involved area, but the perianal area and groin also may be involved. In women the labia majora is the most commonly involved site, but lesions can be present on the perineum, groin, and perianal area. Itching may be the first symptom. Since it can be confused with leukoplakia, any persistent white hyperkeratotic plaque on the genitalia should be biopsied for a definitive diagnosis. Wide excision and lymph node removal generally are required.

Squamous Cell Carcinoma

This tumor usually develops after middle age. In women who have carcinoma of the vulva, lichen sclerosis et atrophicus is a common precursor. Squamous cell carcinoma also may complicate leukoplakia, usually in older adults. In younger individuals it may complicate Bowen's disease. Squamous cell carcinoma also may be present on the male genitalia and is said to be more frequent in uncircumcised men.

BIBLIOGRAPHY

Acute Epididymitis

Berger RE, Alexander ER, Monda GD, Ansell J, McCormick G, Holmes KK. Chlamydia trachomatis as a cause of acute idiopathic epididymitis. N Eng J Med, 298:301-304, 1978.

Berger RE. Editorial. Acute epididymitis. Sex Transm Dis, 8: 286-289, 1981.

Berger RE, Alexander ER, Harnisch JP, et al. Etiology, manifestations and therapy of acute epididymitis: Prospective study of 50 cases. J Urol, 121:750-754, 1979.

Bernstein SM, Celano T, Sibulkin D. Fournier's gangrene of the penis. South Med J, 69:1242-1244, 1976.

Holmes KK. Acute epididymitis. Curr Ther Res, 26:738-744, 1979.

Sufrin G. Acute epididymitis. Sex Transm Dis, 8:132-139, 1981.

Torsion of the Testis

Haynes BE, Bessen HA, Haynes VE. The diagnosis of testicular torsion. J Amer Med Assoc, 249:2522-2527, 1983.

Masses in the Scrotum

Bailey H. Demonstrations of Physical Signs in Clinical Surgery, 13th ed. Williams and Wilkins, Baltimore, 1960.

Acute Prostatitis

Brunner H, Weidner W, Schiefer H-G. Studies on the role of Ureaplasma urealyticum and Mycoplasma hominis in prostatitis. J Infect Dis, 147:807-813, 1983.

Krieger JN. Prostatitis syndromes: pathophysiology, differential diagnosis, and treatment. Sex Transm Dis, 11:100-112.

Mears EM. Prostatitis and related diseases. Disease-a-Month, 26(8), May 1980.

Mears EM. Prostatitis syndrome. New perspective about old woes. J Urol, 123:141-147, 1980.

Simmons PD, Thin RN. A method for recognizing non-bacterial prostatitis: Preliminary observations. Br. J Vener Dis, 59:306-310, 1983.

Infection of the Bartholin and Skene's Glands

Davis JA, Rees E, Hobson D, Karayannis P. Isolation of *Chlamydia trachomatis* from Bartholin's ducts. Br J Vener Dis, 54:409-413, 1978.

Lee YH, Rankin JS, Alpert S, et al. Microbiological investigation of Bartholin's gland abscesses and cysts. Amer J Obstet Gynecol, 129:150-153, 1977.

Pearson HE, Anderson GV. Genital bacteroidal abscesses in women. Amer J Obstet Gynecol, 107:1264-1265, 1970.

Rees E. Gonococcal bartholinitis. Br J Vener Dis, 43:150-156, 1967.

Sarrell PM, Steege JF, Maltzer M, Bolinsky D. Pain during sex response due to occlusion of the Bartholin gland duct. Obstet Gynecol, 62:261-264, 1983.

Nonvenereal Dermatologic Conditions

Akerman AB, Kornberg R. Pearly penile papules. Acral angio-fibromatosis. Arch Dermatol, 108:673-675, 1973.

Attili VR, Hira SK, Dube MK. Schistosomal genital granuloma: A report of 10 cases. Br J Vener Dis, 59:269-272, 1983.

Bingham JS. Carcinoma of the penis developing in lichen sclerosis et atrophicus. Br J Vener Dis, 54:350-351, 1978.

Burket JM. Dark plaque in nether regions. A sign of carcinoma in situ. J Amer Med Assoc, 230:439-440, 1974.

Chapel TC, Rahbari H. Genital bowenoid papulosis-squamous cell carcinoma in situ. Sex Transm Dis, 7:139-141, 1980.

Citron NJ, Wade PJ. Penile injuries from vacuum cleaners. Br Med J, 281:26, 1980.

Drusin LM, Wilkes BM, Gingrich RD. Streptococcal pyoderma of the penis following fellatio. Br J Vener Dis, 51:61-62, 1975.

Ferrer RA, Felman YM, Scham MJ, et al. Nonvenereal anogenital lesions I and II. The City of N.Y. Sex Transm Dis Newsletter, 3(4, 5), 1980.

Fitzpatrick TB, Eisen AZ, Wolff A, et al. (eds.). Dermatology in General Medicine, 2nd ed. McGraw-Hill, New York, 1979.

Fiumara NJ. Psoriasis of the penis: Koebner reaction following oral genital exposure. J Amer Vener Dis Assoc, 3:59-60, 1976.

Fiumara NJ. Nonvenereal sclerosing lymphangitis of the penis. Arch Dermatol, 111:902-903, 1975.

Fiumara NJ, Yaqub M. Pigmented penile lesions (fixed drug eruptions) associated with tetracycline therapy for sexually transmitted diseases. Sex Transm Dis, 8:23-25, 1981.

Friedrich EG, Committee on Terminology, ISSVD. New nomenclature for vulvar disease. Obstet Gynecol, 47:122-124, 1976.

Gochfeld M, Burger J. Sexual transmission of nickel and poison oak contact dermatitis. Lancet, 1:589, 1983.

Hutchins P, Dunlop EMC, Rodin P. Benign transient lymphangiectasis (sclerosing lymphangitis) of the penis. Br J Vener Dis, 53:379-385, 1977.

Jones RB, Hirschmann JV, Brown GS, et al. Fournier's syndrome: Necrotizing subcutaneous infection of the male genitalia. J Urol, 122:279-282, 1979.

Kahn RI, McAninch JW. Granulomatous disease of the testis. J Urol, 123:868-871, 1980.

Lerner AB, Nordlund JJ. Vitiligo. What is it? Is it important?
J Amer Med Assoc, 239:1183-1187, 1978.

Lewis PS. Sexually transferred drug adverse reaction to isosor-
bide dinitrate cream. Lancet, 2:1441, 1983.

Lupulescu A, Mehregan AH, Rahhari H, Pinkus H, Birmingham
DJ. Venereal warts vs Bowen disease. A histologic and ultrastructural study of five cases. J Amer Med Assoc, 237:2520,
1977.

Malloy TR, Wein AJ, Gross P. Scrotal and penile lymphoedema:
Surgical consideration and management. J Urol, 130:263-265,
1983.

McMillan A. Lymphocele and localized lymphoedema of the penis.
Br J Vener, 52:409-411, 1976.

Moss TR, Stevenson CJ. Incidence of genital vitiligo. Report of
a screening programme. Br J Vener Dis, 57:145-146, 1981.

Newell GB, Voelter WW, Mullins JF. Treatment of hidradenitis
suppurativa. J Amer Med Assoc, 233:556, 1973.

Pasricha JS. Drugs causing fixed eruptions. Br J Dermatol, 100:
183-185, 1979.

Shaughnessy DM, Greminger RR, Margolis IB, Davis WC. Hidradenitis suppurativa. A plea for early operative treatment. J Amer
Med Assoc, 222:320-321, 1972.

Stein DS. Transmissible venereal neoplasia: A case report.
Amer J Obstet Gynecol, 137:864-865, 1980.

Stolz E, van Kampen WJ. Sklerosierende Lymphangitis des Penis,
der Oberlippe und des Labium minus. Der Hautarzt, 25:231-237,
1974.

Wilde H, Canby JP. Penile venereal edema. Arch Derm, 108:263,
1973.

Wright RA, Judson FN. Penile venereal edema. J Amer Med
Assoc, 241:157-158, 1979.

Chapter 23

PROPHYLAXIS AND CONTROL OF SEXUALLY
TRANSMITTED DISEASES

Prophylaxis would appear to be an effective means of controlling sexually transmitted diseases. For the population as a whole,
however, the available methods have not been effective, possibly
because of inadequate utilization. Physicians and health agencies
have not actively promoted prophylactic measures, probably because the evidence supporting their effectiveness is so meager.
Given today's safeguards for experimental subjects and the requirements which must be met to demonstrate that a particular measure
is effective as prophylactic, it is unlikely that appropriate studies
will be forthcoming in the near future. The existing data relate to
only a few of the sexually transmitted diseases.

The methods of prophylaxis fall into several categories: behavioral, use of mechanical barriers, local application of chemotherapeutic agents, systemic administration of chemotherapeutic
agents, and immunization. Given the wide variety of infectious
agents that must be dealt with, one can see that the first two measures would have the greatest likelihood of success, if they could be
implemented. The behavioral approach may be the most difficult,
because attitudes are resistant to change. The use of mechanical
barriers, such as the condom, is not popular at the moment in the
United States. The application or administration of chemotherapeutic agents may have harmful side effects, and the wide variety
of sexually transmitted diseases precludes immunization as a practical method.

BEHAVIORAL ASPECTS

Abstinence or the establishment of a monogamous relationship
with an uninfected sexual partner are effective methods of controlling

the spread of sexually transmitted diseases. They are not likely
to be popular, however, within the age group of individuals most
likely to acquire venereal diseases. Attempts at control or suppression of commercialized prostitution also have met with failure.
In 1941 the Surgeon General of the United States wrote to Congress-
man May indicating that venereal disease was at that time the
greatest single cause of noneffectiveness in the Army. With the
passage of the May Act in July 1941, the suppression of prostitution
became national policy. The act was only invoked twice, at Camp
Forrest, Tennessee, in May of 1942, and at Fort Bragg, North
Carolina, in July of the same year. Despite the best intentions,
the May Act was not effective because of the lack of local cooperation combined with the rigid requirements of the federal court in
defining the admissibility of evidence.

The problem of controlling venereal disease among U.S.
troops in World War II illustrates the difficulty of altering behavior,
given widely dissimilar social backgrounds and environmental conditions. In opposition to military policy, some troop commanders
provided brothels for use by U.S. troops. Control of venereal disease was attempted by setting up large prophylaxis stations near
the brothel entrances. The prophylaxis measures at that time con-
sisted of topically applied preparations and condoms. Despite
these efforts, the experience in Oran, Algeria, demonstrated that
the most effective way of diminishing venereal disease was closing
the brothels. This realization followed the observation that the
venereal disease rates dropped markedly after the brothels were
closed for an 18-day period because of a water shortage.

Restriction and control of prostitution as a method of controlling venereal disease is an idea that still periodically resurfaces.
In 1978 the governing body of the City of Rotterdam passed a proposal to concentrate the city's prostitutes in a large motel located
in the harbor area. The plan met with considerable resistance
from the residents of that part of the city as well as complaints
from the prostitutes that such an establishment would not constitute
a cozy atmosphere. It is unlikely that such measures, although
well intentioned, are effective in the reduction of venereal disease.
In the United States the transmission of venereal disease is probably more common through sexual contact with casual acquaintances
than through sexual contact with prostitutes.

Another behavioral method, postcoital urination, also is of no
proven benefit in preventing sexually transmitted diseases.

MECHANICAL BARRIERS

The condom is the major effective barrier device for the prevention of sexually transmitted diseases. It is the most widely used contraceptive in many industrialized countries, including Sweden, Norway, Denmark, the United Kingdom, and Japan. If the condom is correctly in place during sexual activity, it is the most effective mechanism available for preventing sexually transmitted diseases such as gonorrhea. Evidence of its effectiveness in the prevention of nongonococcal urethritis and certain other sexually transmitted diseases is not as convincing.

Condoms have not been widely utilized by individuals attending venereal disease clinics, and in some parts of the United States they may be purchased only in a drugstore. A conference devoted to methods of increasing condom utilization in the United States suggested a number of remedies:

1. Repeal of state and local laws prohibiting the advertising and display of condoms and restricting their sale to certain outlets
2. Removal of the National Association of Broadcaster's ban on contraceptive advertising
3. Efforts to change the attitudes of the media concerning the acceptance of condom advertising
4. Increased application of innovative marketing techniques and commercial condom merchandising
5. Presentation of information on educational programs to correct erroneous images of the condom
6. Development of effective promotion and support of condom distribution in family planning programs
7. Development of internationally acceptable testing procedures based upon the desired performance of condoms in contraceptive use

Beginning in 1970 the Swedish Association for Sex Education (RFSU) undertook a positive advertising and merchandising program to increase the use of condoms. In June 1971 this organization launched a campaign to educate the public regarding the function of the condom as a prophylaxis against gonorrhea. The campaign included public poster advertising and widespread media coverage. The media apparently helped create a more positive attitude toward the condom. There was a marked increase in condom purchases,

particularly by young people and women. Coincident with the rise
in sales of condoms, there was a decline in the number of reported
cases of gonorrhea.

No such campaign has been launched in the United States, and
as late as 1969, many magazines, including those designed exclusively for men, refused to carry condom advertising. Although
condom advertising now appears in some magazines, such ads are
not commonly seen in newspapers and are unheard of on television
or the radio. Yehudi M. Felman, director of the Bureau of Venereal Disease Control for New York City, has pointed out the paradox
of health values in the United States today: while cigarettes, which
are known to cause disease, are prominently advertised in the
press, condoms, which prevent disease, are not considered a suitable subject for advertisements. He also made a plea that the condom be used by sexually active teenagers, pointing out that it has
a number of advantages:

1. It can be conveniently kept in a pocket or purse for quick use
    when needed.
2. It is inexpensive, easily within the limits of most teenagers'
    financial capabilities.
3. It acts as both a contraceptive and a prophylactic, which is an
    advantage to teenagers who may have many different sex part-
    ners.
4. It can be used by the sexually active woman in a doubtful situ-
    ation as a protection against sexually transmitted diseases,
    even if the woman is using another form of contraception.
5. It can actually enhance the sexual pleasure of both partners by
    delaying the man's orgasm. This delaying effect also may be
    considered to be an undesirable feature of condoms by some,
    and may be directly related to the thickness of the condom.
    American standards for condom manufacture permit thicknesses
    of up to 0.09 mm, making American condoms among the thick-
    est manufactured in the world.

Attitudes on condom usage may be changing in the United
States. In October 1979 a national consumer magazine reported
the results of a questionnaire returned by 1874 readers. According
to the respondents, the main advantages of the condom were its
convenience and ease of use, its lack of side effects, and its effectiveness as a contraceptive measure. The disadvantages were
reported to be interruption of lovemaking, awareness of the presence of the condom, reduced sensation in both men and women, and

the need to withdraw promptly after ejaculation. The American market presently offers a large number of latex condoms with a variety of textures, shapes, and colors. In addition, there are a smaller number of skin condoms made from sheep intestines. The latter account for less than 5% of condom sales in the United States. Many individuals believe that skin condoms provide far greater sensation; however, they are two to three times more expensive than the latex condoms.

There are no proven protective effects in terms of the prevention of sexually transmitted diseases to be derived from the use of the diaphragm or other contraceptive devices for women. However, women who use barrier forms of contraception and oral contraceptives are less likely to acquire pelvic inflammatory disease. Women who use intrauterine devices are more likely to acquire pelvic inflammatory disease (Chapter 14).

TOPICAL PROPHYLAXIS

Local prophylactic measures include soap and water, douching agents, contraceptive foams, jellies, creams, and certain other preparations that may be topically applied to men or administered by douche to women following intercourse. In addition, antibiotic-containing tablets have been devised that are inserted into the vagina. At the moment there are no commercial preparations for local prophylaxis of venereal disease marketed in the United States. Some of the spermicidal contraceptive foams, jellies, or creams may have antimicrobial activity and specifically inhibit in vitro growth of <u>Neisseria gonorrhoeae.</u> Jick and coworkers have shown lower rates of gonorrhea among women who use vaginal spermicides.

There is no known value for washing with soap and water. Topical antibiotics or chemotherapeutic agents may have some effectiveness if they are used following intercourse; however, such preparations are not currently available. The use of antibiotics or chemotherapeutic agents topically may be followed by local hypersensitivity reactions and/or the development of resistant flora. It is unlikely, also, that the individuals most often subject to repeated attacks of venereal diseases would be sufficiently motivated to carefully apply the topical agent. During World War II the application of topical ointments containing picrate plus calomel or sulfathiazole plus calomel appeared to have some postcoital protective effect against acquiring gonorrhea. More recently, in a study performed in Nevada, a group of prostitutes appeared to receive some protective effect from the intravaginal preparation containing orthoiodobenzoic acid; however, this material caused vaginal drying or irritation and thus was not acceptable. At present no locally applied preparation can be recommended for the prevention of sexually transmitted diseases except as described for the prevention of gonococcal ophthalmia in neonates.

SYSTEMIC PROPHYLAXIS

Antibiotics used in systemic prophylaxis generally are given immediately following exposure. The idea is to give a single dose of an agent after the sexual contact. Older studies showed that small oral doses of penicillin G reduced the incidence of gonorrhea, and a more recent study with oral minocycline showed similar effects. However, subtherapeutic doses of antibiotics are not now recommended for gonorrhea prophylaxis because of the presence of increased numbers of antibiotic-resistant gonococci, the problem of masking symptoms of the disease, and the possibility of selecting antibiotic-resistant micro-organisms. No single antibiotic is effective for the wide variety of micro-organisms that may be sexually transmitted. Treatment of rape victims and of individuals following a casual sexual encounter with a potentially infected partner is covered elsewhere.

IMMUNIZATION

A vaccine for gonorrhea is currently undergoing development in the United States. But it is unlikely to be available for general use for some time.

BIBLIOGRAPHY

Babione RW, Hedgecock LE, Ray JP. Navy experience with the oral use of penicillin as a prophylaxis. U.S. Armed Forces Med J, 3:973-990, 1952.

Barlow D. The condom and gonorrhea. Lancet, 2:811-812, 1977.

Barrett-Connor E. The prophylaxis of gonorrhea. Amer J Med Sci, 269:4-11, 1975.

Bergman AB. Condoms for sexually active adolescents. Amer J Dis Child, 134:247-249, 1980.

Bettley FR. The medical conduct of a brothel. Br J Vener Dis, 25:56-66, 1949.

Cole CH, Lecher TG, Bailey JC, et al. Vaginal chemoprophylaxis in the reduction of reinfection in women with gonorrhea: Clinical evaluation of the effectiveness of a vaginal contraceptive. Br J Vener Dis, 56:314-318, 1980.

Consumers Union: Condoms. A report based on laboratory tests and on detailed questionnaries filled out by nearly 1900 readers. Consumer Rep, pp. 583-589, October 1979.

Cutler JC. Current concepts of prophylaxis. Bull NY Acad Med, 52:886-896, 1976.

Cutler JC, Singh B, Carpenter U, et al. Vaginal contraceptives as prophylaxis against gonorrhea and other sexually transmitted diseases. Adv Planned Parenthood, 12:45-56, 1977.

Darrow WW, Wiesner PJ. Personal prophylaxis for venereal disease. J Amer Med Assoc, 233:444-446, 1975.

Eagle H, Gude AV, Beckman GE, Mast G, Sapero JJ, Shindledecker JB. Prevention of gonorrhea with penicillin tablets. J Amer Med Assoc, 140:940-943, 1949.

Edwards WM. A study of progonasyl using prostitutes in Nevada's legal houses of prostitution. J Reproduc Med, 11:81, 1973.

Felman YM. A plea for the condom, especially for teenagers. J Amer Med Assoc, 241:2517-2518, 1979.

Harrison WO, Hooper RR, Wiesner PJ, Campbell AF, Karney WW, Reynolds GH, Jones OG, Holmes KK. A trial of minocycline given after exposure to prevent gonorrhea. N Eng J Med, 300:1074-1078, 1979.

Hart G. Role of Preventive Methods in Control of Venereal Disease. Public Health Service, Centers for Disease Control, Atlanta; Department of Health, Education, and Welfare, Washington, D.C., 1976.

Hinman AR. The condom as a prophylactic. Bull NY Acad Med, 52:1004–1011, 1976.

Jick H, Hannan MT, Stergachis A, et al. Vaginal spermicides and gonorrhea. J Amer Med Assoc, 248:1619–1621, 1982.

Keith L, Berer GS, Moss M. Cervical gonorrhea in women using different methods of contraception. J Amer Vener Dis Assoc, 3: 17–19, 1976.

McCormack WM. Sexually transmitted diseases: Women as victims. J Amer Med Assoc, 248:177–178, 1982.

Ohno T, Kato K, Nagata M, Hattori N, Kanekawa H. Prophylactic control of the spread of venereal disease through prostitutes in Japan. Bull World Health Org, 19:575–579, 1958.

Redford MH, Duncan GW, Prager DJ. The Condom: Increasing Utilization in the United States. San Francisco Press, 1974.

Rendom AL, Covarrubias J, McCarney KE, et al. A controlled, comparative study of phenylmercuric acetate, nonxynol-9, and placebo vaginal suppositories as prophylactic agents against gonorrhea. Curr Ther Res, 27:780–783, 1980.

Sternberg TH, Howard EB, Dewey LA, Padget P. Venereal diseases. In Coates JB, Hoff EC, Hoff PM (eds.). Preventive Medicine in World War II. Volume V. Communicable Diseases. Office of the Surgeon General, Department of the Army, Washington, D.C., 1960.

Willcox RR. The prophylaxis of nonvenereal conditions: With its application to venereology. J Amer Vener Dis Assoc, 1:113–117, 1975.

Chapter 24

PENICILLIN REACTIONS, MANAGEMENT OF
ANAPHYLAXIS, AND PENICILLIN SKIN TEST

Penicillin is one of the most frequently used drugs in the
treatment of venereal diseases, and for this reason a short outline
review of the following topics is in order: penicillin reactions, the
management of penicillin anaphylaxis, and the use of the penicillin
skin test to predict penicillin allergy.

CLASSIFICATION OF PENICILLIN REACTIONS

Allergic Reactions to Penicillin

1. <u>Immediate reactions</u> usually take place within 30 min following parenteral administration of penicillin. An "immediate"
   reaction may take place up to 2 hr following administration of
   oral penicillin. The clinical symptoms are those of anaphylactic shock, angioedema or laryngeal edema, and urticaria
   (Table 24.1).
2. <u>Accelerated reactions</u> may take place from 30 min to 2 days
   following administration of penicillin. They are present as
   urticaria, flushing, or asthma.
3. <u>Delayed or late reactions</u> occur 2 or more days following the
   initiation of penicillin therapy. They may present as serum
   sickness, fever, and various exanthematous rashes. Unusual
   reactions include hemolytic anemia, granulocytopenia, neuritis,
   or nephritis.

Procaine Reactions

1. They may be seen following intramuscular injections of procaine
   penicillin G. They may be confused with anaphylaxis.

Table 24.1   Effects of Immediate or Anaphylactic Reactions to Penicillin[a]

	System	Signs and Symptoms
1	Respiratory	Nasal congestion and itching, dyspnea, wheezing cough, rash, tachypnea
2	Cardiovascular	Hypotension, syncope, tachycardia arrhythmia, cardiac arrest
3	Skin	Pruritis, urticaria, asymmetrical edema
4	Gastrointestinal	Nausea, vomiting, diarrhea, abdominal pain
5	Eye	Itching, lacrimation, conjunctival inflammation

Time of onset: Peak reactions occur within 5–60 min

[a] Adapted from J. F. Kelly and R. Patterson, Anaphylaxis. Course, mechanisms, and treatment. J Amer Med Assoc, 227: 1431–1436, 1974.

2. The reaction is due to elevated blood procaine concentration from inadvertent injection of the procaine penicillin into a vein.
3. Symptoms begin within a few minutes following the injection of the procaine penicillin.
4. Symptoms include vertigo, tinnitus, marked anxiety, violent behavior, visual and auditory hallucinations, increase in pulse rate and blood pressure, syncope, grand mal seizures, and sudden death.
5. Laryngospasm, urticaria, and wheezing are _not_ part of the syndrome.
6. The syndrome is usually over within 15 min.
7. Treatment: restraint, reassurance, and observation.

MANAGEMENT OF PENICILLIN ANAPHYLAXIS

If 100,000 patients receive penicillin, approximately 660 patients will have an allergic reaction, 55 patients will have anaphylaxis (and in one-half of these, it will be severe), and 1 patient will die from anaphylaxis.

Suggested Treatment for Anaphylaxis

1. Recognition (see Table 24.1).
2. Promptness is essential.
3. If possible, use a proximal tourniquet and local infiltration of epinephrine at the antigen injection site.
4. Management (see Table 24.2).

PENICILLIN ALLERGY SKIN-TESTING PROCEDURE

Indications

Penicillin skin tests should be performed only on patients who give a history of penicillin allergy and for whom there is no effective alternate antibiotic therapy.

Skin Test Antigens

Sodium penicillin G diluted in physiologic saline to 10,000 U/ml and penicilloyl-polylysine (Pre-Pen, Kremers-Urban Co.).

Purpose

To predict current risk of immediate or accelerated allergic reactions (usually anaphylaxis or urticaria). The test should be performed immediately prior to administration of the antibiotic.

Procedure

The physician performing the skin test should be prepared to manage an immediate reaction which can occur rarely in sensitive individuals. First perform a scratch test followed by an intradermal test.

Table 24.2   Suggested Treatment for Anaphylaxis[a]

Reaction	Treatment[b]
A. Conjunctivitis, rhinitis, urticaria, pruritis	A. Epinephrine HCl, 0.3 ml of 1:1000 subcutaneously or IM, and diphenhydramine HCl, 50 mg PO every 6 hr for 24 hr
B. Laryngeal edema	B. Epinephrine HCl, 0.3 ml of 1:1000 IM; diphenhydramine HCl, 50 mg IV; and oxygen followed by diphenhydramine HCl, 50 mg, PO every 6 hr and ephedrine sulfate, 25 mg PO every 6 hr
C. Bronchospasm	C. Epinephrine HCl, 0.3 ml of 1:1000 IM; diphenhydramine HCl, 50 mg IV (one dose); aminophylline 250 mg IV over 10 min; and oxygen; followed by repeat injections of epinephrine and aminophylline 500 mg IV every 6 hr
D. Hypotension	D. Epinephrine HCl, 0.3 ml of 1:1000 IM or IV; diphenhydramine HCl 50 mg IV; oxygen, metaraminal bitartrate, 100 mg in 1000 ml of 5% dextrose in water; intravenous fluids; monitor blood gases, ECG, and urine output; and isoproterenol HCl in normovolemic low cardiac output hypotension. Arrhythmias in the presence of adequate oxygenation should be treated with appropriate antiarrhythic agents.

[a] Adapted from J. F. Kelly and R. Patterson. Anaphylaxis. Course, mechanisms, and treatment. J Amer Med Assoc, 227:1431–1436, 1974.

[b] The value of steroids is debated. Hydrocortisone 500 mg IV or its equivalent may be given every 6 hr for severe bronchospasm, laryngeal edema or hypotension. It is not a first line drug.

The scratch test

Place a drop of each skin test antigen on the forearm. Make
several 1 cm scratches through the drop using a small gauge syringe
needle. Blot the drop after 2 min. Observe for induration between
5 and 15 min. Any induration that persists for 20 min is considered a positive test.

The intradermal test

Use 25-27 gauge needles on two 1 ml tuberculin syringes.
One-half milliliter of each antigen solution is drawn up into each
syringe. Between 0.02 and 0.04 ml of the reagent is injected intra-
dermally, enough to make a 3 mm bleb. (Note that this is <u>much
less reagent</u> than is used in a tuberculin test.) At the end of 15-20
min, measure the diameter of the induration. The test is positive
if there is 5 mm or more of induration. Disregard erythema.

If either skin test is positive, any penicillin or cephalosporin
drug is contraindicated.

NOTES

1. This type of skin test detects the presence of reaginic or IgE
   antibody.
2. If both skin tests are positive, inject a control composed of
   normal saline to evaluate dermatographism.
3. Recent antihistamine therapy may invalidate the test.
4. Moderate corticosteroid therapy (<60 mg of prednisone a day
   or equivalent) will not affect the skin test response.
5. Positive penicillin skin tests during penicillin therapy do not
   imply serious risk if therapy is continued.
6. The incidence of false negative skin tests can be expected to
   be less than 1%.
7. The skin tests will not predict the appearance of a delayed
   penicillin-induced drug rash or other reactions including hemolytic anemia, serum sickness, drug fever, interstitial nephritis, and exfoliative dermatitis.

BIBLIOGRAPHY

Adkinson NF. A guide to skin testing for penicillin allergy. Res
Staff Phys, pp. 55-59, August 1977.

Adkinson NF, Thompson WL, Maddrey WC, Lichtenstein LM.
Routine use of penicillin skin testing on an inpatient service.
N Eng J Med, 285:22-24, 1971.

Galpin JE, Chow AW, Yoshikawa TT, Guze LB. "Pseudoanaphy-
lactic" reactions from inadvertent infusion of procaine penicillin G.
Ann Int Med, 81:358-359, 1974.

Green RL, Lewis JE, Stephen BS, Kraus J, Frederickson EL.
Elevated plasma procaine concentrations after administration of
procaine penicillin G. N Eng J Med, 291:223-226, 1974.

Jaffe HW, Reynolds GH, Wiesner PJ. National gonorrhea therapy
monitoring study. J Amer Vener Dis Assoc, 3:29-31, 1976.

Kelly JF, Patterson R. Anaphylaxis. Course, mechanisms and
treatment. J Amer Med Assoc, 227:1431-1436, 1974.

Levine BB. Immunologic mechanisms of penicillin allergy. A
haptenic model system for the study of allergic diseases in man.
N Eng J Med, 275:1115-1125, 1966.

Rudolph AH, Price EV. Penicillin reactions among patients in
venereal disease clinics. J Amer Med Assoc, 223:499-501, 1973.

Smith JW, Johnson JE, Cluff LE. Studies on the epidemiology of
adverse drug reactions II. An evaluation of penicillin allergy.
N Eng J Med, 274:998-1002, 1966.

Van Dellen RG, Gleich GJ. Penicillin skin test as predictive and
diagnostic aids in penicillin allergy. Med Clin N Amer, 54:997-
1007, 1970.

Chapter 25

ACQUIRED IMMUNE DEFICIENCY SYNDROME

The acquired immune deficiency syndrome (AIDS) was first
recognized in 1981 when the Centers for Disease Control was noti-
fied of an unusual number of young homosexual men in New York
City and California who became ill with Pneumocystis carinii
pneumonia and Kaposi's sarcoma. Study of these patients revealed
that they had a previously undescribed acquired immune deficiency
syndrome. The increasing numbers of these patients is a cause
for concern.

ETIOLOGIC AGENT

The etiologic agent of AIDS is most likely a virus. The early
suggestions of this came from the epidemiologic data which showed
that the disease primarily affected homosexual men who had large
numbers of sexual partners, drug addicts, transfusion recipients,
and hemophiliacs—a disease distribution resembling that of hepatitis B. The current research has been directed at the retroviruses,
RNA tumor viruses known to cause cancer in animals. Retroviruses derive their name from the mirror-image manner in which they
copy the genetic code by means of the enzyme reverse transcriptase.
One of the retroviruses, the feline leukemia virus, produces immunosuppression in cats. Retroviruses also cause certain types
of human leukemia. The human T-cell leukemia-lymphoma virus,
a retrovirus designated HTLV-1, is most commonly found in Japan,
but also in the West Indies, South America, Central Africa, and
the southeastern United States.

Dr. Luc Mantagnier's group at the Pasteur Institute and Dr.
Robert Gallo's group at the National Institutes of Health have both

reported that a retrovirus related to the human T-cell leukemia-lymphoma virus may be the cause of AIDS. The French virus is designated as the lymphadenopathy-associated virus (LAV) and the American virus as the human T-cell leukemia virus III (HTLV-III). These viruses may be identical. Both selectively attack the T-helper lymphocytes. Antibody to these viruses is absent in the general population but is present in varying proportions in patients with AIDS and in some asymptomatic homosexuals. Possibly other factors are required to initiate AIDS in infected individuals. These remain to be identified.

EPIDEMIOLOGY

The infectious agent of AIDS appears to be transmitted by sexual intercourse in homosexuals and, less frequently, in heterosexual individuals. Another mechanism of infection is via blood or blood products. Individuals at risk for this type of transmission include intravenous drug users who share needles or injection paraphernalia, recipients of transfusions from blood donated by infected individuals, and hemophiliacs who have received anti-hemophilic factor and plasma factor concentrates contaminated with the infectious agent. These blood products are prepared from thousands of donors and are at risk for inclusion of a number of infectious agents including hepatitis B virus, non-A, non-B hepatitis virus, and cytomegalovirus.

Approximately 90% of AIDS patients are between the ages of 20 and 49 years, and 93% are men. The racial distribution of AIDS patients is 58% white, 26% black, 15% Hispanic, and 2% other. Homosexual or bisexual men make up the largest proportion of AIDS patients (71%), followed by intravenous drug users (17%), Haitians (4%), and hemophiliacs (1%), while the remainder of the patients (6%) have been recipients of transfusions, sexual partners of AIDS patients, and of unknown source. AIDS patients have been found predominantly in the large cities of the following U.S. states: New York, California, New Jersey, and Florida. AIDS patients have also been identified in several countries of Western Europe, Central and South America, and Central Africa. There is speculation that the disease originated in Central Africa and gained entry into the United States through homosexuals vacationing in Haiti. Perhaps molecular epidemiological techniques will provide a more accurate story.

The increasing frequency in which AIDS patients are being diagnosed is alarming. In late May of 1984, 4534 cases of AIDS had been reported in the United States to the Centers for Disease Control. At that time, approximately 100 cases per week were being reported in comparison to 30 cases per week at the same time the year before. There is some indication that this increasing number of patients will continue for some time since estimates of the incubation time of AIDS have been in the range of months to years rather than days to weeks. In transfusion-related cases of AIDS, patients received blood 15 to 57 months (median 27.5) before the diagnosis of AIDS.

CLINICAL MANIFESTATIONS

At present, it is difficult to describe the typical AIDS patient. As more information is collected about this group, there will undoubtedly by subsets of patients depending on the route of infection and possibly facilitating factors that might make an individual more susceptible. It is probable that the most flagrant cases of AIDS are being identified at present, and milder forms of the disease are going unrecognized.

Most investigators agree that AIDS patients have a prodromal period of illness prior to meeting the surveillance definition of AIDS that is described below. Whether or not individuals with these prodromes all go on to develop AIDS has not been settled. They fall into at least four categories. The first is comprised of individuals without any symptoms or evidence of illness who have laboratory evidence of immunologic dysfunction. The second group is those patients who have generalized, persistent lymphadenopathy, usually with laboratory evidence of immunologic dysfunction. The third group is those individuals with the persistent, generalized lymphadenopathy syndrome who have, in addition, systemic symptoms of one sort or another. The fourth group is those patients who meet the surveillance criteria for AIDS.

<u>Persistent, Generalized Lymphadenopathy</u>
<u>Among Homosexual Males</u>

The syndrome of persistent, generalized lymphadenopathy has been defined by the Centers for Disease Control according to the following criteria: 1) lymphadenopathy of at least three months' duration, involving two or more extra-inguinal sites, and confirmed on physical examination by the patient's physician; 2) absence of any current illness or drug use known to cause lymphadenopathy; and 3) presence of reactive hyperplasia in a lymph node, if a biopsy is performed.

In Mathur-Wagh's series of 42 homosexual or bisexual men followed for 15-30 months (median 22), 19% developed AIDS. This distressing development was associated statistically with previous heavy nitrate inhalant use, the presence of night sweats, leukopenia and the triad of constitutional symptoms, splenomegaly, and leukopenia. Some of the constitutional symptoms that the lymphadenopathy patients develop include fatigue, malaise, anorexia, diarrhea, weight loss, hepatomegaly, and splenomegaly. Lymphadenopathy often regresses in patients who develop AIDS.

Surveillance Definition of AIDS

AIDS is defined as being present in individuals who develop a disease at least moderately predictive of a defect in cell-mediated immunity, such as Kaposi's sarcoma (in a patient less than 60 years old) or Pneumocystis carinii pneumonia, along with the absence of any known cause of underlying immune deficiency or other disease or therapy that would reduce resistance, such as immunosuppressive drug therapy or lymphoreticular malignancy.

Individuals meeting the surveillance criteria as defined by the Centers for Disease Control have, as their presenting manifestation, signs and symptoms relating to either Kaposi's sarcoma, Pneumocystis carinii pneumonia, or some other opportunistic infection as shown on Table 25.1. Pneumocystis carinii pneumonia and the opportunistic infections are the most common manifestation of AIDS, and the frequency of these complications in AIDS patients is as follows: 26% have Kaposi's sarcoma, 51% have Pneumocystis carinii pneumonia, 7% have both, and 16% have other opportunistic infections. These complications of AIDS are not all equally distributed among the patient groups in whom AIDS appears. Table 25.2 shows that Kaposi's sarcoma is most commonly found in homosexual or bisexual men and that Pneumocystis carinii pneumonia is the most common complication of AIDS in all groups in the United States but strikingly so in intravenous drug users and patients with hemophilia. Kaposi's sarcoma is common in all groups of patients from Central Africa, but the most common opportunistic pathogen in the Central African patients is the cryptococcus.

Table 25.1   Infections Suggestive of Underlying Cellular Immune Deficiency[a]

Parasitic Infections

Pneumocystis carinii pneumonia (on histology or on microscopy of "touch" preparation or bronchial washings).

Toxoplasmosis, causing pneumonia or CNS infection (on histology or on microscopy of a "touch" preparation). Serology is generally not helpful.

Strongyloidosis, causing pneumonia, CNS infection, or disseminated infection (on histology).

Cryptosporidiosis, intestinal, causing diarrhea for over one month (on histology or stool microscopy)

Fungal Infections

Aspergillosis, causing CNS or disseminated infection (on culture or histology)

Candidiasis, causing esophagitis (on histology, microscopy of a "wet" preparation from the esophagus, or endoscopic findings of white plaques on an erythematous mucosal base)

Cryptococcosis, causing pulmonary, CNS, or disseminated infection (on culture, antigen detection, histology, or India ink preparation of CSF)

Bacterial Infection

"Atypical" mucobacteriosis (species other than tuberculosis or lepra) causing disseminated infection (on culture)

Viral Infection

Cytomegalovirus, causing pulmonary, gastrointestinal tract, or CNS infection (on histology)

Herpes simplex virus, causing chronic mucocutaneous infection with ulcers persisting more than one month or pulmonary, gastrointestinal tract, or disseminated infection (on culture, histology, or cytology)

Progressive multifocal leukoencephalopathy presumed to be caused by a papovavirus (on histology)

---

[a] Modified from H. W. Jaffe et al. Acquired immune deficiency syndrome in the United States: The first 1,000 cases. J Inf Dis, 148:339-345, 1983.

Note: "Disseminated infection" refers to involvement of lungs and multiple lymph nodes. The required diagnostic methods with positive results are shown in parentheses.

Table 25.2[a] Percentage Distribution Acquired Immune Deficiency Syndrome (AIDS) by Disease Category and Hierarchical Patient Characteristics[b] (June 1, 1981 to February 27, 1984)

	Homosexual/ Bisexual Men (N = 2546)	IV Drug Users (N = 623)	Haitians (N = 153)	Hemophiliacs (N = 23)	Other Unknown (N = 227)
Kaposi's sarcoma	33%	4%	11%	0%	15%
Pneumocystis carinii pneumonia	45%	70%	40%	96%	67%
Both KS and PCP	9%	1%	1%	0%	1%
Other opportunistic infections	13%	25%	48%	4%	16%
Total (N = 3572)	100%	100%	100%	100%	100%

[a] From the USPHS, Centers for Disease Control.
[b] Cases with multiple characteristics are tabulated only in the group listed first.

There are no doubt good reasons why AIDS should have different expressions of disease in different groups at risk. One suggestion is that patients who are infected by the intravenous route have a larger dose of infective agent and therefore become more immunosuppressed and have as their complication _Pneumocystis carinii_ infection. Those patients infected through oral or rectal mucosa routes may have a smaller innoculum and thus are less immunosuppressed. They therefore have more time to develop a neoplasm such as Kaposi's sarcoma which carries with it less of an immediate mortality.

The immunologic abnormalities in AIDS patients are thought to be the result of selective damage to T-helper cell function by retrovirus infection. Table 25.3 outlines changes found in the cellular and humoral immune systems of patients with AIDS. These changes are not presently considered to be diagnostic of AIDS in that they

Table 25.3 Immune Changes in Acquired Immune Deficiency Syndrome[a]

Cellular

Delayed hypersensitivity skin test anergy
Lymphopenia, reduced total T cells
Reduced number and percentage of certain T-helper cells
Variable number and increased percentage of certain T-suppressor cells
Reduced T-helper/T-suppressor cell ratio
Reduced T-cell proliferative responses to mitogens and antigens
Abnormalities in natural-killer-cell function
Reduced production of gamma-interferon

Humoral

Normal B-cell numbers
Increased serum IgA and IgG
Elevated circulating immune complexes (acquired immunodeficiency syndrome with opportunistic infection)
Inability to mount a _de novo_ serologic response to a new antigen

---

[a] Modified from M. S. Gottlieb et al. The acquired immunodeficiency syndrome (UCLA Conference). Ann Intern Med, 99:208-220, 1983.

are found in some asymptomatic homosexual men as well as patients with the persistent generalized lymphadenopathy syndrome. It is not known if the immunologic test results are predictive of patients who may be expected to go on and develop AIDS. Longitudinal studies are currently underway to assess this question.

DIAGNOSIS

The current method of diagnosing AIDS depends on the patient meeting the surveillance definition of AIDS as described by the CDC in the preceding section. One might expect the development of a virologic or serologic method of diagnosing AIDS if one or both of the current viral candidates, LAV or HTLV-III, is in fact the etiologic agent of AIDS. It is also possible that the diagnosis of AIDS may ultimately depend on a constellation of serologic, immunologic, and clinical criteria.

Immunologic tests to detect the immunologic dysfunction in AIDS patients described in Table 25.3 should only be performed after careful consideration of what use will be made of the results. If these tests are performed on otherwise healthy homosexuals or patients with the lymphadenopathy syndrome and they are abnormal, there is little that the patient and the physician can do but worry, since there is no defined prophylactic therapy. The presence of normal tests does not ensure that a patient will not develop AIDS in the future if he is among the high risk groups. Many physicians believe that routine use of the immunologic tests is to be discouraged until further research informs them how to best utilize the results.

Table 25.4 lists some of the presenting complaints and physical signs of patients who have the persistent, generalized lymphadenopathy syndrome or AIDS. In addition to the lymphadenopathy syndrome, other diseases may also be related to AIDS. These include autoimmunethrombocytopenia and hemolytic anemia, non-Hodgkins lymphoma, and multifocal leukoencephalopathy.

TREATMENT

At the moment, there is no effective therapy for patients with AIDS. Physicians can treat the accompanying neoplasms or opportunistic infections as they arise in the affected patients. For some of these, the therapy is of little benefit. This is particularly true

Table 25.4   Some Signs and Symptoms of Patients with Persistent Generalized Lymphadenopathy Syndrome and AIDS

Persistent, Generalized Lymphadenopathy Syndrome Patients

1. Lymphadenopathy in two or more non-inguinal sites persisting for 3 months or longer
2. Weight loss
3. Diarrhea
4. Fever and/or night sweats
5. Anorexia
6. Splenomegaly and/or hepatomegaly

Acquired Immune Deficiency Syndrome Patients

General: Fatigue, malaise, fever, night sweats, weight loss, diarrhea, lymphadenopathy may be present or there may be a history of preceding lymphadenopathy.

Dermatologic: Painless macules or nodules that may vary in color from pink to purple (bruise-like) present on the skin and mucous membranes (Kaposi's sarcoma). Progressive, chronic, ulcerating lesions on the skin and mucous membranes (chronic mucocutaneous herpes simplex).

Pulmonary: Fever, dry hacking nonproductive cough, shortness of breath (Pneumocystis carinii pneumonia). Fever, cough with or without sputum production (atypical mycobacteria such as M. avium-intracellulare).

Gastrointestinal: Pain on or difficulty in swallowing (oral thrush or Candida esophagitis). Unremitting diarrhea (Cryptosporidiosis).

Central Nervous System: Meningitis or encephalitis or mass lesion effects (Cryptococcosis, toxoplasmosis, cytomegalovirus infection).

---

with patients who have cryptosporidiosis or M. avium-intracellulare infections. Patients with Pneumocystis carinii pneumonia may have adverse reactions to trimethoprim-sulfamethoxazole and, in general, require pentamidine or pentamidine methanesulfonate for therapy. The latter drug is available in the United States from the Centers for Disease Control.

Although it appears that some patients with the lymphadenopathy syndrome may improve spontaneously, AIDS patients in general do not. According to reports by the Centers for Disease Control in February of 1984, 84% of the AIDS patients diagnosed before 1981 had died.

One of the major problems facing AIDS patients is the sense of isolation and hopelessness that they feel at having a disease for which there is no immediate cure. There may be weeks to months when a patient is being treated for one of the complicating neoplasms or opportunistic infections or simply waiting for some complication to occur. It is for this reason that physicians should be cautious about evaluating the immunologic function of an otherwise normal homosexual man. Should abnormal tests be found, all that can be offered is the hope that nothing further will develop, and the patient is left with months of anxiety, worry, and the impulse to repeat expensive tests to see if they are improving.

In order to meet the desire for information and support for these patients and the accompanying risk groups, several organizations have established toll-free numbers and information services. Two in the United States are listed below.

<u>AIDS Hotline</u>

(800) 342-AIDS (Daily 8:30 a.m. - 5:30 p.m. ET)
(202) 245-6867 (Callers from Alaska and Hawaii may phone collect.)

<u>National Gay Task Force</u>

80 Fifth Avenue
New York, NY 10011
(800) 221-7044 (Monday through Friday, 3 p.m. - 9 p.m.)

PROPHYLAXIS

AIDS may pose a threat to health care workers, but to date this has not been a problem. As of July 1983, only four of the 1831 reported AIDS patients were health-care personnel not known to belong to groups at increased risk for AIDS. None of the four gave a history of taking care of an AIDS patient, and none had known contact with blood of an AIDS patient. Table 25.5 contains precautions for the public in general in relation to AIDS patients.

Table 25.5   Advice for the Public in Relation to AIDS Patients[a]

Although the cause of AIDS remains unknown, the Public Health
Service recommends the following actions:

1. Sexual contact should be avoided with persons known or suspected to have AIDS. Members of high risk groups should be
   aware that multiple sexual partners increase the probability of
   developing AIDS.
2. As a temporary measure, members of groups at increased
   risk for AIDS should refrain from donating plasma and/or
   blood. This recommendation includes all individuals belonging
   to such groups, even though many individuals are at little risk
   of AIDS. Centers collecting plasma and/or blood should inform
   potential donors of this recommendation. The Food and Drug
   Administration (FDA) is preparing new recommendations for
   manufacturers of plasma derivatives and for establishments
   collecting plasma or blood. This is an interim measure to
   protect recipients of blood products and blood until specific
   laboratory tests are available.
3. Studies should be conducted to evaluate screening procedures
   for their effectiveness in identifying and excluding plasma and
   blood with a high probability of transmitting AIDS. These procedures should include specific laboratory tests as well as
   careful histories and physical examination.
4. Physicians should adhere strictly to medical indications for
   transfusion, and autologous blood transfusions are encouraged.
5. Work should continue toward development of safer blood products for use by hemophilia patients.

---

[a] From CDC, MMWR, 31:577–580, 1982.

Advice to Clinic Workers Handling
Specimens From AIDS Patients[a]

The precautions that follow are advised for those handling
persons and specimens from persons with opportunistic infections
that are not associated with underlying immunosuppressive disease

[a] CDC, MMWR, 32:450–452, 1982.

or therapy; Kaposi's sarcoma (patients under 60 years of age); chronic generalized lymphadenopathy, unexplained weight loss and/ or prolonged unexplained fever in persons who belong to groups with apparently increased risks of AIDS (homosexual males, intravenous drug abusers, Haitian entrants into the United States, hemophiliacs); and possible AIDS patients (hospitalized for evaluation). Hospitals and laboratories should adapt the following suggested precautions to their individual circumstances; these recommendations are not meant to restrict hospitals from implementing additional precautions.

A. The following precautions are advised in providing care to AIDS patients:
1. Extraordinary care must be taken to avoid accidental wounds from sharp instruments contaminated with potentially infectious material and to avoid contact of open skin lesions with material from AIDS patients.
2. Gloves should be worn when handling blood specimens, blood-soiled items, body fluids, excretions, and secretions, as well as surfaces, materials, and objects exposed to them.
3. Gowns should be worn when clothing may be soiled with body fluids, blood, secretions, or excretions.
4. Hands should be washed after removing gowns and gloves and before leaving the rooms of known or suspected AIDS patients. Hands should also be washed thoroughly and immediately if they become contaminated with blood.
5. Blood and other specimens should be labeled prominently with a special warning, such as "Blood Precautions" or "AIDS Precautions." If the outside of the specimen container is visibly contaminated with blood, it should be cleaned with a disinfectant (such as a 1:10 dilution of 5.25% sodium hypochlorite [household bleach] with water). All blood specimens should be placed in a second container, such as an impervious bag, for transport. The container or bag should be examined carefully for leaks or cracks.
6. Blood spills should be cleaned up promptly with a disinfectant solution, such as sodium hypochlorite (see above).
7. Articles soiled with blood should be placed in an impervious bag prominently labeled "AIDS Precautions" or "Blood Precautions" before being sent for reprocessing or disposal. Alternatively, such contaminated items may be placed in plastic bags of a particular color designated solely for

disposal of infectious wastes by the hospital. Disposable items should be incinerated or disposed of in accord with the hospital's policies for disposal of infectious wastes. Reusable items should be reprocessed in accord with hospital policies for hepatitis B virus-contaminated items. Lensed instruments should be sterilized after use on AIDS patients.

8. Needles should not be bent after use, but should be promptly placed in a puncture-resistant container used solely for such disposal. Needles should not be reinserted into their original sheaths before being discarded into the container, since this is a common cause of needles injury.

9. Disposable syringes and needles are preferred. Only needle-locking syringes or one-piece needle-syringe units should be used to aspirate fluids from patients, so that collected fluid can be safely discharged through the needle, if desired. If reusable syringes are employed, they should be decontaminated before reprocessing.

10. A private room is indicated for patients who are too ill to use good hygiene, such as those with profuse diarrhea, fecal incontinence, or altered behavior secondary to central nervous system infections. Precautions appropriate for particular infections that concurrently occur in AIDS patients should be added to the above, if needed.

B. The following precautions are advised for persons performing laboratory tests or studies on clinical specimens or other potentially infectious materials (such as inoculated tissue cultures, embryonated eggs, animal tissues, etc.) from known or suspected AIDS cases:

1. Mechanical pipetting devices should be used for the manipulation of all liquids in the laboratory. Mouth pipetting should not be allowed.

2. Needles and syringes should be handled as stipulated in Section A (above).

3. Laboratory coats, gowns, or uniforms should be worn while working with potentially infectious materials and should be discarded appropriately before leaving the laboratory.

4. Gloves should be worn to avoid skin contact with blood, specimens containing blood, blood-soiled items, body fluids, excretions, and secretions, as well as surfaces, materials, and objects exposed to them.

5. All procedures and manipulations of potentially infectious material should be performed carefully to minimize the creation of droplets and aerosols.

6. Biological safety cabinets (Class I or II) and other primary containment devices (e.g., centrifuge safety cups) are advised whenever procedures are conducted that have a high potential for creating aerosols or infectious droplets. These include centrifuging, blending, sonicating, vigorous mixing, and harvesting infected tissues from animals or embryonated eggs. Fluorescent activated cell sorters generate droplets that could potentially result in infectious aerosols. Translucent plastic shielding between the droplet-collecting area and the equipment operator should be used to reduce the presently uncertain magnitude of this risk. Primary containment devices are also used in handling materials that might contain concentrated infectious agents or organisms in greater quantities than expected in clinical specimens.

7. Laboratory work surfaces should be decontaminated with a disinfectant, such as sodium hypochlorite solution (see A5 above), following any spill of potentially infectious material and at the completion of work activities.

8. All potentially contaminated materials used in laboratory tests should be decontaminated, preferably by autoclaving, before disposal or reprocessing.

9. All personnel should wash their hands following completion of laboratory activities, removal of protective clothing, and before leaving the laboratory.

During the latter part of 1983, it appeared as if the numbers of cases of AIDS were doubling every six months and estimates were that by 1985, 20,000 persons would be affected. It is to be fervently hoped that these predictions will be incorrect and that an etiologic agent and effective therapy will be uncovered.

BIBLIOGRAPHY

Anderson MG, Key P, Tovey G, et al. Persistent lymphadenopathy in homosexual men: A clinical and ultrastructural study. Lancet, 1:880-882, 1984.

Auerbach DM, Darrow WW, Jaffe HW, Curran JW. Cluster of cases of the acquired immune deficiency syndrome. Amer J Med, 76:487-492, 1984.

Brynes RK, Chan WC, Spira TJ, Ewing EP, Chandler FW. Value of lymph node biopsy in unexplained lymphadenopathy in homosexual men. J Am Med Assoc, 250:1313-1316, 1983.

Centers for Disease Control. Persistent, generalized lymphadenopathy among homosexual males. Morbid Mortal Weekly Rep, 31: 249-251, 1982.

Centers for Disease Control. Acquired immune deficiency syndrome (AIDS): Precautions for clinical and laboratory staffs. Morbid Mortal Weekly Rep, 31:577-580, 1982.

Centers for Disease Control. Prevention of acquired immune deficiency syndrome (AIDS): Report of inter-agency recommendations. Morbid Mortal Weekly Rep, 32:101-103, 1983.

Centers for Disease Control. An evaluation of the acquired immunodeficiency syndrome (AIDS) reported in health-care personnel-United States. Morbid Mortal Weekly Rep, 32:358-360, 1983.

Centers for Disease Control. Acquired immunodeficiency syndrome (AIDS): Precautions for health-care workers and allied professionals. Morbid Mortal Weekly Rep, 32:450-452, 1983.

Centers for Disease Control. Update: Acquired immunodeficiency syndrome (AIDS)-United States. Morbid Mortal Weekly Rep, 32: 688-691, 1984.

Centers for Disease Control. Prospective evaluation of health-care workers exposed via parenteral or mucous-membrane routes to blood and body fluids of patients with acquired immunodeficiency syndrome. Morbid Mortal Weekly Rep, 33:181-182, 1984.

Clumeck N, Sonnet J, Taelman H, et al. Acquired immunodeficiency syndrome in African patients. N Eng J Med, 310:492-497, 1984.

Curran JW, Lawrence DN, Jaffee H, et al. Acquired immunodeficiency syndrome (AIDS) associated with transfusion. N Eng J Med, 310:69-75, 1984.

Downing RG, Eglin RP, Bayley AC. African Kaposi's sarcoma and AIDS. Lancet, 1:478-480, 1984.

Evatt BL, Ramsey RB, Lawrence DN, Zyla LD, Curran JW. The acquired immunodeficiency syndrome in patients with hemophilia. Ann Intern Med, 100:499-504, 1984.

Fauci AS, Macher AM, Longo DL, et al. NIH Conference. Acquired immunodeficiency syndrome: Epidemiologic, clinical, immunologic and therapeutic considerations. Ann Int Med, 100: 92-106, 1984.

Gallo RC, Salahuddin SZ, Popovic M, et al. Frequent detection and isolation of cytopathic retroviruses (HTLV-III) from patients with AIDS and at risk for AIDS. Science, 224:500-502, 1984.

Glauser MP, Francioli P. Clinical and epidemiological survey of acquired immune deficiency syndrome in Europe. Eur J Clin Microbiol, 3:55-58, 1984.

Gottlieb MS, Groopman JE, Weinstein WM, Fahey JL, Detels R. The acquired immunodeficiency syndrome (UCLA Conference). Ann Intern Med, 99:208-220, 1983.

Harris C, Small CB, Klein RS, et al. Immunodeficiency in female sexual partners of men with the acquired immunodeficiency syndrome. N Eng J Med, 308:1181-1184, 1983.

Ioachin HL, Lerner CW, Tapper ML. Lymphadenopathies in homosexual men. Relationship with acquired immune deficiency syndrome. J Am Med Assoc, 250:1306-1309, 1983.

Jaffe HW, Bregman DJ, Selik RM. Acquired immune deficiency syndrome in the United States. J Infect Dis, 148:339-345, 1983.

Jaffe HW, Choi K, Thomas PA, et al. National case-control study of Kaposi's sarcoma and Pneumocystis carinii pneumonia in homosexual men: Part 1, epidemiologic results. Ann Intern Med, 99: 145-151, 1983.

Kalish SB, Ostrow DG, Goldsmith J, et al. The spectrum of immunologic abnormalities and clinical findings in homosexually active men. J Infect Dis, 149:148-156, 1984.

Levine AM, Meyer PR, Begandy MK, et al. Development of B-cell lymphoma in homosexual men. Ann Int Med, 100:7-13, 1984.

Ma P, Soave R. Three-step stool examination for cryptosporidiosis in 10 homosexual men with protracted watery diarrhea. J Infect Dis, 147:824-828, 1983.

Malebranche R, Arnoux E, Guerin JM. Acquired immunodeficiency syndrome with severe gastrointestinal manifestations in Haiti. Lancet, 2:873-878, 1983.

Mathur-Wagh U, Spigland I, Sacks HS, et al. Longitudinal study of persistent generalized lymphadenopathy in homosexual men: Relation to acquired immunodeficiency syndrome. Lancet, 1:1033-1038, 1984.

Metroka CE, Cunningham-Rundles S, Pollack MS, et al. Generalized lymphadenopathy in homosexual men. Ann Intern Med, 99: 585-591, 1983.

Miller B, Stansfield SK, Zack MM, et al. The syndrome of unexplained generalized lymphadenopathy in young men in New York City, Is it related to the acquired immune deficiency syndrome? J Amer Med Assoc, 251:242-246, 1984.

Navin TR, Juranek DD. Cryptosporidiosis: Clinical, epidemiologic, and parasitologic review. Rev Infect Dis, 6:313-327, 1984.

Pape JW, Liautaud B, Thomas F, et al. Characteristics of the acquired immunodeficiency syndrome (AIDS) in Haiti. N Eng J Med, 309:945-950, 1983.

Pitchenik AE, Fischl MA, Dickinson GM, et al. Opportunistic infections and Kaposi's sarcoma among Haitians; evidence of a new acquired immunodeficiency state. Ann Intern Med, 98:277-284, 1983.

Pitchenik AE, Shafron RD, Glasser RM, Spira TJ. The acquired immunodeficiency syndrome in the wife of a hemophiliac. Ann Int Med, 100:62-65, 1984.

Rame FS, Membership of APIC. In-hospital needlesticks and other significant blood exposures to blood from patients with acquired immunodeficiency syndrome and lymphadenopathy syndrome. Amer J Infect Control, 12:69-75, 1984.

Scott GB, Buck BE, Leterman JG, Bloom FL, Parks WP. Acquired immunodeficiency syndrome in infants. N Eng J Med, 310: 76-81, 1984.

Vilmer E, Rouzioux C, Brun FV, et al. Isolation of new lymphotrophic retrovirus from two siblings with haemophilia B, one with AIDS. Lancet, 1:753-757, 1984.

Wong B, Gold JWM, Brown AE, et al. Central nervous-system toxoplasmosis in homosexual men and parenteral drug abusers. Ann Int Med, 100:36-42, 1984.